How Karen Conquered Cancer

Copyright © 2007 Mark J. Volpe
All rights reserved.
ISBN: 1-4196-6066-7
ISBN-13: 978-1419660665

Visit www.booksurge.com to order additional copies.

How Karen Conquered Cancer

Her Husband's Story

Mark J. Volpe

2007

How Karen Conquered Cancer

This book is dedicated to the diligent work and enduring research of Katie Hincher, RN, Dr. Larry Cripe, Dr. Martin Tallman, Dr. Jennifer Schwartz and all of their highly esteemed colleagues around the world who are working tirelessly to rid all humanity of leukemia and lymphoma.

A special thanks to Mary Lynn Webster.

PROLOGUE

If you are one of those people who go to the Indianapolis 500 or a NASCAR race just to see the wrecks and carnage, then this book probably isn't for you. While many people have fought with courage and dignity in their own personal battles to beat cancer, there are certainly numerous stories about remarkable people who survived, and the law of averages tells us there are even more people who fought the battle to its fullest and still lost. These are odds that no human, despite his or her own inner strength and modern medical technology, find impossible to beat.

This is the true story of a remarkable woman, the mother of three who was struck with leukemia in the prime of her life. She fought the fight with faith, family, friends, courage, hope, love and perseverance. There were moments of despair, but a dedicated group of magnificent doctors led by Dr. Larry Cripe of the Indiana University Hospital and Dr. Martin Tallman at Northwestern Memorial Hospital spearheaded a remarkable recovery and the achievement of remission. After two years of remission, everything looked good and she appeared to be out of harm's way. We quickly find out, as much as we would like to believe otherwise, that we are very mortal and not as in control of our own destinies as we would like to think.

There is more to this story than Karen's battle with leukemia. It is the story of the couple's courtship, marriage, the birth of their children, some questionable medical care, a fanatical Cleveland Browns fan who listens to Bruce Springsteen religiously, a problem pregnancy, a small business run by this remarkable patient, all surrounded with the interplay of a wonderful family and the support of numerous friends and neighbors.

Parts of this chronology were written while the author waited to board airplanes or watched his sons at soccer, hockey and baseball practices. There were even some portions that were penned during his daughter's gymnastics meets, while other typing occurred in a more ideal setting under a beach umbrella surrounded by the serenity of the seashore. Toward the end, many pages were typed while the author sat at his wife's bedside during those long hours spent in a variety of hospital rooms.

If your spirits need a lift, if you doubt that there is still something good going on out in the world given the events of 9/11, the Oklahoma City bombing, the death of Princess Diana, the tsunami tragedy, and the continuing conflict in the Middle East, then read this courageous story. Good things really do happen!

God listens to those who believe. Prayers do get answered, and some day soon, maybe not in this lifetime, there will be a cure for cancer of the blood. But until then, there are ways to win and outrun the deadly disease, yet with an understanding and acceptance, of course, that "God's will" ultimately controls our lives. At the end of the day you can't just stand there and allow the illness to take over and control the outcome. Even though we're only human, we can make a difference as to whether someone with this awful disease celebrates life or dies. This is the type of story a director like Ron Howard would make into a movie, or Oprah would recommend as a must-read.

Some of the names of the people involved in this story have been changed to protect the guilty and in some cases to protect those who were simply incompetent. Throughout this story, there are interactions with many different medical doctors, some of whom proved to be marginal at best. The opinions of other doctors eventually proved wrong; and even the prognosis from some of the most highly respected doctors in the world ended up being inaccurate. Medicine, we soon learned, is an inexact science.

This is a husband's story, based on his unique witnessing of events that would forever change him, his relationships and reinforce his faith. All too often, the personal struggle of the supporting spouse (who is also a main caregiver) with the disease is often forgotten. In telling Karen's story, it was never intended to be an autobiography of sorts, but early on during this incomprehensible saga I came to realize that helping save my wife's life was the defining purpose of my own life.

Yet, in the end, this story belongs to a remarkably courageous woman named Karen Volpe, born and raised in Ohio, stricken at the age of 41 with a rare form of leukemia while living what was an otherwise normal life in central Indiana. It's a tribute to Karen, and in many ways this is actually a love story that needs to be read from cover to cover. Not only the love of a husband for his wife, but an entire family and community who showed an outpouring of love for Karen by providing overwhelming compassion and support.

There is no cookbook for survival. It is my hope this story can be a powerful source of hope and inspiration to others with cancer and their friends and families who may find themselves in a similar set of circumstances.

Never give up on the power of prayer and always refuse to lose!

CHAPTER 1

CarePoint

My Grandma Schultz passed away on April 2, 2002. She died in New Hampshire where my aunts, Dorothy and Diane, the twins, had been caring for her during her final days. Her mother, my great Grandma Vitarelli, was the strongest person I had ever met—until Karen. She lost her husband during the depression and had to raise nine children on her own, struggling to get by. The first bar I was ever in, at age five, was Grandma Vitarelli's fine establishment, the Dixon Street Grille, in Dubois, Pennsylvania.

I did manage to talk to Grandma Schultz over the phone for a few minutes a couple of days before she died. When I called, my Aunt Diane answered and she said there was no way I could to talk to my grandma because she was somewhat sedated, incoherent and unable to speak with me.

Then I heard this voice in the background say, "Is that Mark? Give me the phone! I want to talk to him."

My aunt obliged and I was able to have a brief phone conversation with grandma. It was very hard; we both knew we were saying goodbye, and in my heart I knew it was very likely to be the last time I'd ever speak with her. She so wanted to go and not be a burden to anyone. She had lived very quietly on her own in a simple apartment in Cleveland Heights, but pancreatic cancer had taken her at the age of 93. For many years my mother, whom I occasionally refer to by her first name of Marilyn, visited regularly with Grandma Schultz and made sure her basic needs were met. All of our children attended their great grandmother's funeral.

This event marked the end of an era for me as I had lost the last of my four grandparents. During the calling hours, Aunt Diane told me a wonderful story about grandma's last days. She had awoken from a dream and said, "I have seen the most beautiful place ever. My mother was there and so was my husband. There was this baby and I couldn't figure out who it was."

Aunt Diane and her mother concluded it was probably a child great Grandma Vitarelli had lost soon after the baby's birth, back in the early part of the century when my grandmother was still a little girl.

I was honored to do a reading at the funeral Mass and my voice cracked a little as I looked out at my estranged sister and her children. Her husband had slithered in behind them and took his place in the pew. They would hardly even speak to my wife, Karen, when she came over to greet them before Mass. My oldest son, Will, and I both served as pallbearers. I was proud of William as he helped carry the coffin uphill in the slippery grass off to grandma's final resting place next to her husband, Bill, who was one of two great grandfathers Will was named after. I consoled my mom as she said goodbye and asked whether she was all right and she said, "Yes, I have to be!"

A few weeks later I was walking back to the parking lot as Will's baseball practice was winding up when my cell phone rang. Marilyn was very calm on the other end, but I could sense some stress in her voice.

She said, "We have a problem here! It's your dad's heart. He just went in for a stress test; he had a lot of tightness in his chest and barely made it home from his morning walk."

Mom went on further to say my brother, Paul, was with him, but there was no way they could come over to watch our kids while Karen and I took a little junket out to our condo in Las Vegas. Paul had to play hardball with dad to make him stay in the hospital. Dad wanted to keep his weekly itinerary intact with an out-of-town meeting down in South Carolina, so Paul confiscated his cell phone, car keys and even his wallet. Thanks to modern medical technology, the doctors were able to clear the blockage.

Karen and I still went to Las Vegas, where I had a speaking engagement at an energy conference. Luckily, Karen's mother, Pat, was able to fly out on a cheap, last-minute Southwest Airlines flight from Cleveland via Chicago on Sunday to watch the kids. We were all at Chicago Midway at the same time because ATA out of Indianapolis routed us north before we headed west. If we had some slack time, we would have been able to see Pat for a quick visit. My friend, Stan Crisci, picked up Pat at the airport in Indianapolis.

I felt horribly guilty taking off to Vegas with my wife while my dad underwent the medical procedure. Everything went smoothly, but I still felt bad and I kept in contact with my sister-in-law, Tammy, to keep tabs on the situation.

Karen and I had a great time on the Strip. We sat around at the pool during the day at the timeshare we had purchased a year earlier at a place called Club de Soleil, just off the Strip. When we originally heard the sales pitch I immediately decided that it sounded good, but the price tag would be too much for one week per year. Then they told us they were in the final marketing stages of the resort, trying to get rid of the last 15 units, and they had lowered the price considerably.

Karen loves a good deal and the resort was also offering free accommodations for a week just about anywhere in the world you would want to go if you signed on and bought that day. Karen and I talked about it and we agreed to buy a two-bedroom unit.

When we told them I had a boatload of vacation each year, they decided to give us the prize that would have been awarded to the couple buying the last unit. The prize was an entire portfolio of accommodations, cruises and airfare all around the world. In total there were around 30 packages we could use, give away to family and friends, or even donate to various fundraisers. We couldn't resist a good deal, and besides, free accommodations in Rome were part of the package. Karen had been to Rome when she backpacked Europe back in 1982 and she had always wanted to go there with her husband. So, we signed the papers.

Later that evening, Karen and I waited in line to get tickets at the last minute to see Dany Gans at the Mirage. Dany Gans had been a career minor league baseball player, and he was now the toughest ticket to get in Vegas. During his hour-and-a-half show he did song impersonations of at least 30 different performers. He was amazing as he did Frank Sinatra, Celine Dion, Billy Joel, Carol Channing, Tony Bennett and even a pretty poor rendition of Bruce Springsteen. We had great seats down in the fifth row, way to the right. If you ever get the chance, pay the $100 per ticket and go see Mr. Gans, he's worth the price of admission. Karen won $400 on the slots while I was doing my presentation at the conference.

It was late May and school had just let out. On the Sunday following the end of the school year, the entire family strapped on roller blades, with the exception of Mitchell, our youngest of three, who rode his little bike, and we all headed down the Monon Trail for some physical activity. It was a beautiful Sunday afternoon and the trail was crowded. We started out near City Hall in Carmel, Indiana and headed south a few miles. As we cruised along, Will complained of mechanical difficulties with his skates. Will is without a doubt the best skater in the family. During the previous winter he had played competitive ice hockey.

Karen had the backpack with all of our drinks and sandwiches for lunch. About three-fourths of the way through our adventure, Will had another mechanical breakdown and Karen, the much stronger skater, ended up pulling him the rest of the way back. Our middle child, Samantha, was even a little bit tired near the end of our journey. We all stuck our feet in the fountain near City Hall in Carmel, then headed home and grilled some dinner.

Will's baseball team, the Diamondbacks, was not the greatest team ever assembled. There were a number of players who had little clue regarding the fundamentals of the game, and this frustrated Will because his level of play far exceeded most of the players on the team. Will definitely has the skills; it's just a matter of time, once his body grows he'll be a decent player. He has great coordination and has always taken well to good coaching, especially from a very special hockey coach named Neil Placek, who drafted Will for several of his teams. Neil is a generous and giving man. He took a genuine interest in not only Will, but also our entire family.

During the following week, I noticed that Karen seemed somewhat fatigued and I attributed this to her approaching a woman's least favorite time of the month. Our neighbors, Amy Jackson and Kimmie Wetzel, also noticed that Karen seemed less energetic than normal and was spending an inordinate amount of time on the couch. The other unusual thing I noticed was that Karen kept watching the same movie over and over on HBO. She was very intrigued with *Pay It Forward*. This movie was fascinating and starred Kevin Spacey and Helen Hunt. The movie focused on a young boy who had developed a concept of doing good deeds as part of a school project, and then those people who benefited from the good acts would do the same. It reminded me of a well-intended pyramid scheme, and in the end the young boy who inspired the concept ended up getting stabbed when he interceded on behalf of a little boy the local gang was bullying. Karen seemed to really enjoy this movie, watching it at least four or five times during the week, although I also remember her watching *An Officer And A Gentleman*.

I couldn't get one of the scenes in that movie off my mind. Richard Gere discovers that his buddy had committed suicide because his buddy's girlfriend had told him she had an abortion, even though she wasn't even pregnant. I could not understand how a man could become so distraught over these circumstances that he would take his own life. I knew it was a movie, but in real life, similar tragedies occur every day. Sometimes people decide to solve an otherwise temporary problem with a totally inappropriate permanent solution.

On Friday night, July 7th, we met a bunch of our neighbors at the Macaroni Grill, and then went to the Carmel Community Players' production of Agatha Christie's mystery, *Murder on the Nile*. The play was performed outside, under the stars, in a large gazebo adjacent to Carmel's City Hall. Karen was having a good time, but she was cold in the night air, so I gave her my jacket.

She also complained about being bloated and couldn't believe how tight her skirt was, saying, "I don't understand this at all, I wore this same skirt last week and it fit fine. This is disgusting how bloated I am."

We went home and she went straight to bed, while I stopped at the Jacksons' home for a nightcap on their deck before calling it an evening.

Remember the saying things happen in threes? First, there was the passing of my grandmother, and then my dad's heart problem.

The next morning Karen woke up and complained of a stomach ache. We had slept in until 10:00 and she seemed very concerned.

"I think I need to go to the urgent care facility on Allisonville Road. This feels weird," she said.

The kids were just starting to wake up, so I said, "Can you handle driving over yourself?"

She said, "No, I'd prefer that you take me."

We told the kids to get some cereal or some pop tarts, watch TV—we were just running a quick errand and would be right back. As we drove to the urgent care center, I could tell that Karen's level of discomfort was gradually increasing.

We pulled into CarePoint, and I dropped Karen at the door and parked the car. They checked us in quickly, and when I walked in, Karen was already in one of the examination rooms. The nurse put a blood pressure cuff on Karen's arm and pumped it up a couple of times.

She quickly took it off and said, "I'm going to get another one, because this one obviously isn't working."

When she returned I could tell Karen was very distressed; her pain was increasing and her breathing was staggered. She refused to lie on her back because this made things worse. When the nurse returned and reapplied a new blood pressure cuff, she pumped it up, looked at Karen and said, "If this is really your blood pressure you shouldn't be conscious."

A few seconds later Karen became white, and the doctor described her condition as cyanotic. They immediately called the EMT, saying she needed to get to a hospital emergency room right away.

It seemed like seconds later, I heard the sirens and two trucks from the Fishers Fire Department and the EMT squad was there.

The firemen said to me, "Where do you want us to take her?"

I said, "Carmel St. Vincent."

It seemed like the logical choice because it was the closest hospital. Also, it was a Catholic hospital where I knew we had insurance coverage because I had gone to the same ER with a severe case of poison ivy a year earlier.

The technicians put her on a gurney and administered an oxygen mask. Once they had her loaded up, I started driving rather briskly, north and then west, to St. Vincent's so I could be there when she arrived. As I drove I started to doubt and had trouble recalling whether I was clear on Carmel St. Vincent versus the bigger St. Vincent Hospital on 86th Street in Indianapolis, so I doubled back to CarePoint. The large fire truck was still there.

I yelled to the firemen, "Do you know which St. Vincent's they're heading to with my wife?"

He said, "No, but I'll radio them and find out."

The young fireman radioed the EMT squad and then yelled to me, "St. V Carmel," as I took off.

I was somewhat confused and fearful for Karen.

As I drove west on 116th Street, I thought I saw the EMT transport ahead of me about half a mile past Allisonville Road. I was surprised that the siren wasn't on, and that they were driving along rather casually. I managed to catch up, and stayed right behind them hoping I could get a glimpse of Karen inside, but it was too dark to see her. I said an Our Father. Something in the pit of my stomach suggested that something was really wrong, but I tried to remain optimistic.

When I arrived I parked quickly and ran to the back of the truck. Karen was still conscious and she had a puzzled and slightly panicked look on her face. They took her into the ER while I handled the registration details. I saw Karen only once very quickly after they did an ultrasound where they determined that her abdomen had filled up with blood. They could not see exactly what was wrong. They suspected a ruptured ovarian cyst, but wouldn't know for sure without some exploratory surgery.

Luckily, Dr. Sarah Bradley, an OB/GYN, had just delivered a baby and was available to do the surgery. Karen signed the consent forms and the nurses could not believe that she was still awake with her blood pressure being so low. After they whisked her away to surgery, I went outside to make a couple of calls on my cell phone.

The first call I made was to Kimmie Wetzel, and I asked her to just check on the kids, but to not tell them what was going on. I did not want my kids to get alarmed and scared over what I thought would be some minor surgery. Then I called Karen's mom, Pat, and I explained the situation and that I'd be in touch when I knew more.

"I just hate it that you live so far out when things like this happen," Pat said.

As I hung up the phone I thought to myself, "I've got a great paying job, it just happens to be in suburban Indianapolis, not Mars."

I paced around outside while Karen was in surgery. It was beautiful day. I made a few calls to check on the kids; I called my parents and Karen's dad, Tom, to let them know what was going on and that we expected everything would be fine. Finally, after about two hours, Dr. Bradley came out and let me know that a cyst on her left ovary had burst and filled Karen's abdomen with two liters of blood. She had removed Karen's left Fallopian tube, which didn't upset me too much because we were done having babies.

Dr. Bradley said it was difficult to irrigate around all the organs, but she felt comfortable that they were able to collect most of the blood, and that Karen would be home in a couple of days. Karen's biggest problem would be dealing with the incision and that it would take awhile for her to heal. I called everyone with the good news, and about an hour later I was able to see Karen in recovery as she came out of the anesthesia. She seemed fine, so I went home to check on the kids, and then I went right back to the hospital. By now she was admitted and she was conscious.

"What do you think we should do about the party we were going to have tonight?" I asked her.

She said, "Go for it. It's easier to have the party than to call everyone and cancel; besides, I'm fine."

We had been working on finishing the lower level of our home for about nine months, and we were finally to the point where the big screen TV was installed and we were ready to host a party even though our builder, Alvin Jones, still had a minor punch-list of things that needed to be finished. Alvin was a big boxing fan, and we had purchased the pay-per-view package off the satellite dish that would allow us to see Lennox Lewis fight Mike Tyson. Alvin invited some of his friends, and a number of people in the neighborhood came over to see the fight. Alvin brought over all sorts of food, and we grilled some beef and pork prior to settling in to watch the fight.

Once the fight was over and everyone had left, I headed back to the hospital after I had cleaned up the minor mess. Everything seemed fine. She was stable, but her breathing was a little labored. Around 2:00 a.m. I went back home and got some sleep, but it was more like a nap.

I was very restless and concerned about her persistent breathing problems.

CHAPTER 2

St. Vincent

When I got back to the hospital on Sunday morning Karen's problems with her breathing persisted, and she was listed as stable. She was in the intensive care unit due to these complications, not a normal surgical recovery room. She was also on morphine to deal with the pain related to the incision in her abdomen. Karen was not aware of what was going on, because the morphine had put her into such a funk. She had very little recollection or realization of what was going on around her, especially those events immediately following her surgery.

Some time early Sunday morning, they performed a basic chest x-ray and the results showed what appeared to be congestion, or to what my untrained eye looked like clouds in both of her lungs. Dr. Reisman was the cardio-pulmonary specialist in charge of Karen's case. At this point, I called Pat and let her know that Karen was in the ICU. She told me she was on her way west from Ohio in a few hours. One of the nurses told me Karen was receiving several blood products intravenously, that her platelets were low and she was getting transfusions of whole blood.

I asked what the platelets were for and she said, "She's having trouble clotting. We're giving her these transfusions of blood products and her body is just gobbling them up like a little Pac-Man."

To me this all seemed most odd.

I also remember looking at her blood chemical results and seeing that her white count was elevated to 19,000 and had been at 13,000 the day she was admitted. This was not uncommon for a person who just had surgery. I looked further down the page and noticed her platelets were at 45,000 and a normal range was between 150,000 and 450,000. This was consistent with the information I had just been told by Karen's nurse. I also noticed another number at the bottom of the page regarding a metric called "Blast." The normal range was between zero and five, but Karen's number was 95 and a review of her medical records from Saturday showed her Blast in the 40s with a note next to this number indicating this was a measure needing further review.

I thought to myself that this was nothing of any great consequence, because it was found at the bottom of the page indicating this was the measure of a factor that was not greatly significant.

I would learn later that this number was very important.

Another noteworthy item I found in Karen's medical records, which we did not get a full copy of until a year later, was written by the pathologist who had reviewed Karen's blood work. He wrote the following into Karen's medical records after analyzing a sample of her blood drawn on Saturday, June 8th at 9:20 p.m.

DIFF REVIEW-PATH
DFREV-PATH COM-1   Thrombocytonopenia may be congenital, hereditary-sex linked or autosomal, or acquired. Acquired thrombocytonopenia may be secondary to plastic anemia, marrow infiltration by leukemia, lymphoma, carcinoma or other malignant

	conditions, granulomatous disease, viral infections, ionizing radiation, myelosuppresive drugs, thrombosuppreseive drugs such as thiazides, alcohol, estrogen, nutritional deficiencies including iron, floate and B-12 lack, paroxysamal noctural hemoglbinuria, isoimmunity, D.I.C., T.T.P., postransfusional, etc.
DFREV-PATH COM-2	SLIDE REVIEWED. MANY BLASTS ON SCAN, RECOMMEND HEME CONSULT, BONE MARROW EXAM
DFREV-PATHOLOGIST	ANDREW C CHESTER, MD: Pathologist

Even though the analysis appears to be a cut-and-paste recital from a textbook, it is related to key factors presented under the microscope, which in this case was the indication that the pathologist saw "MANY BLASTS" on the scan. The hematology consult eventually took place days later, but there was never even a single mention of performing a "BONE MARROW EXAM" at any point in time at St. Vincent's. What cannot be readily ascertained from these records is exactly when the pathological review of Karen's blood was actually performed and actually entered into her records. The blood draw was taken the first day she was admitted, but it could have been well into the week before the pathologist actually performed the analysis and added the potential underlying cause of Karen's affliction to her records. The possibility of this analysis being done over the weekend on Sunday seems remote, and a more likely scenario would have the review occurring on Monday or even as late as Tuesday.

In any event, it wasn't soon enough.

Dr. Reisman would spin his wheels for several days before finally finding a consult that would come up with a plausible diagnosis.

I turned my focus to the breathing problems, and Dr. Reisman called in a respiratory specialist who immediately ordered Karen to use a meter dose inhaler that resembled a pipe. She breathed through it for 10 or 15 minutes at a time, at least three times that day. This was administered in an aerosol form that resembled dry ice and introduced a drug to help alleviate the moisture in her lungs that also puzzled Dr. Reisman. He told me that this type of condition generally results in elderly post-surgical patients, but not a woman in her early forties who was in otherwise good health just a few days prior.

The rest of Sunday was spent trying to get Karen's breathing back in check using a nebulizer, which is an apparatus that helps the lungs expand and contract by applying pressure as the patient exhales. My recollection is that Pat arrived later in the day on Sunday.

Our neighbors were meeting our children's needs. They were totally absorbed in the joy of school being out, and I told them that Karen was having some minor problems. However, I was confident that the doctors would figure things out and that she'd be home by the end of the week.

When Pat arrived I was very grateful that she was there, not only because she was Karen's mother, but because she is a registered nurse still active in administering to the needs of patients at an oral surgeon's office in Akron. Pat could tell Karen was totally out of it and suggested a switch from the morphine to Percocet.

Pat spent the night with Karen. I slept at home with the kids, but I barely got any meaningful sleep. I was very concerned about my wife's condition. I prayed that she would show some progress toward recovery on Monday.

Right before I came home one of the hospital staff's personnel, who had no clue as to how to clean the room and handle bloody items like Karen's gown, came in and made a big mess. This incident upset Pat. This poor person was so damn clueless it was almost comical.

Karen's father, Tom, arrived the next day and the respiratory therapy continued. It seemed to be helping. Tom started to complain to me that the level of care his daughter was receiving was inferior. He implored me to life-flight Karen to the Cleveland Clinic, saying, "We're not even trying. We've got to do something, man!"

I said, "This puzzle will come together and when it does we will get Karen wherever she has to go to get well, but I'm not just going to put her on a plane to Cleveland. What if she has a problem like cardiac arrest at 30,000 feet? Then what are we going to do?"

He stated, "At least then we can say we've tried. We're not doing anything."

Later in the day Tom was on the phone to his oldest daughter Kathy, who was also en route, and I overheard him say to Kathy that Karen was on a ventilator. This wasn't the case. Karen was using the nebulizer and definitely was able to breathe on her own. I knew a ventilator was only used when a patient was in a coma or otherwise unable to breathe on their own. When Kathy arrived I made sure she understood that her sister was not on a ventilator.

Monday was a wasted day at best and one we could not afford. From the moment Karen initially came into the emergency room at St. Vincent's on Saturday up until early Monday morning, it is my opinion that she received a reasonable standard of care given the symptoms she originally presented at admission. Her low blood pressure and the bleeding in her lower abdomen were handled appropriately by Dr. Sarah Bradley. It was not reasonable to expect, given these symptoms, that St. Vincent's would have been able to readily determine the root cause of Karen's problems over the weekend. But as Monday wore on, we barely stayed afloat, taking on water all day long. Karen made no discernable progress toward recovery and the fact that Dr. Reisman still seemed puzzled concerned all of us. I called my parents and talked to my mother at length to let her know what was going on and to get some guidance. My mom is very smart.

"You'll get this figured out," she told me with confidence.

At that point my dad packed up and headed toward Indy to help. I also consulted with my friend, Lori Spence, an attorney at the Midwest ISO where I worked, regarding the competency of St. Vincent's and she said, "I hate the place!" She had numerous stories to back up her lowly opinion of the facility. I knew in my heart that we had to do something fast, but I felt that there were clues, and as I prayed, I felt the Lord tugging at me to continue to be patient and to not act in haste. Late in the day Monday, Karen's youngest sibling, Tommy, arrived and he and Kathy spent the night with Karen.

I left the phone off the hook and was finally able to get some quality sleep into early Tuesday morning. Then, in the middle of the night, I heard a hard pounding at the front door that vibrated the whole front of the house, and could hear Marty Wetzel's deep voice saying, "Mark, wake up, wake up. It's the hospital; you've got to get there right now."

I put on my clothes and drove over at 3:00 a.m. When I got there, Kathy explained that Karen had flat lined, as in no heartbeat, for about seven seconds according to the recordings on her monitor, and according to Kathy the nursing staff seemed clueless as to what to do. The resident that was attending on the graveyard shift explained to me that it was a phenomenon that caused people to "vagile" and it happens due to shifting body fluids.

Karen told me she heard everything and was aware of the confusion swirling in her room. Everything seemed to be in order when I got there, but Kathy was alarmed, and we wondered whether they had a crash cart nearby just in case a patient went into cardiac arrest. In the middle of the night, one lone resident was on duty with responsibility for numerous patients. I was starting to get an education of how the American healthcare system worked, especially the understaffed graveyard shift. I went home and got some shuteye, but was back at the hospital early at 7:00 on Tuesday morning.

By now my dad had arrived, and it was great to have my father to consult with and bounce things off. Tommy and Pat were both helpful, offering constructive suggestions and guidance. I remained steadfast in my conviction that St. Vincent's would put the puzzle pieces together and we would eventually know what to do to help Karen.

At one point Kathy approached me and said, "Mark, we've got to do something. You seem very prayerful, but I don't think this place has a clue."

I was confident that things would come together, and I was against doing anything rash. At the same time Scott Zigmond, a friend from church at St. Louis de Montfort, stopped by and told me that St. Vincent's had all of the most modern facilities and technically was as good as it gets. He was a medical equipment sales representative for General Electric.

He said, "If I had a family member in need, there's no doubt in my mind that this is where I would bring them."

I had a lot of input, but some of the information contradicted itself so there was no obvious solution. We were new to Indianapolis, so we had very little knowledge of the local hospitals. My attitude continued to be eerily calm and patient. It was not like me to wait and see, but I was still confident the situation would reach a resolution.

This was all so confusing!

How was I to know that if I took her somewhere else in Indianapolis, I wasn't making a bad situation worse? It was so hard, because I had conflicting local information from two people I trusted. Usually I read and react quickly, but something inside me said to continue to hold my ground, that Dr. Reisman would figure this out soon. Yet, the clock was ticking and my in-laws were not happy with the pace. I wasn't pleased either, and as I prayed to the Lord for guidance something yanked at me to stay the course.

At one point Tuesday, Karen was lucid enough to say to me, "Yesterday was nothing but socializing."

I knew that we had to do something, so we brokered a meeting with the head administrator of the hospital, Dr. Stephen Priddy.

At this point Karen's cousin Alice arrived. When I first saw her outside the hospital she was talking with Tom and he was trying to bring her up to speed on Karen's case. In the back of my mind I had concerns about Karen's blood; I thought it might be an extreme case of anemia, possibly meningitis, or maybe some sort of rare viral infection that had manifested itself via poor blood quality.

The meeting with Dr. Priddy took place in a family waiting room just outside the ICU. Dr. Priddy started out by reassuring us that Karen was getting the very best of care, and that they were doing everything possible to figure out what was wrong with her even though she was not making any discernable progress. By now Karen had been under the care of St. Vincent's for 72 hours, and she was regressing. I asked a few questions about her ability to clot and the respiratory therapy she was getting.

Then I said, "I don't want to monopolize all of the Q and A time with my concerns. I want everyone in the room to have a chance at airing their concerns."

One by one Pat, Tommy, Kathy and Tom asked questions.

Of primary concern was a lack of attention to detail, in that several tests, medications, and treatments that had been ordered were so slow in actually happening. We had to be very vigilant to watch out for Karen. The staff didn't seem to have any sense of urgency. Karen's cousin Alice sat in the corner quietly waiting and studying Karen's blood chemical work results for the last 48 hours.

Alice had worked as a nurse oncologist early in her career, but she was not currently practicing. Finally, she asked two questions.

"What is being done to figure out why this platelet count remains so low at 45,000 and what about the extraordinarily high white blood count?" she asked Dr. Priddy.

Dr. Priddy replied that these factors were being examined and he informed us that Dr. Reisman had consulted a hematology-oncologist about Karen's case. The nature of Alice's questions, given her background and the consult Dr. Priddy mentioned, had my mind thinking in terms of some sort of a blood problem consistent with my unqualified theory. I remember just sitting and staring at Alice because she seemed like she was onto something, as she studied the blood chemical results. Her questions conveyed what to me was the third set of clues regarding what was really wrong.

The first indication I received was the nurse's comments on Sunday regarding "PacMan," coupled with me noticing a set of numbers regarding her high Blast factor that was significantly above the norm, which I blew off as being of little consequence despite how out of whack the numbers were. Now Alice's questions again pointed back to the blood.

As the early evening hours drew near, Karen seemed to be stabilizing, and Samantha's second-grade teacher, Lisa Roach, who had heard about Karen's hospitalization, brought us a great dinner that we all ate picnic style in front of the hospital's main entrance. We were in a bit of a celebratory mood, as it seemed as if Karen had turned a corner and was moving along in a positive direction. Her breathing was less labored, and she seemed to be more alert as to her surroundings now that the morphine had been taken out of the equation.

When I left the hospital on Tuesday night, the hospital's nursing staff was very upbeat and felt that Karen had turned the corner, too. I had every reason to believe that Karen was going to be better soon; it was just going to take a little longer than expected to recover from the surgery due to some weird and bizarre blood-related complications. That night I finally got about three or four hours sleep, the most I'd had in a long time.

When I arrived at the hospital at about 6:45 the next morning I was in a very good mood. I ran into Tommy, who was pacing out front talking on his cell phone.

He paused for a second and said, "Dr. Reisman wants to talk to you right away."

"Fine," I said, figuring Karen had made great progress during the night. I looked forward to this update.

Tommy said, "Wait up. I'll go with you!"

When I got to the entrance of the ICU, my dad was very disenchanted with what was going on, and he said, "I'm leaving. I obviously don't have any rights here," and he started walking away. Apparently his name had been omitted from the list of "family only" members who were permitted to see Karen. As Karen's husband this was easy to fix, so I talked to the nurse, added his name to the list and managed to chase him down just as he was getting ready to leave. Tommy waited patiently for me while I straightened out this snafu.

Meanwhile, Tommy tracked down Dr. Reisman, who took us to a dark and secluded portion of the ICU. He had a very serious look on his face. Then he said quickly, "I have had our hematology-oncologist look closely at this case, which has had us all puzzled for a few days. But now we're 99% sure your wife has leukemia."

My heart sank. I immediately had flashbacks to Barb Duckworth, my fellow eighth-grade classmate who lived three houses up the street. Barb had died of leukemia after a two-year battle some 30 years prior.

"What exactly is leukemia?" Tommy asked.

"It's cancer of the blood and we can't treat it here. You have your choice of three different facilities here in Indianapolis where you can transport her for treatment," Dr. Reisman replied.

He was all business, so I took a hard swallow and said, "Okay, what are our choices?"

Reisman said, "You can take her to either St. Vincent's on 86th Street, which is what we would prefer, Methodist Hospital or the Indiana University Medical Center."

He said we had about three hours to figure it out; he was finishing up paperwork and arranging transport, but that he needed an answer quickly.

The word of this bad news spread quickly. Lots of cell phone calls were made; my dad was very sullen and I went to the chapel to say a quick prayer. What happened over the next hour and a half was truly remarkable. I have to give credit to Tommy and his brother, Kevin, who had just arrived that morning, for taking quick action on behalf of their terribly ill sister.

Pat and I went in to tell Karen about her situation. Karen had trouble grasping the full depth of what we were telling her as we tried to break it to her gently that she had cancer of the blood. She looked concerned, confused and startled. At this point Karen knew that decisions were being made on her behalf, but she was still having trouble dealing with the reality that she more than likely had cancer, and use of the word *leukemia* didn't help make it any clearer to her. Things were happening very quickly and it was difficult for her to assimilate everything at once.

Her dad didn't believe the news and was positive that there was some sort of mistake. If the situation were the same for me and I had just found out that my Samantha, God forbid, was stricken with leukemia, I might be stuck in the same boat. But for me personally, I immediately accepted the verdict as it confirmed my uneducated and creeping inclination that there was something wrong, very wrong, with Karen's bloodstream, although admittedly cancer had never really crossed my mind.

Tommy and Kevin took the bull by the horns and immediately started combing the Internet, making personal contact with several parties in northeastern Ohio to find out which one of the three facilities in Indianapolis would be best at giving Karen a shot at finding a cure. While Tommy queried the Internet, Kevin called his brother-in-law, Chris Connors, at Sherwin-Williams in Cleveland because Chris served on the boards of several hospitals in the Cleveland area. Chris was literally pulled out of a meeting and then he made several calls to doctors in the University Hospital system in Cleveland. Kevin also contacted a pediatric oncologist he knew from Ohio State for some input. After about an hour and half, a common thread to the information-gathering effort became apparent, as Tommy and Kevin had consulted with numerous independent sources.

A single name kept coming up as the man who could best serve our needs and save Karen's life, which teetered in the balance. Tommy and Kevin, working independently of one another, had both come up with the name, Dr. Larry Cripe at the Indiana University Medical Center, or IUMC.

When we met in the family waiting room, I remember four people being in the room: John Volpe, Kevin Coyne, Tommy Coyne and myself. It was very important to me that this decision be one of consensus, that there is no looking back with any regret or second guessing, regardless of what happened down the road. We all agreed that Dr. Cripe at IUMC would be the man with whom we would place all our chips. This was a well thought-out, business-like decision, even though it was made in less than two hours. The one negative we heard about Dr. Cripe indicated that he was slightly impersonal, but what really mattered to us was that his patients often walked out alive after being under his care.

I give all the credit for this decision to Tommy and Kevin. They made the calls, and knocked on all the doors necessary in order for us to make an informed decision under extreme circumstances. This wasn't like buying a car; this was critical. Living versus dying was on the line, not just trying to decide whether to buy an extended warranty. Dr. Reisman eventually poked his head in the room and asked what the verdict was, adding that if we were staying with St. Vincent's there would not be a transport fee of $300 because we were staying within the same hospital system.

"The fee is of no object to us; we're taking her to Dr. Larry Cripe at the Indiana University Medical Center," I said.

"Fine. I'll finish up the paperwork and we'll have her moving in that direction in an hour," he replied, rather curtly.

St. Vincent had just lost a patient's business, but they also hadn't done anything to gain our confidence. I believe Dr. Reisman is a good doctor, but this case had them puzzled for way too long.

With the decision made, I then went in to inform Karen that she would be taken to another hospital in about an hour. I don't think the whole cancer thing had sunk in yet. She was still very confused and putting it in even the simplest of terms didn't help, as she had been through so much. Her poor body had deteriorated rapidly. She had been on morphine for a few days, so her ability to comprehend what we were saying was lacking, even though she seemed able to comprehend what she was being told.

Karen was able to pipe up and say, "If I'm going somewhere downtown, I want my navy blue Victoria's Secret long-sleeve top and bottoms for the ambulance ride."

Some things never change; even under the most extreme situations she was still very concerned with fashion. If it were me, I probably would have said, "So long as I'm in front of the TV to see the kickoff at 1:00, I don't care where you take me."

At this point we were relieved that the mystery had been solved, and we were able to get out of St. Vincent's with Karen still breathing. Kevin had likened the facility to a nice veterinary clinic, just barely competent enough to keep Karen alive. We were going to a premier, research-oriented teaching hospital with a fantastic reputation for treating cancers of the blood. Tommy reminded me, as we got organized for the transport, that the Indiana University Medial Center was where Lance Armstrong chose to be treated for his testicular cancer. Pat was relieved that we were leaving St. Vincent's and were moving Karen to a place where she could be treated properly.

As we began to move Karen out of the ICU toward the elevator, I went to Kevin and gave him a hug. I teared up a little and whispered, "Help me!"

On our way downtown, I could hear Karen gabbing away, complaining about how hot she was while I made small talk with the driver. As we approached the hospital, I saw a small park-like area that had sculptures of a family and a big stone sign that read, "CANCER SURVIVORS PARK." I said a Hail Mary to myself and vowed that Karen, Mark, Will, Samantha and Mitchell would one day have a picnic lunch in that park with our cancer-free wife and mother.

A couple of tears rolled down my face again. I knew we were in for the fight of our lives. Seeing this place reminded me there was always hope. Now I had to dig down and find the courage and faith to endure the fight. I knew Karen had the will to fight. I had seen it before when she decided that she would bring our healthy Mitchell into the world seven years earlier. I knew she would never give in.

The Irish never say die; they are stubborn and will continue to fight.

And as for us Italians, well, we fight, too, but we just have anyone who gets in our way removed one way or another.

CHAPTER 3

Kitzbuhel, Austria

It was a cold and sunny day back in February 1987. Ed and I hadn't seen each other for two or three years, but when he picked me up to head for Cleveland Hopkins Airport it was just like our old drinking days. We grew up on Oak Road in Stow, Ohio, in the late '60s. Even though Ed was a year older than me, we were good friends dating back to our days playing in the band at Holy Family Catholic School. We only lived six houses apart, and throughout our days at Walsh Jesuit High School in the mid-'70s Ed, his next-door neighbor, Brad Winkler, and I were thick as thieves.

Growing up near Kent State University, we had numerous adventures to the bars in Kent, especially JB's and Ray's Place, to hear bands such as the Immortal Porpoises and my personal favorite, The Numbers Band, also known as 15-60-75. Of course we drank beer, and in the early '80s after high school, Ed shared an apartment with a couple of guys on beautiful Akron Boulevard in Kent, not far from the campus watering holes. Eddie had called me two months earlier in December 1986 to ask me whether I wanted to join him on a ski trip to Kitzbuhel, Austria. I remember the call vividly.

"Hey, Volpe, we're going skiing to the Alps in Europe this February, so I want you to send Nora Haas a check for $984," Eddie said.

I gave the invitation about three seconds thought before I said, "Sure." I had just quit my first job out of college after five years with Marathon Oil Company in Findlay, Ohio. I had graduated in 1981 from Ohio Northern University with a bachelor's degree in business administration, majoring in accounting and pre-law studies. In accepting Eddie's invitation to be a ski bum for a week or so, I did it knowing that I may never have a better chance to do something like this for a long time. In fact, when Ed called, I was packing up my worldly possessions from my fabulous bachelor pad.

My parents had told me I was welcome to return home and live with them until I found a new job. They didn't mind the fact that I had just quit my job. I had never been much trouble, and to them I seemed to have a plan. Having a plan is always a good way to get along with your parents. I was also working on a post-graduate degree. I had just vested in Marathon's 401(k) retirement plan, and the Internal Revenue Service had a 10-year income averaging tax code advantage ending in 1986 that made it financially advantageous to quit your job, retire or die and cash in the 401(k) plan while paying a minimal amount of taxes to liquidate the funds. So, as a bachelor with a nice stash of cash, and having no real responsibilities, quitting what I saw as a dead-end job and then heading off to Europe to ski and drink real beer for a week, seemed like a no-brainer.

In Findlay, the relationship with my girlfriend, Matilda, and I was going absolutely nowhere fast. Ending the relationship gracefully seemed difficult. We had been seeing each other for about nine months, and many of our friends, most of them newly married, whispered that we made a great couple and should consider getting hitched. Leaving town and heading home to live with one's parents seemed like a good way to hint to Matilda that it was over. It wasn't as if I had found a new job. I had only sent out about a dozen resumés prior to quitting my billing analyst job at Marathon. My last job at Marathon, processing invoices for their refinery operations, was a task that a modestly trained monkey could perform. It was time to leave Findlay, Ohio.

In February, the day of the big trip abroad arrived, and on the way to the airport, Ed and I picked up a six-pack of Bud Light, which we polished off in the parking lot after the 45-minute ride to Cleveland. We had a six-hour transoceanic flight ahead of us, and drinking on a plane can be expensive, so we slugged down the road pops and caught up on the latest news. Once we got into the airport, we checked our luggage through to Frankfurt, Germany, and headed for the gate to meet the rest of the entourage.

Our ski adventure organizer, Nora Haas, her parents Leigh and Andrew, her Aunt Charlotte, her cousin, Carla, and best friend, Karen Coyne, were all assembled at the gate awaiting the first leg of our journey to Boston before the big flight to Heathrow International in London. I introduced myself to the Haas family members, having known them casually for many years, as they were also fellow parishioners at Holy Family Church. Nora was a year younger than I and came from a very large family.

Nora then introduced me to her friend, Karen, who didn't seem real thrilled to see either Ed or me, although she seemed to be more irked with him than me, as she constantly gave Eddie a steady glare. She was dressed rather nicely, but man, was she ever mad, and there I was unshaven, unemployed and living with my parents.

What a way to make a first impression!

I was wearing a bright orange Cleveland Browns hooded sweatshirt. I had to wear the sweatshirt because I was still mourning the Browns' loss in the American Football Conference title game to John Elway and the damn Denver Broncos.

"The Drive" will always haunt me, as it does every diehard Browns fan. I had been a Browns season ticket holder for several years despite the fact that I lived 120 miles from downtown Cleveland. Even though I didn't have a job, I was ready to head to Pasadena to the Super Bowl versus the New York Giants if it hadn't been for Elway's heroics. I could only sit there in my seat and squirm while Elway marched his team down the field, in 15 plays, for the tying score. Actually, I still believe to this day that Rich Karlis's field goal to allegedly win the game in overtime was no good.

So there I was all dressed in orange, just the kind of guy you would want to have father your children. I was the original George Costanza, unemployed and living with my parents. I know I didn't make much of a first impression on Karen, but I don't recall really caring one way or the other either.

Ed was talking to Karen, and I could tell she was still noticeably perturbed with him. Then it dawned on me: Karen and Ed were an item. Ed had failed to mention this fact to me on the way to the airport, but I remembered a phone conversation I had a few months earlier with our mutual friend Brad Winkler. Brad had said that Ed, even though he lived in Milwaukee, had been carrying on this long-distance relationship with Karen in Cleveland.

So finally, at the airport, the light bulb went off. When we skied out west at Lake Tahoe a few years earlier with a bunch of high school and college friends, Ed's motives were different than they were now. He was chasing after this fetching young lady named Karen Coyne, whom he had been dating for some time. A few months later, I found out that Ed was supposed to have picked up Karen and her luggage at her office in downtown Cleveland, but he either forgot or blew her off, choosing to catch up with his buddy instead. Karen's younger brother, Tommy, a freshman at John Carroll University, had to take the rapid transit from University Heights into town at the last minute to take his sister to the airport. This wasn't such a bad deal for Tommy. He was able to use Karen's new Mustang convertible for two weeks while she traversed the Alps. Free wheels are important when you're a college kid!

It's a pretty quick flight to Boston and we didn't have a long layover in Beantown. I don't remember much of the flight across the Atlantic. It was early evening when we left Boston for London, and the flight wasn't very full, so I stretched out across six seats, making a little bed for myself. Once we were fed the wonderful airline food, I fell asleep for a few hours. When I awoke we were on our descent into London. It was early in the morning in England and we were only allowed off the plane for a half hour. I found a much-needed cup of coffee at a small cafe. It was my first time leaving North America. Karen, Ed, Nora and I walked the concourse and then boarded our flight for Frankfurt. Ed and Karen seemed rather chummy, probably having had plenty of time to kiss and make up on the long flight.

Upon our arrival in Germany, everybody sailed through customs except for me. Maybe it was the fact that I have a somewhat dark complexion, coupled with an unshaven face, sunglasses and slightly bloodshot eyes. The well-armed Germans finally let me through after figuring out that I was just an American going on a ski trip. After we gathered our ski gear and luggage, we boarded a touring bus for the last leg before reaching our final destination.

The German Autobahn was pretty cool. Our bus was only permitted to travel 48 miles per hour, while over in the fast lanes the high-speed Mercedes and Porsches flew by at over 140 mph. We were on the bus for about five hours before reaching the quaint little village of Kitzbuhel, Austria. It was late at night in the dead of winter. After checking in, as exhausted as we were, one would think that well-educated people with a little common sense would get some rest before hitting the slopes early the next day. None of us were ready to hit the sack. We found a bar playing American rock-n-roll, and true to form, we closed the place before getting some shut-eye.

Our accommodations were pretty nice and the food was extraordinary. We had a full breakfast every morning before venturing out to the slopes, and in the evenings, we had a great meal. I would always order one of the least popular entrees like the venison or duck, knowing that the girls would be unable to finish their dinners. They would offer me whatever was left of their chicken or beef, allowing me to sample lots of superb European cuisine.

The skiing was fabulous. Ed, Nora and Karen were all accomplished skiers. I had just taken up the sport a few years earlier, so I struggled at times to keep pace. In fact, it was Ed who had given me my first ski lesson on the beginner hills at Brandywine in northeastern Ohio. I had always been afraid to ski in my high school years for fear of breaking my legs prior to baseball season. Even though I was a marginal player at Walsh, unable to hit a lick, I still loved the game and took it pretty seriously in spite of my lack of talent. For much of the time in Austria, I skied with Nora's father, Dr. Andrew Haas. He was pretty hardcore about his skiing, seldom taking any breaks. Gradually, my skiing improved over the course of the week, as I was forced to keep pace with the veteran skiers. We had a great time and we all enjoyed the post-skiing activities.

Our tour guide, Hans, would take us to little bars in the village to debrief after a day in the Alps. The terrain was difficult and the skiing was terrific. Hans introduced us to a traditional local beer called Old Fursteinburgh. This was a fine beer and Hans had one rule: You had to drink your beer left-handed; otherwise, you were free game to be called "Buffalo." Once you were caught and pointed out with a jabbing left elbow, you had to chug the remaining contents of your brew. This is a great way to get hammered really quickly.

I also recall one evening after dinner we went out to one of the local bars. Naturally, I had a few and I asked Karen to dance. I went to dip her on her back and then pull her back up, but I missed catching her, and Karen fell backwards hard, lying prone on the floor with her big blue eyes wide open, looking up at me. I thought she was hurt, so I hesitated to pull her up.

She looked up at me and exclaimed, "Pick me up, you idiot!"

Karen seemed okay, because later in the night she was on stage with the lead singer taking her turn on vocals to some obscure song from the early '60s.

One other night we managed to get into an exclusive after-hours club. It was probably 2:00 or 3:00 in the morning when we arrived. Once we got in, we couldn't help but notice that the bar was filled with gorgeous, well-endowed, blonde Scandinavian women. Ed poked me on the shoulder as we entered the bar and said, "Can you say Hello, Heidi?" After awhile Ed was out on the dance floor with this group of beautiful blonde women, shaking it up and dancing his heart out.

Most men prefer Ginger; I'll take Mary Ann.

It didn't take long for Karen to get pissed at Ed again. Eventually, she decided to walk back to the hotel by herself. The next day at breakfast, she told me that a man walking his German shepherd kept calling out to her while following her to the hotel. I felt bad for allowing her to walk home alone, but she made it safely in spite of her encounter with the stranger. As for Ed, he was like the proverbial kid in a candy store. It was hard for me to blame him for being out there on the dance floor with all of those pretty women, but right in front of your girlfriend was probably not the brightest of moves, assuming you want the relationship to continue—even if it was just innocent fun.

One of the other highlights of the trip was the ski safari, when we went from village to village over the course of a day.

Finally, we were nearing the end of the trip and the last few days were full of some memorable events. My last ski run of the trip with Nora was down the famous Hahnenkamm Run, which is a well-known downhill slalom course. Karen decided to go shopping for souvenirs the last day after we were done skiing and Ed threw some money at her, asking her to pick out something for his mom.

This is not how you score points with your girlfriend!

I tagged along with Karen and we had a wonderful time shopping, and she seemed to have forgiven me for dropping her on her head earlier in the week. The multi-course gourmet meal served our last night in Kitzbuhel was exquisite.

We took the tour bus to Munich on the way back to Frankfurt, stopping at the Hoffbrau House for lunch and more beer. I was starting to get a sore throat, but I pushed on as we headed for home. We visited an old castle in Heidelberg and spent our final night partying in this old city that is home to many American servicemen. When we returned to Cleveland, a surprise visitor was waiting for me at the gate. It was my girlfriend Matilda from Findlay.

"Did you open the envelope I gave you before you left on Valentine's Day?" she asked. I looked at her sheepishly and admitted that I had forgotten.

Now it was my turn to get the evil eye at an airport.

Back in Stow, I continued to search for a new job, and took the last couple of courses I needed to finish my MBA. I had a job interview in northwestern Ohio at the Davis-Besse Nuclear Power Plant as a financial systems analyst working for Centerior Energy. Oddly enough, it wasn't very far from Findlay, the place I was trying to get away from. I was offered the job at a salary exceeding my compensation at Marathon, so I accepted and decided to look for a place to live in Port Clinton, Ohio. I had decided to use my 401(k) proceeds as a down payment on a condo or home instead of continuing to rent. While I looked for a home, I stayed in a hotel during the week and commuted back to Stow on the weekends to finish my final MBA course at Ashland University.

On Saturday nights, I would meet Nora and Karen, my fellow ski travelers, at Rocknes, one of our favorite gathering places in nearby Cuyahoga Falls. Nora lived nearby in an apartment on the Cuyahoga River. We reminisced about our trip to Europe, sharing our photos from the trip, and I showed Nora and Karen the real-estate listings I was looking at for my first major investment. Karen liked talking to me, and she was obviously a little perplexed about the relationship she had with Ed. I always stuck up for my long-time buddy and told her that his antics were just Ed being Ed. Everything would work out in time.

As for myself, I half-heartedly continued my relationship with Matilda. She visited me in Port Clinton. I looked for my first house. My search concentrated on the peninsula of Catawba Island. Nearby, the Erie Islands of South Bass, Middle Bass, North Bass and Kelley's were only a short ferry ride away. This was a great summertime vacation mecca for boaters, fishermen and partiers from Detroit, Cleveland and Columbus. I remembered having traveled to the area for short day trips when I was younger. Cedar Point, one of the best amusement parks in the country, known for its roller coasters, was only a half hour away. Even though the winters in this region were brutal, the summers were a blast. However, I could tell Matilda was not thrilled with the relationship and she seemed uninterested in my first venture into real estate.

Finally in May 1987, I found a way to end the relationship without being labeled as the bad guy. We were supposed to attend a wedding of a family friend I had known since the second grade. Matilda called me the Thursday before the wedding to say she wasn't happy with the relationship and that she didn't want to go. Over the phone, I tried to sound so wounded and hurt, but inside I was jumping for joy. I thought about it for 10 or 15 minutes and then I decided what the heck, I needed an escort, and maybe Karen would go with me. We were just friends and I needed a date, so I called her from my hotel room.

I hemmed and hawed over the phone as I explained my predicament, and then Karen finally said, "Well, if you're asking me to go with you to this wedding, I'll be happy to, except my sister, Kathy, has a wedding shower that day so you'll have to pick me up there."

I was elated, relieved, nervous and excited all at the same time. After all, she was still my best friend's girl, but I knew that relationship was on shaky ground.

The day of the wedding arrived quickly, and I dropped by Carnaby Street, a restaurant on Akron's west side, "in the valley," as they say, where the wedding shower for Karen's sister was taking place. All of the women attending the shower were very welcoming as I looked around the private room, anxiously searching for Karen. I kidded with the ladies that the shower looked like more fun than the wedding I was heading off to with Karen. She finally walked up and smiled, introducing me to her mother, Pat, her sister, Kathy, and several other women attending the shower.

We went to the wedding, and before the early evening reception started there was a break, so my mom invited everyone in the family back to the house for drinks prior to the reception. When we walked in Karen looked around and said, "I've been here before, at a Walsh pre-prom party." Initially, I thought she was making things up and then I flashed back to the 1977 party before the Walsh Jesuit senior prom my parents co-hosted with Jim and Sally Klein.

The Kleins were good friends, and their oldest son, Jeff, who had accepted a basketball scholarship to the University of Virginia, was dating my sister, Lynn, at the time. Jeff and I had played baseball at Walsh together our junior year. Right before the season started, we were both running after a pop fly into short center field. Jeff was at short and I played second; we collided ever so slightly, and I ended up getting spiked in the face. The result was 17 stitches in my face and a swollen head that looked like a prizefighter that had just received a good ass-whooping.

Long story short, at that time, Karen was dating one of my classmates at Walsh. Karen brought up having been there 10 years earlier, and before we knew it, my mom had the pictures out. I remembered the prom evening fondly because it was one of those rare occasions when my father, John, allowed me to use his silver 1964 Corvette Sting Ray for the evening's festivities. My parents were also pretty cool at that party because they just looked the other way and went in the house when the majority of my all-male classmates started bringing in beer and wine from the trunks of their cars to the picnic tables set up in the backyard.

Eventually we headed over to the wedding reception. Karen has two vivid memories of the reception. One is the homemade Italian cookies my Grandma Mary Volpe had stacked up in front of her at the table. The second was my insistence to turn on my little battery-operated, 2.5-inch Sony TV to watch the annual running of the Kentucky Derby at 5:00 p.m. We had a very nice time and I really appreciated Karen so graciously pinch-hitting as my escort after Matilda stood me up.

Karen and I went out for drinks after the reception with my brothers, David John (we call him D.J.), and my younger brother, Paul. My sister, Lynn, and her husband also joined us for a nightcap. I remember Lynn asking me what was up with Karen when she was off powdering her nose. Lynn mentioned Karen obviously had a lot more personality than the rather boring Matilda. I explained to her that Karen was dating my good friend Ed and that she was a last-minute date so that I didn't have to show up alone. When I dropped Karen off at her apartment she invited me in.

I think we stayed up talking until past 4:00 a.m. We talked about our trip to Germany and Austria, but she was more concerned about her relationship with Ed. She also asked me about my relationship with Matilda, which from my point of view was about over, in spite of the fact that so many people who knew us thought the relationship was getting pretty serious. Matilda and I had continued to see each other from time to time on weekends once I had taken the job at Davis-Besse, but I think we could both tell that the relationship had run its course and had nowhere to go. When I left, Karen gave me the obligatory good night kiss, and thanked me for such a fun day.

I went back to my hotel and new job on Lake Erie somewhat confused, but still impressed with her. She was Ed's girlfriend and I was not about to do anything else that could be construed as hitting on his girl.

A couple of weeks later, I met Karen and Nora at Rocknes to socialize and stay in touch. Karen had grown even more disenchanted with the way things were going with Ed. Karen, Nora and another friend, Missy, had met up with Ed in Chicago to see the sights and paint the town. According to Karen, her boyfriend was hitting on Missy every chance he got, and Karen was finally fed up. At this point, I decided to make my move.

The next time I was in town, I asked Karen out to dinner. After dinner we headed down to the Portage Lakes for a drink and I got lost on the way. She could tell I was upset about getting slightly off course. I so wanted everything to go smoothly on this first real date. At one point she said, "Mark, it's not a big deal." And then she leaned over and kissed me firmly on the lips. Our first real kiss made me wilt. I dropped her off at her apartment after we had a couple drinks. She invited me in and we made out a little while, and after an hour or so I left. I did my best to be a perfect gentleman and tried to make a positive impression on our first real date.

Once I got out to my Camaro, I jumped in the car and the first song on the cassette was "She's The One" from Bruce Springsteen's *Born To Run* album. It's a powerful song, with a heavy rhythm vamp throughout, led by drummer Max Weinberg: boom, boom, boom, then a quick boom, boom. I love those lyrics, especially considering the kiss earlier in the evening.

With her hands on her hips and a smile on her lips,
Because she knows that it kills me.
With her long blond hair and eyes that shine like the midnight sun.
Oh, Oh, She's the One, She's the One, Oh, Oh.

With one soft kiss,
She turned those long summer nights with her tenderness...

A week later Matilda called me and asked me to meet her for a drink just to talk, and I told her that I was seeing someone else. I had no second thoughts and knew the best thing to do was to just leave the relationship behind me. It was time for both of us to move on, and I wished her the best.

My Grandma Volpe always said whenever a girl had dumped me in the past, which was often, "Don't worry, Sonny, another bus will come along if you missed this one." Grandma was right, except this new bus named Karen was one I wasn't about to miss.

The following weekend when I was in town, Karen invited me over for dinner at her apartment: steaks and shrimp. Our relationship was quickly getting steamier, although Karen still hadn't really broken it off with Ed yet. At one point, we were slow dancing on her balcony and she said to me that she was still so confused. I told her, "No you're not."

A couple of weeks later Ed was in town to attend a couple's shower that Karen was throwing for her sister, Kathy. Ed decided to play golf instead of going to the shower with Karen.

Strike three!

The next day she dropped by his parents' house on Oak Road to tell him the long distance thing just wasn't going to work out. Thank God, she didn't tell him about me. Then she headed down the street five houses and rang the doorbell at my parents' house. I answered the door and she told me to get in her car. I did what she said, jumping in the passenger seat of the Mustang convertible. I could tell that she was excited about something and needed to talk. We went to the local park and talked about how to tell Ed that his girlfriend had been seeing one of his best friends. I didn't know how strongly she felt for me, but I knew I was falling for her. I felt bad for Ed, but things hadn't been working out for Ed and Karen. When Karen and I began seeing each other, everything changed. Besides, we had grown weary of sneaking around the area, running into mutual friends and acquaintances, and feeling awkward. We decided I had to say something to Ed.

A couple of weeks later, I called Ed to tell him I was seeing his former girlfriend. He took it pretty well, and didn't sound angry with me. In fact, he told me that Karen was a great girl, and he wished me luck. Today, Ed and I are still friends, even though we don't stay in touch. He is a successful executive in the tire industry with a beautiful wife and family. In retrospect, I suppose I could have handled the situation more gracefully. Nevertheless, things worked out for all of us.

Karen visited me at my newly purchased ranch house on Catawba Island, right after her sister's bachelorette party. Our relationship was growing more serious. I was crazy about her. I told her that I loved her for the first time in my garage, of all places, right before she left to head back to Cuyahoga Falls.

We went to her sister Kathy's wedding and I met the entire Coyne family, as well as her mom's family, the Smiths from Huntington, West Virginia. It was a great time; in fact, even though I was a newcomer to the scene, Karen's brother Kenny, his friend Greg Scanlon, and I sang Springsteen's "Thunder Road" to Kathy at the reception. Greg and I happen to be big fans of "The Boss." We knew all the words, and Kenny just faked it, although he did know when to shout, *"Show a little faith, there's magic in the night, you ain't a beauty and hey you're all right."*

Later in June, Karen attended my graduation from Ashland University after I finished the final course toward my MBA. We dated throughout the summer, seeing each other every weekend. On one weekend in particular, Karen was in the bathroom at my house for a long time, and every time I knocked at the door to see if she was all right, she would just say everything was fine. About 45 minutes later, she walked out after having peeled off most of the wallpaper, explaining that it had just fallen down. My first home was rather simple, with the previous owner's 1977 earth tone décor scheme from hell. The wallpaper Karen tore down was brown, gold and orange velour. She had always kidded me that you didn't need a towel after showering; you could just rub up against the wall. She bought wallpaper to fix up the bathroom and over time she redecorated other parts of the house in order to bring it up to date. She made herself right at home; I think she was trying to give me a hint.

I knew she was the one, but I had no idea whether she felt the same. In October 1987, it was Sweetest Day weekend, and Karen was cruising up to see me so I went over to the Sandusky Mall to get her a card and a present. I never really had much of a plan, but somehow I wandered into Alvin's Jewelers. After looking at diamond engagement rings for about a half hour, I found one I liked and put it on layaway. I didn't know exactly when I would need it. Karen was the one, but I wasn't really sure she would ever say yes to a guy like me. I knew that in due time, I might propose marriage. I had to wait and see.

However, I did have a tentative plan that I was hatching in my little mind. A year and a half earlier, when my parents were touring western Canada, I told my mom to look into tickets for the 1988 Winter Olympics in Calgary. She brought me back an order form, which I sent in, and a few months later my VISA statement showed $200 in mysterious charges that I eventually traced back to Calgary.

At Christmas, everyone expected us to get engaged, but this wasn't my style. Just about everyone gets engaged at Christmas except for me. Kathy had champagne and the glasses ready to go. She was carting these items around in the trunk of her car, but I had something else in mind. So for her present, I got Karen a new white 10-speed bike, which was exactly what she had asked for. The problem was that she had given the same hint for a present to her father, Dr. Thomas J. Coyne, and he delivered a beautiful white Schwinn. I volunteered to return the bike I had purchased.

This was my chance to test the waters, so I decided to get her a diamond necklace to replace the bike. If she accepted the necklace, I knew she might say yes if I decided to pop the question in Calgary. If she said no to the necklace, that it was too serious, then I would know that the engagement ring probably wouldn't fly any time soon.

My present from Karen was an awesome, slightly distressed brown leather bomber jacket that was made from goatskin. When I showed up to give her the necklace, my hand was trembling slightly as I handed her the small wine-colored jewelry box. She loved it and immediately put it on, and she has worn it often ever since.

A few weeks later, I picked Karen up at Cleveland Hopkins, after she was returning from a business trip to Louisiana. She looked so hot getting off the plane in her pink sweater and white skirt. Karen told me a very upsetting story that happened to her. She ran a training center in downtown Cleveland where they trained and placed less fortunate people who needed a fresh start for careers in the hotel services industry. The types of positions she trained people for included front desk clerks, housekeeping and food services. Karen received great satisfaction in helping those who needed a break getting back on their feet. She went down to a center in Monroe, Louisiana to "train the trainer" for a three-day stint without a rental car. Always being the adventurer, she ventured into town, walking through a dangerous neighborhood. Frustrated when she found nowhere safe, she stopped and headed back to the hotel.

As she was walking, she suddenly realized a bunch of teenage boys were walking behind her, and they were yelling, "Hey, pretty white girl, when we catch up with you, we're gonna slash that pretty face of yours up pretty good. Then you ain't going to look so pretty no more, bitch!"

Suddenly a police cruiser came across the bridge and the police yelled at Karen for being stupid, by walking into such a "hood" alone. One of the officers chastised Karen and said, "White people don't even drive into that area without a gun. Go back to your hotel and stay there."

Monroe is not a very nice place and Karen hated it there. I knew I had to take her away from this calling, even though she received so much personal satisfaction from helping people. I needed to get her into my life permanently. There were other ways for her to give to others without taking such personal risks.

We had stopped at the airport bar to talk and I asked her whether she would go to Calgary to the Olympics with me the following month.

She accepted, and my plan to propose was slowly falling into place.

CHAPTER 4

Calgary

Once again, I'm at Cleveland Hopkins Airport, only this time it's with only Karen. Her mom took us to the airport for the early Saturday morning flight to Calgary via Chicago O'Hare. We were waiting to check our luggage after Pat had dropped us off when Karen's wonderful mom reappeared behind us to tell us to have a great time and give us one last hug. I told her we would have a good time and I vividly remember telling Pat I would take good care of her beautiful daughter. Karen and her mom have a special relationship.

Let's face it, mothers know everything. I know that Pat sensed that her daughter had fallen in love with me and that I might be proposing in Calgary, especially since the anticipated Christmas proposal hadn't happened. Hey, the Browns were in the playoffs again and, as a devoted fan, I had to concentrate on football. This time they lost to Denver in the AFC Championship game when Earnest Byner fumbled just before crossing the goal line to score what would have been the game-tying touchdown. The Browns had followed up "The Drive" with "The Fumble." Byner had played one of the greatest postseason games I had ever seen and unfortunately he will always be remembered for this untimely miscue.

A few years earlier, after more than 29 years of marriage, Karen's parents, Pat and Tom Coyne, went through a difficult divorce. Karen immediately quit her job in Columbus, Ohio, and returned to Akron to help her mother through this tough time. Karen was a 1982 graduate of The Ohio State University, graduating with dual bachelors' degrees in business administration, majoring in marketing and economics. She worked in hotel administration and had quickly found a job, helping train people for hotel-related positions. The training center was based at Stouffer's Renaissance Hotel on Public Square in downtown Cleveland. Karen loved her job and took great care in helping the less fortunate find a vocation that would get them off social assistance programs and allow them to become more self-sufficient. Karen produced great results and found the job most rewarding.

She told me a couple of stories that I have always remembered. The trainees' checks were issued on Fridays. Karen would cash the checks for the trainees, if they didn't have a checking account. This allowed the trainees to pick up some groceries so they could feed their children over the weekend. Once a woman pulled a pen out of her purse to endorse the check and a big black roach, probably a resident from her Section 8 apartment, crawled out of the purse. Without getting startled Karen handed over her pen and said, "Use mine!" She proceeded to act like nothing happened.

On another occasion, Karen told me about a former Vietnam vet that he was let go from the program because of his failure to show up for class. He backed Karen up against the wall and lifted her off the floor. Karen's secretary called security and they responded immediately to diffuse the situation, making sure Karen did not suffer any major physical harm.

Karen never ceased to amaze me with her genuine concern for people. She took great personal satisfaction from her job. She gave people hope. One of my concerns while I considered popping the question was that she might say no to my marriage proposal because of her job. In some ways I felt guilty about the possibility of whisking her away when so many people benefited from her leadership at the Hotel and Lodging Training Center. Karen has even tried on several occasions over the years to track down her former secretary, Mona Johnson, still concerned for her welfare.

On our way west to Calgary, we had to go through security and customs in Winnipeg rather than Calgary. They explained to us in Winnipeg that all international flights bound for Calgary would go through security and customs in a Canadian city other than Calgary. I thought this was a wonderful idea from a security standpoint: the province of Manitoba looked like frozen tundra from the air. After we cleared all the security checks, upon reboarding for our flight into Calgary, the metal detectors went off when I went through the sensors.

The lady working security went over me with the wand and the detector went off as the wand passed over the left-hand pocket of my ski jacket. There was only one item in that pocket: the one carat, solitaire engagement ring I planned on giving Karen. The security guard insisted that I open the pocket immediately. My pulse quickened and I knew I had to think fast; otherwise my plan would be spoiled. I yelled to Karen, "It's nothing...I'll catch up." I quickly unzipped my pocket, pulled out the ring and showed it to the somewhat startled woman, explaining to her rather quickly that the metal jewelry box had set off the alarm and she was about to spoil my romantic plan.

The female security guard smiled and seemed to apologize for doing her job, then hugged me, wishing me luck and sending me on my "marry" way. When I caught up to Karen, she inquired as to what the commotion was all about. I told her the aluminum foil from a piece of gum set off the sensors. Karen looked at me and said, "Right." Hell, if I had put the rock in with my checked luggage it could have ended up in Vancouver or been stolen. Actually, Air Canada was wonderful. Every flight was on time and the Labatts beers on board were free. What a great country!

When we hit the ground in Calgary we grabbed our rental car and drove off to our ski chalet in Banff, about an hour west of Calgary. Some of the Olympic events were near Banff, but we had to travel into the city of Calgary for other events at the Saddledome. Our accommodations were in the Banff National Forest and many nights we had deer actually eating out of our hands at the sliding patio doors. It had a nice little kitchen where we cooked in a couple of nights, and as I recall, it wasn't very expensive, at about $150 per night. The Olympics had been going on for a week already when we arrived. We drove over to Calgary the following Sunday morning for the two-man bobsled. Occasionally, we would get lost or miss a turn, and unlike my nervousness on our first date, Karen and I adopted a slogan we were to use often during the trip. We'd just shrug off whatever happened and say, "The Adventure Continues."

There was no assigned seating for the bobsled event so we walked up and down the track and eventually found a good spot up near the starting line. The warm Chinook winds blew hard and due to the lack of snow, there was a lot of dirt and debris on the track. The race was stopped because the West German and Soviet Union teams kept complaining about the bad track conditions. Eventually, the event was postponed until the next day.

We had tickets the next day, which was Monday, to see Team Canada play Sweden in hockey. On the way into Calgary we stopped at the bobsled run to see the resumption of the postponed event. Upon arriving, there was another delay due to the bad conditions. As we walked around we ran into members from the Jamaican bobsled team. These dreadlock-laden men had sold T-shirts to finance their training and trip to the '88 games. ABC television had put together stories on the Jamaican bobsled team and "Eddie the Eagle," the British ski jumper who had a penchant for rough landings, so we were familiar with these short-time international celebrities. Unfortunately, none of the pictures Karen took of the Jamaicans came out. Such is life! We left the bobsled venue and traveled into Calgary to find our way to the afternoon hockey game between the host Canadians and the Swedes.

Our seats at the Saddledome were excellent, right behind Team Sweden's bench. The fans from Canada made a lot of noise cheering on the home team, but it was to no avail as the final score was a 2-2 tie. During one of the intermissions, Karen made a sign with the help of a vendor and a borrowed black magic marker that said, "We'd Rather Be Watching the Cleveland Browns." You'd think that the Canadians wouldn't find this sign amusing, but amazingly many people liked the sign, including several Seahawk fans from Seattle. After the game we had some dinner and visited the Olympic Park, where many medal ceremonies took place. It was refreshing to see people gathered peacefully from all over the world to participate in the games. Passing the flame from the Olympic torch to each other's small replica of the torch was pretty cool.

On Tuesday we did not have any event tickets so we used the opportunity to ski the Canadian Rockies. We ventured out to Sunshine Village for a day on the slopes. On the way up in the gondola, Karen was talking to a couple of children from Quebec who were most intrigued with her English. While she gabbed I plotted. I had shown the solitaire engagement ring to only one person prior to leaving for Calgary. The one person I let in on my secret in advance was my mom. I told her that I was going to propose on skis. She was very excited about my plan to ask Karen the big question, but she was skeptical about me dropping the ring in the snow. After a couple of runs down the major bowls at Sunshine, I saw the perfect spot to propose.

The next time down I drifted off to my left toward a more private area of the slopes and I fell down on purpose.

Karen came up from behind me and said, "Honey, why did you fall down over here?"

"So I could be on my knees to ask you if you'd marry me," I replied.

There I kneeled, holding out the ring toward her, grabbing it tightly between my thumb and index finger to ensure against dropping it in the snow. Every time she reached toward me to see what I held onto so tightly, I instinctively moved my hand. Little did I know that she had trouble seeing the ring due to the glare of the sun shining directly into her gorgeous blue eyes.

Then she realized that it was a ring and she jumped on me with big alligator tears in her eyes. I asked her if this meant "Yes" and she nodded. At this point I could hear some guy yell from the chairlift, "Do it in the snow, go for it!" Seconds later the guys doing all the yelling were over near us explaining that they were volunteers at the Winter Games who had the day off to ski. They hadn't seen their wives in weeks and they didn't think it was fair that we were rolling around in the powder on top of each other. Karen told them we were newly engaged, at which point they congratulated us and took our picture. In fact, we also took their picture to commemorate the moment. While we rode the chairlift back up to the top of the hill I asked Karen what kind of wedding she was envisioning and she immediately responded, "A big one!"

On the way down to the bottom of the hill we ran into an older couple that had been married many years. I think they were from Arizona, and they were very happy for us. Karen was very happy and so was I because we had never discussed the subject. Besides, I had broken with tradition and had never gone to her father to ask for his daughter's hand in marriage. Karen didn't seem to mind.

Later that evening we went to a beautiful rustic restaurant near Lake Louise for dinner. Karen spent some time on the phone calling her mom, dad, sister and Nora to tell them her news. This was before cell phones were so commonplace. I'll never forget Karen telling me that Nora just cried. Nora and Karen were very close friends, dating clear back to high school at St.Vincent-St. Mary's. They backpacked Europe together in the summer of 1982 along with Karen's sorority sister from Ohio State, Margaret Evans. While we dined, Karen noticed people at a large table adjacent to ours who seemed familiar. It turns out that they were from Akron, Ohio, and they even knew Karen's mom. You see everybody at Summit Mall in Akron. It was just kind of weird that we were so far from home and we had run into people we knew.

The rest of the week in Calgary was awesome. We saw the men's and women's giant slalom at Nakiska. Alberto Tomba of Italy was impressive in winning the gold medal. It had finally snowed in the mountains and Karen and I put away a couple of bottles of wine while watching the world-class skiers. We ran into another couple that told us about an outdoor, mineral spring-fed spa that wasn't far from where we were staying in Banff. We spent about an hour and a half in this gigantic public hot tub that could have been very romantic if we hadn't been with 150 other people.

Besides getting engaged, the highlight of the trip was being able to see the women's short program in figure skating over in Calgary at the Saddledome. Karen spotted a very pregnant Dorothy Hamill wearing a beautiful full-length mink coat standing in the aisle down 10 rows from our seats. Before I knew it, Karen had cruised down to get a quick photo and an autograph. Down on the ice, Katarina Witt versus Debbie Thomas was the big battle for the gold medal. What you don't see on TV at home are all the girls who skate hours before the real contenders hit the ice. These little girls were, in a word, *terrible*. I remember Karen digging her fingernails into my arm as this poor little girl from Korea smacked head first on the ice for the third time during her performance. It was painful to watch and Karen made it even more torturous. Debbie Thomas and Katarina Witt were both outstanding and very pretty.

When we arrived home on Sunday, Pat threw a little engagement party to welcome us home and celebrate our big news. We had started back to Ohio on the morning on the final day of the 1988 Winter Games and were actually at the engagement party as the torch went out at the closing ceremonies.

Another torch had been lit!

CHAPTER 5

Catawba Island

Now that I was engaged and planned on forming a family, a more fervent devotion to my newly rejuvenated career seemed to be the right course of action. Working at the Davis-Besse Nuclear Power Station in Oak Harbor was a lot of fun. There were consultants and contractors from all over the country working at Davis-Besse, and when the plant was shut down for maintenance the daily costs for having the facility off-line amounted to $750,000 per day in order to purchase replacement power. The work environment there was reminiscent of a MASH unit. During outages there was constant pressure to get the plant back on-line, on time and within budget.

Back in 1985, the plant had to be shut down for 18 months after nearly exposing the reactor core. Pretty serious stuff given what had happened at Three Mile Island and Chernobyl. My responsibilities were to maintain the cost control system that tracked the ongoing costs of running the plant. During these outages, the expenses could get out-of-control pretty quickly, with as many as 1,500 additional high-priced consultants on-site. I worked for a great guy named Dave Rauske, who commuted back and forth from Rocky River on Cleveland's west side each day. I had taken a job with Centerior Energy, and Dave was a contractor who was the lead person responsible for maintaining and supporting the cost control system. Centerior was a new company that had formed due to the merger of Cleveland

Electric Illuminating Company and Toledo Edison. There were many problems due to the clashing of cultures between the two utilities. I was lucky because I had no roots or allegiance to either company. Dave was a great guy and he taught me many things about the cost control system. Most of our programming support was based in Independence, Ohio, which is a suburb just south of Cleveland. I worked out in the field with our users, who ran the accounting division for the plant.

I made friends with several of my colleagues at Davis-Besse. In the systems area there were some great people, especially Mary Ann Sciarrapa, Julie Young, Michelle Kreh, Jim Bambrick and Dan Kudlac. Our supervisor was Vivian Chiemilewski, who was great to work for, because she was a hands-off manager who just let me do my job. This was culturally very different than the management style at Marathon, where I felt like I was being babysat all the time and then being shafted into a job in accounting, where I was stamping invoices and processing payables like a chimpanzee. I felt redeemed in that I had found a higher-paying job as a financial systems analyst.

More importantly, I had found the woman of my dreams. I had just bought a house and was finishing my MBA. Life was good! I had picked myself up out of the rut and was moving forward.

Catawba Island, where I bought my first home, is located about 15 miles east of Davis-Besse. The nearest city of any consequence is Port Clinton. Catawba is technically a peninsula, connected to the mainland of Ohio. The winters can be pretty brutal, but the summers rocked. Most Americans don't know that the state of Ohio includes four islands known as the Erie Islands. These islands are 50 miles east of Toledo and 80 miles west of Cleveland, just a few miles out into Lake Erie. The most popular is South Bass Island, best known for Put-N-Bay. The bars, boats and wineries are a magnet for people who party. Rental bikes and golf carts buzz about the streets.

Live music is everywhere. The Danger Brothers, who also play at the HeiniGate parties after Ohio State football games, and the famous Pat Dailey, were the island favorites. The other islands are Middle Bass, home of Lonz's Winery, and the more desolate North Bass Island. Another fun island that is more family-oriented is Kelley's. Midwesterners love the area for a quick weekend getaway.

This was home for now, and Karen was in charge of planning the wedding. It was March 1988 and the details were starting to come together. My contributions to planning the big day were minimal. As the groom, I had three responsibilities: the honeymoon, the tuxes and the band. Actually, I can take little credit for the music as my dad handled this important detail.

Karen and her mom did all the real planning, although I do remember venturing to the Grand Ballroom high atop the Cascade Plaza Holiday Inn in downtown Akron, which became our immediate favorite site for the reception. It was a beautiful room and George Bush had just held an event there in conjunction with his bid to become President in November. The date was set based on the availability of the church, band and the big ballroom.

October 15, 1988, would be the big day.

In the meantime, Karen would come up to Catawba on some weekends and on others I would head over to Akron. We were both Catholic and we were getting married at Karen's home parish, which was St. Sebastian's in Akron. St. Sebastian's is a huge, beautiful church with a grade school. I played in many CYO basketball games early on Saturday mornings at St. Sebastian's gym as a sixth, seventh, and eighth grader at Holy Family. St. Sebastian's always kicked our butts.

In order to get married in the Catholic Church, couples contemplating marriage are required to attend a marriage preparedness course called Pre-Cana. You meet several times with the priest who will be performing the ceremony, in our case, Father Ray Horley. Most Catholic priests are the first to admit that they really know very little about marriage. They know about the sacrament of marriage, but the best mentors are obviously couples who have been in a good Catholic marriage for many years. Our sponsor couple, guiding us through this process, had been parishioners at St. Sebastian's for years, and they had several grown children. Karen and I found our sessions with our sponsor couple to be very productive. We knew what we were doing; after all, we were not teenagers who had just decided to get hitched after two weeks of going steady.

We were both well educated, had decent professional careers and came from the same type of strong Catholic, family-oriented roots. Karen Patricia Coyne was the Irish-Catholic and I was Mark Joseph Volpe, the Italian-Catholic. On our wedding day I would be 29 years old and Karen was 28, so we were pretty mature and ready to settle down. I also found out pretty quickly that Karen would not tolerate any innuendo or jokes about divorce.

On a Saturday afternoon in April, Karen was visiting me at Catawba and I spent most of the day watching the *NFL Draft* on ESPN. This did not go over well, and we had our first real fight. I thought she was going to give the ring back, but eventually we ironed things out. Slowly but surely it was starting to sink in that the Browns were not the most important thing in the world. I really needed to start to focus on Karen, my love for her and the family that we planned to create, with the help of the Lord, of course.

The time had come to get rid of the Camaro in favor of a sport utility vehicle. I traded in the sports car for a tomato-colored Isuzu Trooper. Paul worked in sales at Family Pontiac, GMC and Isuzu, made me a great deal on the one remaining 1986 model. The only problem was I had never learned how to operate a car with "four on the floor." Pretty bright, me buying an SUV that I couldn't even drive. Karen had learned to drive a stick and luckily for me she taught me the basics in the neighborhood behind the dealership. She actually drove the car off the lot. I had no clue, and as she taught me, I ground the gears and stalled the part-car/part-truck several times, but eventually I got the hang of it.

In May, I received my MBA having finished my final classes at one of Ashland's satellite campus sites, so we ventured back to Findlay where many of my Marathon friends met Karen for the first time. Up on Catawba, Karen and I had made friends with two other couples. Brad and Cindee had met at the nuclear plant, and John and Barb were contractors working at the plant in the metrology lab. We grew to be good friends: dinners, parties, and trips to Put-N-Bay on the little 18-foot boat, co-owned by John and Brad.

Early in June on a sunny Sunday afternoon we ventured over to Put-N-Bay from Catawba. Paul and his new girlfriend, Tammy, were visiting for the weekend. John and Barb handled the boat, while Paul, Tammy, Karen and I enjoyed the spray of Lake Erie and a couple of cold beers while we made the short voyage over to the party-oriented island. Since it was Sunday, things were starting to slow down at the bars after a weekend of vigorous partying.

At about 5:00 we decided to head back to Catawba so Tammy and Paul could hit the road. As we headed around the west side of South Bass to head back the six or seven miles to

Catawba, I noticed a wall of ominous gray clouds to the west about 15 miles away. The storm looked like it had just hit at Davis-Besse and was heading our way. As we drew away from South Bass, the shallow waters of Lake Erie became increasingly choppy and the wind picked up considerably.

Suddenly, I realized that even though John had the boat at full throttle we were hardly moving. The temperature dropped quickly, about 20 degrees in 10 minutes. I knew we were in trouble. Paul looked really scared and his girlfriend, Tammy, was petrified. Barb handed out lifejackets and we pulled the boat cover over us to keep the rain, which was increasing in its intensity, out of the boat. Karen kept her cool the entire time. I wasn't in a real panic, because I could see Catawba about a half mile to our left. There was nowhere on the shoreline to dock the boat even if we could have made it there.

Nothing but rocks!

We tried to forge ahead, but the boat was hardly moving forward. John looked back at the prop because the engine sounded muffled. The engine was running, but we were getting nowhere as the storm hit us hard. John went back to look at the prop, and he discovered that it had become stuck in a fisherman's net that we had somehow snagged. He grappled with the net and was finally able to cut us loose. By this time the storm had hit us full force and the mighty lake tossed the boat back and forth like a toy in the bathtub. I thought for sure we were going to end up in the lake. We kept trying to throttle our way back toward the docks, but made little headway. Finally, the storm let up even though the rain continued, and we were able to limp our way back to shore.

The whole ordeal was probably an hour and a half to two hours. It was pretty dark by the time we reached the shore. Brad and George, another friend from Davis-Besse, were at the dock with towels and blankets. After we regrouped and got rid of the shakes we headed back to my house.

Karen asked me if I was scared and I said, "Sure, but I knew I could make it to shore."

"That's nice, honey, but what about me?" she said.

Then it dawned on me: I had to stop my selfish ways of thinking. I had to start thinking in terms of us. We were forming a team and I needed to change my mindset. I remember Tammy calling her mom to tell her a little white lie as to why she would be home a little later than planned. Tammy was pretty shaken up; years later I found out that she couldn't swim very well. We all went back to our weekly routines and even though it was a scary experience. I don't think it would do justice to refer to the situation as a near death experience. You never know, even though everyone except Tammy was a decent swimmer, there's always the possibility of hypothermia setting in due to the churning of Lake Erie, which is very shallow around the islands at only 30 feet deep. Paul and I swore never to tell our parents about it, but now that this book is out the proverbial cat is out of the bag.

Planning a wedding is easy, if you're the groom. We met with a travel agent, who recommended that we honeymoon in Barbados. So we booked the trip to leave on the Sunday after the wedding and return the following Sunday, an unbelievable leap for me as I agreed to miss not one, but two Browns games. Must be love! The only other details I helped with were procuring a limousine and assigning seats at the reception. For example, we would take a table of eight and split it between her sorority sisters from Alpha Phi at Ohio State and my fraternity brothers from Sigma Pi at Ohio Northern. Our neighbors from where we grew up were seated together as were our co-workers. We saw this as a great way to complete the merger by getting those from each side to co-mingle. In order to make sure nobody was totally uncomfortable with our plan, we tried to have at least some familiar faces at the same table.

Karen, Kathy and Pat did all of the real planning. My mom helped by making sure the invitation list from our side was organized. My invitation list included co-workers, friends, frat brothers and my new neighbors on Catawba.

The family living across the street on Catawba was the Carroll family: John, Mary Lou and their children, Colleen, Leigh, and Chuck. They were very welcoming and helpful. I think they were excited about having a new couple with plans on starting a family across the street. John worked for the Air National Guard and was also a volunteer fireman. Mary Lou was an office manager for a local contractor, while Colleen and Leigh were enjoying high school. Chuck was a tall and somewhat gangly fifth grader.

A few weeks before the wedding, a friend of mine at Davis-Besse named Michelle Kreh asked me whether Karen and I would be interested in providing a home for one of several abandoned puppies a friend of hers found on the side of the road the previous Saturday night. I told Michelle that the timing really wasn't very good because of the upcoming nuptials, but that I'd check with Karen. As I walked away I asked her what the dogs looked like and Michelle said they were yellow Labs.

I thought to myself how I could understand leaving a litter of kittens by the side of the road, having always been a big cat hater, but yellow Labs?

Michelle was slightly pushy and there were only two puppies left. She asked me if I wanted to see the male or the female at lunch. I shrugged because of her tenacity and said, "The little girl!"

I knew Karen found the dangling anatomy of a male dog to be rather gross. I remember distinctly meeting Michelle, driving to a local ice cream stand to see the yellow puppy. When I saw the young Lab, I immediately fell in love with her and took her directly to the house. I needed to drive 100 miles that afternoon for some meetings with the software programmers in Independence, Ohio, over near Cleveland. Karen had come out to Catawba to begin the moving process.

We never lived together prior to getting married, but Karen was slowly bringing her things out. When I walked in with the dog she was out running errands, so I put the new puppy in a moving box and attached a printed note that said, "Can I please live with you? I promise to be a good dog. P.S. Can I have some milk, please?" I also signed the note with a little paw print. Hours later when I arrived back from work Karen was clutching the dog and gleefully pleading with me to keep her.

She said, "I have no idea who put her in the house. She's so cute…can we keep her, please?"

I just had to grin and tell her, "Sure we can!"

"Really," Karen said.

So I immediately replied, "I'm the one who wrote the note."

After considering several names I smiled and suggested Calgary, thinking she would nix the idea, but she loved it. I always planned that the first addition to our family would be a little boy, but Calgary, the little yellow Lab, was a great way to start. There was one couple that we had met on Catawba who thought we were very religious people, having named our dog Calvary.

The weekend before the wedding arrived and it was time for the traditional bachelor and bachelorette parties. I obviously wasn't invited to the party for Karen, but a photocopy of my head was affixed to the body of a well-carved, muscle-bound man that the girls used as nametags. Karen and her friends were at a local drinking establishment when a young lady, who was not attending the party, came up to Karen, looked at her nametag and said, "Hey, that's Mark Volpe." I have no idea who this person was and I am very grateful she turned around and promptly left. I know it wasn't Matilda. She lived far away and didn't like hanging around bars.

My bachelor party started with a round of golf, followed by loads of Italian food at Vaccarro's. Then we headed over to her brother Kenny's house to watch some films and drink some shots. I was standing on the porch, drunk off my ass, when one of Karen's other brothers, Kevin as I recall, picked me up and threw me in the backseat of his car. It was time to go see some athletic young dancers. We had 20 guys in the club; all were drunk and raising hell. I think I enjoyed myself, but I have very little memory of this portion of the day. I do remember getting up the next morning very hung over. I stayed at my parents' home and when I got up I was a hurting unit, dehydrated big time.

My mom was making my brothers and me breakfast. I couldn't even attempt to eat. I gulped down some orange juice, but I was in major pain. I should have been in bed sleeping it off, but instead we were topping off the bachelor party with one last trip to Cleveland Stadium, as a single man, to see the Browns take on the Seattle Seahawks.

On the way up to the stadium I started to feel sick. My brothers stopped at the 7-Eleven convenience store to pick up beer and other tailgate supplies. I went in the back by the dumpster and threw up the orange juice I had just guzzled down. Paul felt bad for me and asked me if he could get me a Coke or something and I nodded. I managed to get back in the SUV for the rest of the trip up I-77 to the Flats area along the Cuyahoga

River where we tailgated. I sipped the Coke and held a garbage bag close by just in case I vomited again.

Once we got to the tailgate party I started to feel a little better, then the Coke started to make me sick again, with all of the carbonation not settling. So I lost it again, and my brother Paul walked up to me and grinned.

"Now, that's what I call a real Browns fan: one minute throwing up orange, and the next minute throwing up brown," he said.

Not many people can lay claim to being able to vomit in their favorite team's colors, not even a Steelers fan. The Browns lost as I sat there with the garbage bag in my lap to ensure against puking on fans sitting in front of us.

The evening of the rehearsal dinner was finally here. Things went very well given the fact that we had 19 people in our wedding party. The two families were getting along handsomely as both clans knew how to throw a party, and my dad toasted the rich ethnic traditions of both the Coyne and Volpe families on the eve of the wedding. After Karen and I handed out our gifts to our wedding party, my niece, Francine, who was our beautiful little flower girl, came up to me with a present and said that it was from Karen. Then I handed her back a little box from my pocket that she happily took over to Karen. I opened mine first, and I was amazed to see a handsome Seiko watch. Karen told me that she would like me to wear this new watch on special occasions.

Probably my most prized possession is the 14-carat gold Lucien Picard, Seashark model, a fine retirement watch that my deceased grandfather, Vincent Volpe, left me in his will when he passed away in 1967. I seldom wore this special heirloom for fear of losing it, and now I had a superb timepiece given to me by the woman who would be my wife. Even though I had always planned to wear the Lucien Picard on my wedding day, I now had a new, very special watch to wear instead.

Karen opened her present next and was especially pleased with the pair of diamond earrings that I had picked out for her to wear on our wedding day. In a short period of time she went from no diamonds to the pendant I gave her for Christmas, to the engagement ring and now the earrings. I asked her what was left and she replied, "Even bigger earrings!" The first two diamond purchases had left my finances a little depleted so these minor-sized earrings were small, but adequate.

I remember a joke from Johnny Carson's monologue a few years earlier when he said, "The only reason the Lord created Akron, Ohio, was so that Cleveland could have someone to look down on." Well, on October 15, 1988, the weather in Akron could not have been more picturesque. It was 65 degrees and sunny with a beautiful bright blue sky. The leaves had just started to turn and there was a slight breeze.

It was a perfect day for football, and a great day to get married.

I was in the front of the church with my groomsmen ready to go. The parents were about to be seated. Paul came up to me with an envelope from Karen.

It was a Sweetest Day card.

She signed it, "Love you forever. I'll see you in five minutes."

I almost lost it right there. It was kind of ironic that a year earlier on Sweetest Day, I had bought the engagement ring. It was about five minutes before noon and Father Horley had not suited up in his vestments.

"Father, don't you think it's time to get ready?" I asked.

He was shocked because he had never seen a Catholic wedding start on time, especially a large wedding with 19 people in the wedding party.

As Karen came up the aisle with the brass quintet playing "Trumpet Voluntary," it appeared as though her mascara was running a little due to a few tears. She stopped to give her mom sitting in the second pew a kiss, right before her dad handed her over to me. Throughout the customary recital of our vows I tried to be very serious, this was a major contract. Karen couldn't keep from kissing me at every opportunity. The tapes show that she kissed me three times during the vows alone.

Right after we said our vows and moved to the left side of the altar to sit next to one another as husband and wife for the first time, she whispered, "Are you sorry you married me?"

At which I replied, "Not yet!"

Then a few minutes later she told me to look at the inscription inside the ring. I figured it would say "Karen and Mark 10/15/88," but much to my surprise it read, "THE ADVENTURE CONTINUES." I just smiled and told her that it was pretty neat. Over the following years it was a very rare occasion that would cause me to take off the gold ring, with its five little inset diamonds and unique inscription.

After the ceremony, we greeted our guests at the back of the church and took a few pictures. I got in trouble when I got in the limo. The first thing I did was turn on the little TV: "Miami of Florida 7, Notre Dame 0," I announced the score out the sunroof.

Karen said, "You're unbelievable!"

Then it was off to a nearby retirement community called Rockyknoll that had a pretty landscape for the outdoor pictures. On the way, all the cars in the wedding party went through Mal's Drive Thru—first things first, beer and champagne. The reception wasn't until late afternoon, so in the meantime the wedding party made three stops: first over to Tom's home, where Karen's family grew up, for a quick visit, then over to Stow to my parents' home to have a bite to eat, and then back to her mom's condominium for a quick nap before the reception. On the way from the condo to the reception Karen sat between Ed, her former boyfriend, and one of our ushers and me.

She looked over at me and said, "This is just too weird."

Ed was very cool about the whole thing and was genuinely happy for us. I will always be grateful to him for asking me to be his roommate on the trip to Kitzbuhel.

Our reception was awesome, mostly because of the 14-piece orchestra that played a great array of music that I personally picked out. Back in high school at Walsh, I played tenor saxophone in the jazz band. I was raised on a heavy dosage of Frank Sinatra, Glenn Miller, Tommy Dorsey, Four Freshmen and Five Saxes, so I knew the lay of the land when it came to the sound of the big bands, even though I had evolved into a huge Springsteen-loving rocker.

As Karen and I were dancing together, she whispered in my ear, "This is the greatest day of our lives, there's no way that we can top this."

I told her, "Just wait until the birth of our son, that'll be the greatest day of our lives."

She just smiled and kept dancing. I'm a very lousy dancer, so Karen generally leads given that I have no clue as what to do on the dance floor.

Later in the evening, I decided to put Karen on my shoulder and literally carry her out of the ballroom. This was a move I saw another guy do on his wedding night. It was a more civilized way of clubbing your woman over her head and then dragging her back to your cave. Karen has a few memories from the day, but to her it was mostly a blur. The kick line of ladies singing the chorus of Sinatra's "New York, New York" was hysterical. Everyone had an awesome time.

Karen's cousin Ricky was given the responsibility of driving our Isuzu Trooper filled with our wedding gifts to her father's house. We found out weeks later that it took him three hours to make the trip because he got lost.

Our honeymoon in Barbados was pretty typical. We drank lots of rum punch, went out to dinner, met other honeymooners, toured the impoverished Caribbean island and did what couples are supposed to do on their honeymoon.

Karen was physically exhausted from the wedding day and spent most of the time in the shade wearing a sun hat, making sure that her beautifully freckled body didn't get too much sun, while I lay out in the extreme heat taking in as much sun as I could stand. The ocean was so blue and much calmer than the Atlantic beaches I was accustomed to. I seldom ventured out into the water; it was a big blue pool, with hardly any waves. Occasionally, one of the natives would get past the security guards and try to sell his trinkets or drugs to the honeymooners at the resort. This was a little annoying after awhile.

When we returned to Catawba, Karen worked at Lazarus department store at the Sandusky Mall in the larger-sized women's bra and underwear department. This ended up having its advantages as the employee discount made our Christmas shopping much more palatable from a financial standpoint. Karen looked for a job more in keeping with her educational attainment, and eventually landed a job as the office manager and accountant at Wilkes and Co., a mechanical contracting firm based in Huron, Ohio. She had joined a Women's Club and one of their civic projects was to staff Santa Claus's little outpost in downtown Port Clinton. She volunteered me to hang out in this little hut for a few hours in the freezing cold. It was actually pretty fun listening to what all the little children wanted from Santa and Karen did stay with me out in the cold, providing services as one of Santa's little elves. One of the other husbands, who had posed as Santa, told me it's fun to invite some of the pretty mommies accompanying their children to sit on Santa's lap too.

The biggest highlight of the long cold Catawba winter was a trip over to Richfield, Ohio, to see Bruce Springsteen and the E Street Band's, *Tunnel of Love* tour. Karen knew when she married me that I was a devoted fan of the Boss. She had heard all my stories about the *Born in the U.S.A.* tour from my bachelor days back in the mid-'80s. I had seen Bruce in Cleveland the first time back in February 1976, right after the *Born To Run* fury, when he was on the cover of both *Time* and *Newsweek* the same week. I still have the ticket stub to that show—the best $6.50 I ever spent.

Back in the summer of 1985, I was playing in a men's softball league and on a bang-bang play at second base, I had my feet cut out from under me as I slapped the tag on some idiot who had decided to try and stretch a gap single into a double. My feet got caught up in his hard slide into the bag, and I went head over heels into the hard-packed clay, separating my left shoulder and lacerating my forehead. I was okay, a little banged up and done for the season, with my arm in a sling. I decided to spend my spare time chasing Bruce's long stadium *Born in the U.S.A.* tour around the great Midwest. I had seen an earlier show at the Richfield Coliseum, but now was the time to hit the road. I saw the E Street Band play Cleveland Stadium. Cleveland is known as the birthplace of rock-n-roll. I have always insisted Springsteen is the greatest American-born rocker ever.

Elvis who?

Then it was on to Chicago's Soldier Field to see a classic show on a hot summer night. My friends from Findlay—Kent Benson, Gary Eymer and I sat behind the stage. I scored two tickets for $20. A Chicago Cubs pitcher named Rick Sutcliffe, who was also on the disabled list at the time, sat right in front of me. Even though the very tall pitcher made it harder to see, I could still see Bruce's hot new wife, Julianne Phillips, watching from the side backstage. I talked to Sutcliffe a little; he was a big fan and later would actually become friends with Bruce. This night was tragic for a group of teenagers driving in for the concert, who were killed in an accident right outside Soldier Field on Lakeshore Drive on the way to the show.

I also ventured up to the Silverdome in Pontiac, Michigan and to the Hoosier Dome in Indianapolis, where Bruce closed the show with "Santa Claus is Coming to Town" in the middle of July.

The *Tunnel of Love* show was sold out in Cleveland, and I had to pay a ticket agent $60 a piece for us to get in, but it was worth it. I knew I could never get Karen to share my love for the Browns, but Mr. Springsteen was another story. When he came out on stage Karen proceeded to jump up to hug me, breaking my glasses all in one swoop. Later on during the concert, Bruce and his new backup singer, Patti Scialfa, were doing a romantic duet of "Tougher than the Rest." Karen leaned over to me, motioning toward the two of them on stage gazing into each other's eyes and she said, "They're doing it!"

"Don't you dare say anything like that about my Bruce, that's blasphemy," I said.

Little did I know, months later Bruce would get caught with Patti on a hotel balcony over in Rome early one morning; the pictures taken by the paparazzi left no doubt. Bruce and Julianne would get a divorce; then he'd marry Patti and soon start a family of his own. Karen made the call, and I knew that when it came to judging character, or at least body language, Karen has wonderful insight regarding people.

After the concert we settled back into our routine where I went to Davis-Besse and Karen made the trek over to Huron each morning. Given that we were both approaching 30, we decided to have children as soon as possible. Karen asked me whether we shouldn't wait until our financial situation was better aligned before starting a family and I replied, "In time we can solve any financial dilemma, but what we can't do is turn back time and change our biological clocks." We immediately started to do everything we could to get pregnant, which isn't all that bad.

For the first year of our marriage we took our dog Calgary on walks, painted the interior of our simple home, built a deck, did some landscaping, visited family on holidays and continued to try and have a baby. One weekend we installed all of the posts for the deck. Karen's brother Kenny and his friend Greg Scanlon came up to help with this labor-intensive part of the project. We had all gone to a club called Players for a few beers after a long, hard day. Not long after we had arrived, Kenny was grabbing some beers and Karen was standing near a group of guys. One of them was standing against a pillar, and he looked pretty drunk as he leaned there taking a little nap. Then, out of nowhere he picked his nose and wiped the contents of his finger on my wife's arm. She was grossed out and I was pretty fired up. As I walked over to the jerk, I was considering punching him before he was fully awake. Kenny grabbed my shoulder and said, "I'll handle this!" A little pushing match ensued and the bouncers made us leave. Karen said, "Can you believe that guy wiped a booger on my arm?"

Despite our efforts to have a child we still hadn't hit the mark. Karen began charting her cycle in order to determine when she was ovulating. Her sister had just given birth to her first child Ryan when she took one look at Karen's chart over the Christmas holidays in 1989.

"You're not doing it at the right time," Kathy said.

We altered our timing and two months later, in late February 1990, Karen called me at the office to confirm her suspicions that we were pregnant with our first child. After receiving the news I stood up at my desk and exclaimed, "Touchdown!" as I elevated my arms gleefully above my head like a referee.

During her first trimester Karen did very well, however, cleaning and cooking raw meat like chicken made her sick. She didn't like to look at the gross chicken and the smell made her nauseous. I took over many nights in the kitchen, while Karen was content to eat multiple bowls of cereal.

Her obstetrician was a short Indian man named Dr. Shindee. He had offices in both Port Clinton and Sandusky. He delivered babies at hospitals in both locations. There weren't a whole lot of OB/GYNs to pick from in this less-populated part of Ohio.

They don't build nuclear power plants near major metropolitan areas. In May 1990, my employer, Centerior Energy, announced that they would be reorganizing, better known as "downsizing," in most business circles. We were given a choice: either leave the company and take a modest severance package, or move to the corporate headquarters in Independence, over in northeast Ohio, with the benefit of a substantial moving package and a little raise. For us it was a no-brainer: we were moving back home. We needed a bigger home, not only because of the baby, but also due to our plans to have as many children as possible by the time Karen reached age 35. We took the move rather than the severance. It was a huge blessing for us, as we would have the support of our family once the baby was born.

We looked at houses in the heat of the summer and decided to build on a lot located at the end of a cul-de-sac on a little lake. Our new street was Crystal Cove Circle in Stow, Ohio. I would have about a 40-minute commute to the outskirts of Cleveland each day. During the summer I also took the Dale Carnegie course on Human Relations and Effective Public Speaking after work on Monday night for 15 weeks. This course was great because it allowed me to hear about other people's life experiences and challenges. It was most helpful in allowing me to make the transition from bachelorhood to fatherhood. Karen was invited to the graduation and she remarked that the course had changed me in that I was more spontaneous and much less rigid. I always tended to be a live-by-the-rules type of guy.

During the late summer we took Lamaze classes to get educated on the miracle of childbirth. As the summer turned to fall, Karen and I were given a due date of sometime around Thanksgiving. We asked Dr. Shindee after one of Karen's exams about the use of an epidural during the birthing process. Dr. Shindee explained to us that he would meet with us to explain about the epidural after our last Lamaze class. One Sunday after church we stopped by Magruder Hospital to check out the facilities, well in advance of the big day.

Little did we know that we'd be back in just two days!

CHAPTER 6

Magruder Hospital

On Tuesday morning, October 30th Karen awoke and went to the bathroom. I heard her say through the door as I laid in bed, "Do you hear that?" and I said, "Yes," as the sound of a small trickle of water indicated to me that she was peeing.

After a brief pause she said, "Guess what…I'm not peeing!"

She crawled back in bed and showed me a wet spot that she thought was due to the fact that the baby was pushing on her bladder. This is pretty common among women who are expecting. So I gave the clear liquid a sniff, just like any good husband would do. It didn't smell at all, and it certainly didn't have the aroma of urine.

In minutes we were packing a suitcase to head off to the hospital. If indeed her water had "broke," we knew we needed to get to the hospital pronto. We called Dr. Shindee and took off for the hospital. I kidded Karen as I boosted her into the Trooper that maybe we should put some plastic over her seat for the ride. She wasn't having any contractions yet, but we knew that if her water really broke loose that we needed to move quickly.

Once we were admitted, Karen was escorted to a very nice birthing room. They gave her Pitocin intravenously in order to induce the contractions. After about six hours the contractions began. We had called Karen's mother and we found out that she was at the hospital in Akron. Karen's brother, Kevin, and his wife, Colleen, were also in a hospital a hundred miles away, as Colleen was about to give birth to their first child as well. Both babies were due around Thanksgiving and oddly enough both babies decided to make an early entrance. Colleen and Karen were able to talk to one other over the phone to wish each other good luck.

Later in the evening Karen's contractions were starting to pick up. Karen's mother naturally wanted to be there for the birth of both new babies. Things had progressed pretty rapidly for Colleen, while Karen seemed to be going much more slowly. I told Pat that based on my non-expert opinion she had plenty of time; Karen was still hours away from delivering. It was logistically possible for her to be there for Kevin and Colleen, and then drive two hours west from Akron to Port Clinton in order to make it for her daughter.

At 8:00 in the evening Colleen gave birth to Sean Michael Coyne. Pat got to hold the new baby, then she jumped in her car and drove straight to Magruder, arriving at 11:00 that evening. Having her there was great; I had absolutely no experience with the birthing process, not that I was expected to do anything special. However, we were in a small-town hospital and this fact gave us both reasons to be cautious. I had all the faith in the world in Dr. Shindee as he had a great reputation. Everything to me seemed very textbook, but I always wondered what they would do if something extraordinary happened.

The closest major hospital was in Toledo, about 40 miles away. You would always hear on the news of people involved in major accidents getting life-flighted to St. Charles Hospital in Toledo. Having Pat there was a blessing for me. She is a registered nurse and had given birth to five children, so she was way ahead of the curve. Pat was also very conscientious about her presence, not wanting to overstep any boundaries. She even asked permission to be in the room when the baby arrived. I do remember her getting somewhat frustrated with the nurses, as the night shift crew didn't seem too concerned about the pain Karen was dealing with. Once the contractions heightened, they offered no pain medication, just something to help her sleep.

Earlier in the day Dr. Shindee informed us for the first time that he didn't do epidurals. Karen was going to have our first baby without the benefit of modern medical technology. We were irked that we were not informed of this situation when we had specifically asked about this well in advance. Otherwise, we would have considered another hospital where they weren't stuck back in the days of the Conestoga wagon, out on the plains where the ladies gave birth and were back in the fields hours later.

The only medication Karen was given was an aid to help her sleep through the contractions, which were now increasing and becoming more painful as the clock approached 4:00 in the middle of the night. At one point Karen was asleep and somewhat lucid lying on her side, but she was still able to do the breathing techniques we learned in Lamaze class.

As one of the contractions subsided she said, "Volpe, Volpe, Volpe…shit."

Into the early morning hours her contractions were getting closer together, but she had not dilated enough for us to believe that the blessed moment was very close. Then the nurses informed us that the baby would not be making it out into the world anytime soon. He was posterior, meaning his head was facing the wrong direction and was unable to make it through the birth canal.

I guess in some situations they can help spin the baby around with a suction cup device, but in this case the nurses just said, "Let's just leave them alone, mother and child will have to work this out."

Then one of the nurses said to me at about 6:00 a.m., "You'd better try and get some sleep, it could be a long day."

I tried to shut my eyes. I was very excited, but a little tired from having been up for 24 hours straight. I had just started to doze off when Pat came in and grabbed my arm, saying, "Hurry up, something's happened."

I hurriedly put on my gown and mask and washed up before running down the hall toward the birthing room. Karen wasn't sleeping through the contractions anymore; she was on her back and she was excited.

The first thing she said to me was, "I thought you had kicked me in the butt and when I turned to yell at you I realized that nobody was in the room; it was the baby!"

The young Volpe had figured out that there was no way to get out without flipping around and when this happened Karen called for help and was suddenly feeling the urge to push.

Moments later Dr. Shindee arrived in the room and I said to him, "Isn't that the same suit you had on yesterday?"

He said, "You weren't supposed to notice."

Dr. Shindee immediately appraised the situation and told Karen not to push yet. I was up at the head of the bed coaching Karen, feeding her ice chips and watching the monitor.

Then Dr. Shindee said, "Go ahead and push."

Pat stood back and watched from near the door, but I could tell by her wide eyes that it was getting close. She said, "I see some dark hair."

Then one of the nurses pounded her hand like a catcher and said, "Come on, bring it to me."

Karen pushed again and I could tell we were getting closer. I noticed Dr. Shindee was very active with his hands. I was suspicious that he was doing an episiotomy, but I wasn't about to look or tell Karen. She pushed again, still no bambino.

Finally, Karen said, "Mark, I need you to pull on my feet towards my head. I'm not getting any resistance in these stirrups."

So with the next push, I pulled on her left foot and one of the nurses pulled on the right. Seconds later I looked to the left and I could see this handsome little face with a little bit of gunk stuck in the dent of his chin. Dr. Shindee continued to maneuver the arms and legs out. Then the doctor pulled the young lad all the way out to the point where I could see external plumbing.

I yelled, "IT'S A BOY! IT'S A BOY!" as tears welled up in my eyes. Somehow, I don't remember the traditional slap on the baby's butt to get him breathing. One of the nurses handed me some scissors and with my hands trembling ever so slightly, I cut the umbilical cord. The nurses quickly rinsed him off and wrapped him up.

Then they handed him to Karen as she exhaustedly exclaimed, "Come here you beautiful child!" and she clutched this good-looking baby boy to her chest.

We never were able to agree on a name for a baby girl, but we did have a boy's name picked out. I had lobbied for Vincent after my paternal grandfather, but Karen nixed that idea, saying, "I'm not bringing any Vinny Volpe into this world."

However, it occurred to us that both of our maternal grandfathers were named William. Karen's grandfather, William Stough Smith, had died from cancer during Karen's pregnancy earlier in the summer while we were in Bethany Beach, Delaware. In fact, we drove directly from the beach to his funeral in Huntington, West Virginia. I vividly remember the pastor saying, "Bill lives on in his children and in his grandchildren."

I put my arm around Karen pulling her close to me and thought to myself, "And even his great grandchildren, too."

My mother's dad was named William Schultz. He had also died from cancer, back in 1963. I don't have any recollection of my Grandpa Schultz, however everyone says he was a good man. He was also an accountant who worked for the City of Cleveland. Many of my relatives would comment over the years that I reminded them of Bill. Both of these fine men went by "Bill." But we had decided that if we had a son he would be named, William Vincent Volpe and we would call him "Will." He was born at 8:12 a.m. on October 31, 1990, which also happened to be Halloween.

Karen noticed that Dr. Shindee was doing a little sewing down at the base of the bed, so she asked, "Did you do an episiotomy?"

Dr. Shindee just smiled and nodded back at her.

Even though we were in a little hospital up on Lake Erie, they did have one nice little perk: toll-free calling to family and friends. We spent the next hour or so calling everyone in Akron, Bath, Stow and Huntington, West Virginia. Then we said an Our Father to thank the Lord above for this wonderful blessing. Will was the only baby born at Magruder Hospital that day and the staff was happy to see he had two parents present who were actually happily married to one another.

We were very blessed.

I was especially proud that our first child was a son. I was the oldest, with three other siblings. However, I was the third one to get married. I always thought that D.J. and his wife Paula, who had been married for a couple of years, would have the first Volpe grandchild, but Karen and I were the first to have a child that would carry on the family name. Finally, at about 11:00 a.m., I headed back home to our ranch home on Catawba Island for some sleep while Karen rested comfortably. Will's APGAR test scores were very high. He was a healthy baby, with great skin color and even some muscle tone, weighing in at seven pounds, seven ounces. They had cleaned the gunk out of the dent in his chin—it looked just like his dad's chin. His eyes were blue just like his mom's, but they warned us that this could change. All I could think about was what a lucky man I was to have a son. Now I understood the emotions other men felt at that very proud moment. I was also very proud of my bride. She was such a trouper to go through this process out in the middle of nowhere with only her mom and myself. The lack of an option for an epidural was perplexing, but everything worked out.

Later in the afternoon I went back to the hospital to see Karen and Will. They were both doing fine. Karen was attempting to nurse Will for the first time, and even though this didn't go smoothly at first, Will eventually caught on.

About 5:00 p.m. I got up to leave and Karen said, "Where are you going?"

"To the A&P to get candy, beer and cigars," I said.

There was no way I was going to stay at the hospital and let the neighborhood kids, many of whom Karen and I had been the little league coaches for earlier in the summer, soap the windows of our house. I wanted to be there to give out candy, hand out some cigars and drink a few beers. We had always thought with Karen's due date being in mid-November that there was a possibility that we would have a Thanksgiving baby. Instead, with Will's early arrival, we had our own little goblin on Halloween. I always loved Halloween and it seemed fitting that my son would have All Hallows Eve as his birthday. After all, I was an April Fools Day baby, born back in 1959.

As I left the hospital Karen said, jokingly, "You don't love us!"

I smiled and left anyhow, heading straight to the grocery store to buy Kit Kat bars, Michelob and Garcia Vega cigars. It was a festive night as I handed out candy, cigars and beer. There was a small sign in the front yard denoting Will's arrival and blue balloons were affixed to the mailbox. I only gave the cigars and beer out to the adults, and when a very obnoxious 12-year-old named Will came by with a group of his friends, I gave him five Kit Kat bars and said, "We just had a boy today named Will."

The neighbors and friends were wonderful. About 11:00 p.m., I went back to the hospital to see Will and Karen. It was so cool, there were three of us now—we were a family.

Two days later Karen, Will and I came home from the hospital. John Carroll had put up a message on the sign at the Catawba Island Volunteer Fire Department. It read, "Welcome to the World—William Vincent Volpe." All sorts of family came to visit us on Catawba for the last time before our move.

Two weeks later, on November 13, 1990, my grandmother, Mary Volpe died after having some arrhythmia problems with her heart. She never got to hold her great-grandson. Weeks before Will was born she was having trouble with her heart and my mom said she seemed very down, almost resigned to dying.

My mom told her, "Hey, don't you want to be around to see this new baby. It might be a boy, the first Volpe great-grandson."

I guess that it was enough motivation for her to hang on for a few more weeks, because two weeks after Will was born she passed away. At the funeral home in Akron, Will's presence seemed to give the calling hours a bit of a lift—it was a joyful event in a way.

One Volpe had passed on after a long, fulfilling life and there was a new promising, young life just starting, Will was waiting in the wings to carry on the family name. There was something special about the way this had played out.

God does have a plan.

I was so proud of our William and my wife. I also know, despite my dad's own personal loss of his mother, that the new grandson, who shared his same middle name of Vincent, provided some solace for him.

There were all of these old Italian ladies, friends of grandma, passing Will around at the funeral home and looking at the new great grandson that Mary never got to see. I'll never forget my sister telling me about putting pictures of each of the great grandchildren, including Will's official baby picture, in the little purse that was to be buried with her. On the day of the burial I was kneeling at the casket saying my last goodbyes when my dad walked up next to me holding the little guy.

It was one of those few moments that make even a grown man cry.

Six weeks later William, Karen and I moved to 5393 Crystal Cove Circle, our new home in Stow, Ohio. The move was very unfair to Karen in a lot of ways. She was up there on the island alone with Will while I worked the new job in Independence. She had to clean the house and help the movers with the packing, all while trying to take care of the new baby. All of the furniture had been packed away and she nursed William for the last time on Catawba, with only the toilet in the guest bathroom to sit on. I wish it could have been different, but with these corporate moves, all too often the lady of the house gets dumped on. She was there for a few weeks without me, out on an island somewhat alone some 85 miles away.

In the end, I think it was worth it because we were headed home.

CHAPTER 7

Crystal Cove

Our new home in Stow on the little lake was very pretty. It was about 2,700 square feet, with a first-floor master suite and a beautiful view of the water. When we moved in, the basement was a dirty mess and the house was hardly ready for us to move in, but we moved in anyhow the day after closing. Our builder was a brazen young guy named Tony Troppe. This was his first venture on his own into residential building. The home was very nice, but it took him forever to actually finish it. It was well into the summer of 1991 before he hooked up the air conditioning, after Karen marched in on him at an open house down the street and demanded that he get the air conditioning going because we had a baby that was unable to sleep in the heat.

The first party we had there was for William's baptism in February. Karen's brother, Kenny, was the godfather and Karen's good friend, Margaret Evans, was the godmother. It was the first of many festive family gatherings we would have at the house.

During the summer we took on many projects to make our house a home. Karen had received a quote for thousands of dollars for custom draperies, so she decided to make them herself. She did a masterful job and saved us a bucket-load of money. Once spring broke we tried planting grass, however, the hard packed clay made growing grass nearly impossible for most of the summer. We set our sights on landscaping and the big project was building a multi-tiered monster deck.

Will was the center of our lives. We still loved our dog Calgary, but she got less and less of our attention once we had our William. He soon took his first steps, and he had the most beautiful little face. One morning while I was at work Karen called me and initially she sounded rather upset.

She yelled into the phone, "They're brown, they're brown! His beautiful blue eyes turned overnight from blue to brown and it's your fault!"

Karen has riveting blue eyes, while mine are basic brown. I had always known that this was a possibility and the doctors explained to us that this was sometimes the case. The eye color could change by the time a child turns a year old. I remembered looking at his little blue eyes the day he was born and noticing a slight brown marbling near the pupils, so I wasn't at all surprised that the little guy's eyes had changed overnight.

As Will got a little older he became harder to hold and one time when he wanted down he slammed the back of his head right against Karen's nose. She had broken it at a party a few years earlier when she was kicked in the face by a drunken, rowdy dancer. A young intern took it upon himself to give her nose a little twist to put it back into place. The next day Karen woke up with the "raccoon eyes" look. Her mom was horrified, but eventually the swelling subsided. This time, Karen had minor rhinoplasty surgery months later to repair the damage Will had inflicted.

William had a great time playing with his cousins, Sean and Ryan. A few months after Will was born, Kathy had a second son named Adam, whom we referred to as the "First Man."

I made my daily trek back and forth from Stow to Independence. The job at Centerior was going along fine where my responsibilities for maintaining the cost control system stayed true to course. I did manage to hire in from Davis-Besse a brilliant young programmer named Dave Placko. He helped out immensely with a big accounting code conversion project and he also helped me with the big deck project that first summer. Dave was a bachelor who eventually left Centerior for a big-dollar job with a software developer in Seattle. I was glad to see him get the level of compensation he deserved. He was the most gifted programmer I had ever met.

One day Karen got a wrong number from a little old lady named Gertrude, who was all alone in the world with no family. Karen packed a care package together and went to visit this total stranger living out her final days at a meager nursing home. It meant so much to the elderly woman. Karen was very busy as a mom, but she took the time to go see this poor woman. It was acts like these that made me realize how thoughtful and special Karen was, to take the time to visit a virtual stranger who had nobody.

Eventually Karen started working for a large telemarketing firm in Montrose, Ohio, called Infocision. She supervised telemarketing programs to raise money for conservative causes such as Oliver North's election campaign for the U.S. Senate. She was very good at what she did, but the late hours were tough on us. Karen's mom lived alone and she watched Will until I could pick him up after work. We pulled together and did what we had to do. We were slaves to the house. I must admit that we bit off more than we could chew, but I didn't want to move again once more children arrived.

We were into the daily grind, and then one day, out of the blue, Karen told me, "I'm pregnant." Unlike the first time, I was in total disbelief. How could this be? Just a month earlier, Karen had emergency gall bladder surgery. We had gone out to dinner with Karen's father and at the restaurant Karen did not feel well. On the way home she had her head out the window of the car—it was freezing, but she was boiling. I was puzzled and alarmed, so I rushed her to the hospital, driving 80 mph down Route 8 to Akron City Hospital. The next day her gall bladder was removed.

At one point well into the pregnancy Karen put my hand on her tummy to feel the little baby girl's kicking. This time we decided to peek so we'd know the sex of the child in advance.

"This little person in here is not going to be one who tiptoes through life," Karen said.

"How do you know?" I said.

"Trust me, moms know!" she answered.

Karen was seven months pregnant and was asked by Tammy, the girl who had been dating Paul from the boating incident on Lake Erie, to be in their wedding. I found the pregnant version of Karen absolutely beautiful. Weddings are all about starting a family.

A few months later, on August 19, 1992, our second child, Samantha Leigh Volpe, was born. Dr. McVay was in his sixties and nearing the end of his career, and in a world of odd coincidences had also delivered me some 33 years earlier at the same hospital. This pregnancy had gone pretty well. Karen was very tired and worked right up until the time Samantha came along. Being pregnant during the summer in the Midwest, where humidity rules, can be tiresome for those carrying around the extra weight the final months before the child arrives.

This time we were at Akron City Hospital, a much larger and seemingly more sophisticated hospital than the simple, little Magruder Hospital in Port Clinton. An epidural was administered, but it only numbed up one side. When they reapplied the epidural, Karen suddenly had trouble breathing. In addition, they bruised Karen's back and then had the audacity to send us a bill for $963 for these alleged services.

Big hospitals aren't always better. In any event, the important thing was that we had a beautiful baby girl that we love to call Sam. She had huge blue eyes that never changed, other than getting bigger and bluer each day.

We continued to work on the house by finishing off the lower level into a family room. Karen and I continued to work. I began playing catch and pitching Will Wiffle balls. He learned the game of baseball at the very young age of two. Sam was just a wonderful little baby, so full of energy and those huge blue eyes. People would stop us in malls just to admire those major ocean blue peepers.

Once Sam learned to talk she would just say to strangers who would make remarks regarding her eyes, "I know, I know… I have such pretty blue eyes."

We did what new families are supposed to do, and were more devoted to getting to church regularly on Sundays in order to set an example for our children. We hosted many family gatherings. Karen and I loved to entertain and our home was perfect for all occasions, with about 40 people out on the deck for Sam's first birthday party. Those early family Christmases were so special. I fondly remember having all of Karen's family over the day after Christmas. There were lots of new babies, tons of toys and some great beef tenderloin, of course.

At Centerior my job responsibilities took a minor shift in focus as I was assigned, on a part-time basis, to work as an internal consultant on a Software Quality Assurance Project. However SQA, as it was formally known, slowly became a full-time job. We were charged with examining the software development process, the focus being on designing the software business functions correctly, before launching into the programming code. In other words, we were to make sure the business functionality was designed upfront before starting into construction to avoid designing a system on the fly. The underlying functionality is defined upfront, similar to how the Japanese design quality into the automobile manufacturing process. Everything is well-defined ahead of time—quality is built into the process, resulting in a superior product at a lower cost.

I worked with 12 of the best and brightest people from the Information Systems unit at Centerior for nine months on the project. We used metrics and a new unit of measure for assessing software projects called "function points" to ascertain the true magnitude of the software development process. We took an inventory of function points for several of the major software applications to gain a better understanding of what we had already developed. After months of work, we were told by our management steering committee that we could not afford, as a company, to devote the resources to the initial implementation and ongoing expenditures for maintaining the SQA program.

During this time I worked closely on developing the metrics portion of the program with an academic type named Mark Coleman. He was very well-educated and knowledgeable. When we got the word from upper management that the project was dead, he said, "They just don't get it, do they?" The company needed to spend money to save money; the SQA program costs would return savings and efficiencies in a matter of months.

After the project was canned, I was a little pissed off. I decided that if the upper management in IT had such a narrow view of the world that I didn't want to work for them anymore. Leaving the company didn't seem like a good idea. The compensation was decent and the benefits at a large electric utility were very good. I checked the career opportunity board to see if there were any internal postings that were of interest. I found an opportunity in systems planning where they were looking for someone to help with the capital expenditures database. I applied and got the job. It was nice to finally be free of the information systems world. The experience was great, but when you provide computer services in the IT area you really don't get into any true day-to-day decision-making that is at the core of the business.

The director of the systems planning area was a very good guy named Stan Szwed. He gave me additional responsibilities in developing the departmental budget. This was a great change for me. I had an MBA and more than 12 years of financial systems experience to build on. Most of the professionals in the department were electrical engineers, so over time I was able to get a better technical understanding of electrical systems planning and operations.

In the intervening months during early 1993, Karen's mother, Pat, had met a very classy man named John Bird. John's wife, Dorothy, had died a few years earlier from cancer and Pat's friend, Maria, whose husband had also died from the same illness, knew John from a support group for people who had lost their spouses to cancer. Maria and other friends had decided to play "Yenta the Matchmaker" with John and Pat. The Birds were the proud parents of 12 children and long-time parishioners at St. Hilary's Catholic Church in Fairlawn, Ohio. Years earlier, Karen had been classmates with Julie, one of John's daughters. In addition to raising a dozen children, John had a long career in journalism and advertising.

After dating for some time, Pat and John were married at St. Sebastian's in July 1993. John was several years older than his bride and at the reception the priest who married them remarked during grace that, "Even though the wedding was at St. Sebastian's, all the baptisms would be at St. Hilary's."

The entire family was very happy for John and Pat. They traveled to Hawaii for their honeymoon and had wonderful plans for their senior years traveling, playing golf and, most importantly, visiting the multitude of grandchildren, most of which hadn't even been born yet.

One night, during the winter of 1993, Karen and I ventured to downtown Cleveland to see Bruce Springsteen's *Ghost of Tom Joad* tour. It was an entirely acoustical set in a small venue, the State Theatre, as I recall. This evening saw a more serene and serious side of Bruce. At the beginning of the show he announced, "This is going to be a little different kind of show, no singing along, no shouting, and if anyone around you is bored and just talking, turn to them and tell them to shut the hell up." Some people still gabbed as Bruce played most of the ballads from *Tom Joad*, including the local favorite, "Youngstown." We both enjoyed all of the songs he did off the not-so-popular *Nebraska* album.

As we walked out I heard a guy say, "I was just waiting for Clarence to come out from the side and let it fly with one of his patented saxophone solos, but it just never happened." Bruce hung around afterward and talked with some of the people who had seats down front—we were up in the balcony. I'd have loved to have been down there close, to at least be anywhere near the modern-day poet.

I tried to stay in shape, however it's hard when you're working a desk job, sitting in traffic, trying to raise a family and not playing ball anymore. I took up an offer from Karen's three brothers to play in a men's indoor soccer league. At one of the early games, I came in off the bench and after clearing the ball up the field I started to trot toward midfield when I felt a sudden pop in the back of my left calf. I turned around and started to yell at the referee when I realized that there was nobody behind me except my own team's goalie out in front of the net. I hopped off on one leg and jumped over the boards unable to return to the game. I managed to drive myself home even though I could hardly hold down the clutch on the Trooper. I made my way inside. Karen was in bed with the flu, so I iced down the injury.

The next day I went to see Dr. Ross, who was our family doctor. He examined my injury and told me that he was confident that I had torn my calf muscle.

"In six weeks you'll be fine," he stated with certainty.

I pointed to the severe swelling and what looked like a divot above my ankle bone and said, "Are you sure this isn't a ruptured Achilles?"

"No," he said. "This is exactly what happened to me on the tennis court last summer—with rest and therapy, you'll be fine."

So, I went home and rested. For the next several weeks I trudged through the snow on crutches back and forth to work. Eventually, I made it off the crutches and started into a rehab program, but there was still a lot of pain, major swelling, a great deal of bruising and discoloration. My lower leg also seemed jagged, swollen and disfigured. I pressed on through the summer.

Seven months later, in the fall, after gimping around on one good leg, a high school friend of Karen's named Brian Wynne was over for dinner one night and he noticed that I was still laboring with the old injury. Brian is a doctor and he suggested I get an MRI. He referred me to Dr. Chris Clunk, who was the orthopedic surgeon for the University of Akron football team. A day or so after the MRI, I received a call from Dr. Clunk informing me that I had a ruptured Achilles' tendon. I needed extensive reconstructive surgery. The surgery was scheduled for early January 1994.

I was under the knife for five hours and I was bedridden for a month before I could return to work on crutches. The rehab was long and painful. During the surgery, Dr. Clunk relocated the tendon that allowed my left big toe to pick up a marble. The tendon was disconnected from where it was attached to the toe, dragged through a hole he drilled in my heel and then wrapped around the scar tissue of the damaged Achilles' that further reinforced the weakened tendon. This procedure is more commonly referred to as a total reconstruction of the Achilles' tendon.

This was a pretty tough time on a young family. Will was a little over three years old and Samantha was still brand new at only a year and a half. Karen continued to work the long evening hours at Infocision. It was an exhausting period and was, in a way, a bit of a struggle. Samantha and Will would spend the late afternoon hours at Pat's condominium until I could head down from Independence to pick them up. Pat was wonderful and often made us dinner before we would head back to Crystal Cove, about 20 minutes away.

We had some wonderful neighbors on Crystal Cove across the street named Blanche and Dick Green. Their children were grown and gone. Dick was semi-retired, still doing a little writing and consulting. Blanche is a character; she drove a brown 1983 Mazda RX7. Seeing a grandma drive around in this cute little sports car was quite the sight. They loved Calgary, and our children were always welcome at their home. Dick had a nicely manicured lawn and beautiful landscaping. The Greens were members of St. Stephen's Methodist Church, where my good friend Brad Winkler's parents had attended services for years.

We thought the world of the Greens, and as the years wore on both Dick and Blanche had health problems of their own, with Dick's eyesight beginning to fail despite his travels to Boston for surgery. One thing that Dick and Blanche decided to do before his sight diminished further was to visit Walt Disney World. I found it remarkable that of all the things on the planet one would choose to see before being unable to see further, they chose the astounding brilliance and imagination of Walt Disney's playground for children of all ages.

Right next door lived the Derringers. They were also enjoying the rewards of retirement, but their oldest daughter, Sue, and her son, Garrett, still lived with them. Sue was not very attractive—her feet reminded me of Fred Flintstone's feet, except her toes looked like she was wearing black fur slippers. Talk about hairy toes!

We felt bad for her son Garrett; he had some sort of a physical defect that was a form of elephantitis. As the story goes, a couple of years earlier Garrett and Sue were in the checkout line at the grocery one day. A lady in front of them in line realized that she had forgotten paper towels. Her son ran to fetch an eight-pack of towels, and when he arrived back at the checkout line he lofted the package from the back of the line. The paper towels fell short of the mark and hit Garrett's arm, resulting in a severe break that never healed.

The Derringers sued and won a substantial sum. A few years later, Sue was on her way to work and was involved in a minor traffic accident. She managed to get a doctor's opinion that allowed her to collect disability for about two months. She told us that she wasn't really hurt, but that she was just milking the system.

Sue always wondered why we were reluctant to let Garrett play on our swing set and sky fort. It was a fear of being sued.

Mrs. Derringer, the alleged lady of the house, smoked little cigars, causing our Will to ask me one day, "Daddy, why is that man smoking?"

On a hot summer day, Will and Sam were playing on the swing set and Garrett had come over to play. We reluctantly allowed him to play even though I was somewhat hesitant because of a potential lawsuit.

Garrett called out to me, "Dad, can you help me down?" and I politely ignored him. He called out again, referring to me as "Dad" a second time, asking for help down from the sky fort that Will and I had built the previous year.

I mumbled as I walked over just loud enough for Karen to hear, "Not on my drunkest, horniest, out-of-my-mind night would I ever be your daddy!"

I've never seen Karen laugh so hard in the handful of years that we had been married.

Later that summer my dad and Karen were talking, and Karen had always thought that the children didn't spend enough quality time together with Grandma and Grandpa Volpe. We only lived a few miles apart, but we never seemed able to get together for any meaningful time. My dad decided to put together a long weekend or something longer. A week or so later Karen told me he had made a reservation for us to spend an entire week at Virginia Beach. We made the long trip over to Virginia in my dad's minivan. I remember a detour through the hills of Pennsylvania. Karen and I both just about lost our cookies as we swerved our way east. We had a wonderful time, and the trip certainly served its purpose. It was mid-September and school was back in session, so we basically had the beach to ourselves. It wasn't too hot and we seldom had to wait for a table at restaurants.

On the way out of town at the end of the week, my parents went in to see a realtor for about an hour. My dad had expressed an interest in finding a nice beachfront vacation property. He had been there a few times before and was stationed nearby at Fort Eustis back in the late '50s while in the U.S. Army's Transportation Corps.

On the way back, somewhere in Maryland, we had stopped for lunch. As we headed back toward I-70, just after accelerating away from a stop light, the rear hatch of the minivan opened, leaving beach towels, toys and the like all over the road. Luckily, the car behind us was most patient and didn't honk at us while my dad scurried to pick up the mess. I wasn't very quick on my feet due to my injury. My mom and Karen were laughing so hard. It was hilarious to them, but my dad didn't see any humor in the rather embarrassing moment.

Karen eventually decided to leave Infocision to spend more time with her family. She had been getting offers to come in full-time, but Karen wanted to spend more time with the family. She took a job as the accountant for a small Catholic grade school in Columbus, Ohio. She drove down one day a week and kept the books on our PC at home. The U.S. mail and fax machines also helped get the job done. This wasn't ideal. The perfect situation would be for Karen to find something she could do entirely from the comforts of home, where she could be with the kids.

Tammy and Paul had been married for a year and at first lived in an apartment. When they bought their first house, Tammy went out and got some estimates for window treatments. The three windows she wanted done had a price tag of $3,000 or some outrageous amount that only the rich and famous could afford. Karen had taken a sewing class in high school and she taught herself how to design, construct and install custom draperies.

Tammy asked Karen for some help getting their house decorated. Men think sheets are fine, but for the ladies blinds and real window treatments are a must. Karen made some very nice jabots that Tammy loved.

Soon thereafter Karen lost her job with the school in Columbus due to board politics. Karen seized the opportunity and with the encouragement from family members, she decided to take her talent for decorating and design to a higher level. This would be a real business, not just favors for family and friends, where she could make some bucks to buy groceries while at the same time staying at home with Samantha and William.

Karen's Kurtains, a sole proprietorship, was born. At first, Karen advertised in the small weekly paper, but after the first few happy clients were landed, word of mouth and networking allowed Karen to build a huge client base. A sewing room in the lower level of our house was set up so Karen could work at night after the kids were put to bed. After the dinner hour, Karen would head off to visit with potential clients on what we fondly referred to as "curtain calls." My contributions to the business included an occasional referral, building cornices and helping on the installation of her finished projects. There was a huge demand for Karen's services.

She had a sterling personality and an eye for the business, even though she had no formal training in art or interior decorating. It was commonplace for the lady of the house to love Karen's work, and the man of the house didn't mind writing a check for amounts that were a fraction of the cost compared to the costs of the high-priced, high-overhead custom designers. One of the things Karen could do that I could never get over was her ability to compliment the customer whose taste in fabric selection left a little to be desired. She was a regular at the local Joann Fabrics store and even the sales people at Joann's drummed up some business for Karen. A simple business card, innovation and perseverance paid off.

This business was all Karen's.

She was enthusiastic and energetic. Her tenacity and spirit of entrepreneurship rubbed off on me and inspired me to do more with my career. Early on Karen was always supportive of my career and swore that she would follow me anywhere—even Erie, Pennsylvania, she joked.

This endeavor was important to the overall standard of living for our young family. Karen was at home where she needed to be. Will started playing sports. He was on his first baseball team, or should I say t-ball team, at age four. One night, Will somehow managed to puncture his foot with a toothpick. The toothpick was stuck in his foot and was lodged so tightly that Karen thought it best to take him to a local trauma center to have it removed.

Poor little William was saying over and over, "I'm going to die, I'm just gonna die."

Karen said, "No, you're not."

She held his little foot in front of her face while she drove to the trauma center. I stayed with Samantha until I got Blanche Green to come over and watch her. When I got to Karen and Will at the urgent care, they had already done an x-ray and determined the toothpick was not entwined in between any of the small bones comprising the foot. One pull with the needle-nose pliers and the toothpick was out. He picked up the errant toothpick as he walked down the steps to the lower level in his stocking feet. Somehow the toothpick caught in his sock and with his own weight, he accidentally ended up with the toothpick tightly stuck a half-inch into the ball of his foot.

I thought we were done having babies; after all we weren't young parents, with both of us approaching our mid-thirties.

Karen told me she wanted to have another baby. I pushed back on the idea, mostly because I was tired. The new job responsibilities brought on additional pressure and the Achilles injury had taken a toll on me physically. At one point Karen agreed that maybe we were pushing it, and at that point I thought the decision was made to not have a third child.

"I'd really love for Samantha to have a little sister," Karen said.

"I'll decide the sex of this child," I joked back.

A few weeks later, after consulting with her sister, Karen said to me, "I've changed my mind, and I've always pictured myself having three kids." Tired of vacillating back and forth on this question, I said, "Fine!" Previously, Karen had put it very bluntly, "Men need to have sex and women need to have children." We proceeded to take off our clothes, lock the door and do it on the bedroom floor right in the middle of a warm September afternoon.

As I got up off the floor and headed toward the bathroom, I smiled back at her and said, "By the way, that one's a boy!"

CHAPTER 8

Akron City Hospital

It was November 1994 and Karen's third pregnancy was proceeding according to plan. She continued to work hard in her small, but profitable business. The demand for Karen's services picked up right before the Thanksgiving and Christmas holidays, as many of her customers would be entertaining over the holiday season and they would want their homes to have that extra lift from the redecorating finesse Karen's Kurtains provided.

There was a lot of new home construction in the area, and once families started to spend more time inside, the demand for Karen's time also increased. Karen loved the holiday season and would spend an extraordinary amount of time shopping, generally at Summit Mall with her mother. On one Friday afternoon visit to the mall, our young Will, now a vibrant four-year-old, fell asleep. Karen carried the little guy on her hip, having left the portable stroller in the back of the GMC Jimmy.

The following Sunday I was watching the Browns on TV. They were just thrashing the Philadelphia Eagles at Veterans Stadium. I was enjoying watching Michael Dean Perry sack Randall Cunningham repeatedly.

I was walking down the hallway during a commercial, and I heard Karen cry out, "Mark, come here right now, I need you."

I very slowly and somewhat tentatively pushed open the door to the little half bathroom off the kitchen. Karen was crying while still sitting on the john.

She looked up at me and said, "I don't want to flush my baby down the toilet."

At that I peered down into a toilet filled with crimson colored water.

Obviously there was some vaginal bleeding. I helped Karen over to the bedroom and had her lay down. I went back to the bathroom and flushed the contents away, wondering if our chances of having a third baby had just vanished.

As Karen lied there sobbing in bed, I was initially in a slight panic, not knowing exactly what to do. At first, I thought Karen had a miscarriage. We called her new obstetrician's answering service. Dr. McVay, who had delivered Samantha three years earlier, subsequently retired and died soon thereafter from leukemia. Karen's new doctor was Dr. Rachel Burns. She had a wonderful midwife named Laura, who was the point guard for dealing with Karen's pregnancy at her recent checkups. Everything up to this point had gone fine. Dr. Burns was out of town attending a conference, and another doctor, whose name I don't remember, was on call. When she called back she spoke with me on the phone calmly.

She was very reassuring and told me that some "spotting" occurs in one out of every five pregnancies without there being any real trouble. However, she wanted us to come down to the emergency room at Akron City Hospital for an ultrasound and a physical exam to see what was going on. I relayed everything I had just found out to Karen. She was still lying in bed, very upset, but the news about the spotting being somewhat commonplace gave us both some hope.

We prayed a Hail Mary and called my mom, explaining the situation, and asked her to watch Will and Sam while we went downtown to the emergency room.

The bleeding had subsided, but there was still some occasional leakage. We didn't say much on our way to the hospital. Karen insisted I took a lot of time to get going, instead of going to the hospital right away, in order for me to see the end of the Browns game. This was not the case. We had two little children that needed adult supervision, and we couldn't just up and leave. My initial reaction was to run straight to the hospital, but now I tended to be a bit analytical in these types of situations. I want to get as much information as possible before making any rash decisions. Italians are known for being somewhat hot tempered and prone to knee-jerk reactions. I'd like to think that in time I became a little more even-keeled.

Upon our arrival Karen was taken to the maternity and obstetrics floor. The attending doctor was Dr. Robert Marino. I knew of Dr. Marino; he was an honors student from Walsh Jesuit High School. He was a year younger than me. After the typical high-level physical exam, including blood pressure check and listening to the heart, we answered a few questions, including, "Had Karen ever had a miscarriage or an abortion?" The answer to both of these questions was an emphatic "No!"

We were quickly whisked off to the ultrasound unit to try to ascertain more precisely exactly what we were dealing with.

The ultrasound technician was wonderful. Karen lied back on the bed and the technician squirted a gel-like substance on her abdomen that helps create the medium that allows the images to be seen on the small black and white monitor.

She set our minds at ease and was very comforting. Karen remained still, straining to look at the screen. I held her hand as we both tried to understand and decipher the visual images we were seeing on the little black and white monitor. The technician explained that the oval or circular image was the uterus, and then we could make out near the bottom of the oval the vertebrae, leg bones and even the skull.

The wonderful woman looked around the room and said to us very softly, "I'm just a technician and I'm not supposed to do this because I could lose my job, but if you look right here you can see the baby's heart pounding away. This baby is still alive and looks fine to me." We could see a strong little heart muscle continuing to pulse. This brought us great joy and tears to both our eyes, because this meant there was still hope, all was not lost—there was a little life in there struggling to survive. They did some measurements of the fetus and from this data we could determine Karen was 13 weeks along. They also pointed out that at the bottom of the uterus there was some pooling of blood. We waited for Dr. Marino to see us. Karen would stay overnight for observation.

Another young resident confirmed what we had seen on the ultrasound. He stated that the probable cause for the bleeding was that the placenta, which provides nourishment and oxygen through the umbilical cord to the fetus, had partially torn away from the uterine wall. This resident was on his obstetrics rotation, which coincidentally was his intended area of specialization. He told us that if there had been an abruption or tearing away of the placenta from the uterus, that there was a way to continue the pregnancy and maximize the odds of having a normal healthy baby.

Naturally, this doctor had our full and undivided attention. The resident further stated that if Karen went on full bed rest for the next three or four months and concentrated on lying on her left side as much as possible, that this would have the effect of pushing the placenta against the uterine wall, thus allowing for continued maximum sustenance through the mother to the fetus.

Karen and I were optimistic. We understood that there were risks and there were no guarantees, but there was no doubt in our minds that we would do everything humanly possible to give this baby a chance.

We had been at the hospital for three or four hours. Once Karen had settled in her room, I headed home to check on Will and Sam. When I returned to the hospital, Karen told me Dr. Marino had stopped in. Karen was very upset because Dr. Marino had told her that this was a very risky pregnancy.

He advised against the bed rest solution and said, "If you get up and walk around you'll eventually miscarry and then we can perform a DNC. You're young enough; you have plenty of time to get pregnant again and have another baby."

We were horrified at the suggestion!

In a politically correct manner, Dr. Marino was suggesting that Karen should get up and continue with her normal daily activities. We took what he was saying to mean just let nature take its course and don't do anything extraordinary. This made no sense. What Dr. Marino was suggesting was obvious: the abruption would get worse and eventually Karen would miscarry because the fetus would die due to a lack of nourishment.

In our minds, this would be like having a passive abortion. The DNC would be a more active means of discontinuing the pregnancy without calling it a full-fledged abortion in a clinical sense. We were appalled that a doctor would have the audacity to suggest this course of action when we could see that the baby was fine. Furthermore, there was a very viable option that didn't call for any Herculean efforts or complex microsurgery. Maybe as an ethical standard they are required to present all options, but it seemed to us that the medical profession, in the wake of numerous malpractice suits, in order to minimize their risk, present the easy way out and that termination is always a suggested course of action. Karen and I both believe that this was going well beyond the bounds of medicine and that Dr. Marino was trying to "play God."

By now we were more determined to beat these odds and do everything humanly possible to have this child. We decided that bed rest was our only option. We had seen a beating heart and the technician had told us that the baby looked fine. That, coupled with the resident's bed rest scenario, made this the only clear choice. The resident had also explained to us that there wasn't any test available to monitor whether the oxygen flow to the fetus was sufficient to ensure that the baby would be born without being slightly mentally retarded or have some other sort of physical impairment.

Karen wanted so much to have a third child and she had always envisioned us having three children. She felt terrible about the situation.

She said often during the next months, "What if the baby is less than perfect? What will we do?"

And I always told her, "We will just have to love this child more. If the baby needs more, then he or she will get the much-needed love and attention."

It is easy to judge others from the sidelines when other people are faced with an unwanted or difficult pregnancy, and then, as a Catholic, say that abortion is wrong. But when it happens to you, and you are put in the shoes of the one having to make these decisions, it's not that easy.

This was a true test of faith!

At this point I found out what a true "family" was all about. Karen did exactly what the resident had prescribed. She would lie in bed on her left side for hours on end and minimize her daily activities. Kathy and her mom helped out with watching William and Samantha. They also handled the mounting piles of laundry. My parents paid for a housekeeper to come over weekly to clean our house. My new sister-in-law, Tammy, came over and took little Samantha on outings to go shopping or whatever. I didn't miss very much work because everyone in the family did everything they could to make sure Karen remained horizontal. Both families were spectacular, helping us through this challenging time.

Having a first-floor master bedroom came in handy; Karen had an ongoing relationship with the pizza delivery guy. When she called, her instructions were for the delivery guy to come on in. He would take off his shoes at the front door and deliver the pizza right to her bedside. She had the checkbook on the nightstand. Even total strangers helped us. Karen made weekly visits to her obstetrician's office. I think she had more than 20 ultrasounds during this time period.

I joined her as much as possible at these appointments, and from what we could see there was plenty of reason to be encouraged. The little fetus continued to develop just fine from a physical standpoint. Kathy's husband, Roger, even named the little fetus "Brutus" after the Ohio State football mascot. What could not be ascertained via the ultrasounds or any other scientific means was whether the baby's brain was developing normally. At one point, about two months before the due date, Karen called me at work to explain that there was a test that could be performed to see if the baby was going to be mongoloid.

"Two-thirds of the time the test yields a false positive and 70 percent of the time the test itself can start labor prematurely," she said.

Almost immediately I said, "I've thought about it and I don't see the value in having the test. There's no reward worth the risks."

She agreed and we never gave the decision a second thought. What good is a test where 66 percent of the time the results are wrong, and then we have the possibility of labor starting early when we have a young life that needed every chance possible to go full term? I'm no doctor, but it was my feeling that after seven months of brain development, given the abruption, the baby's fate was already determined. Viable babies are born with normal mental capacities at seven months, so why would we consider adding the physical challenges inherent in having a premature child?

What I had learned from this ordeal and our other medical-related dilemmas was the following: even though we have all of this modern medical technology and well-educated doctors, they too are human. They are not above reproach, even though many of them think they are above being questioned. Karen and I had learned to question their advice, and to a degree, once the information had been gathered, to make an informed decision as a couple. Karen and I never once disagreed on any of the decisions we had made in our marriage. We had our convictions and we stuck to them. Our faith also helped get us through this difficult test. Karen continued to take good care of herself throughout the rest of the pregnancy, but she was guilt-ridden that she might bring a child into the world that was less than perfect.

We talked about names for the new baby a lot. Karen knew the sex of the child and asked me if I wanted to know. I'm one who prefers to be surprised, so I insisted that Karen keep this precious piece of information to herself. Then one day it dawned on me. When discussing names for a little girl, Karen never objected to any of my suggestions, therefore I knew the question must have been moot. I pretended the sex of the child was in doubt, but I had figured out we were having a boy. One day I suggested the name Mitchell, having remembered that a couple

I knew from Findlay had decided to name their first child with that strong-sounding name.

"I really like that name," Karen said.

"What about Mitchell Joseph Volpe? That way I'll have someone to pass on my monogrammed stuff," I said.

Karen agreed, and with that we knew the name of our third baby. The decision bolstered our mental outlook—he had a name and his initials would be MJV, just like mine.

Well into her ninth month, Karen could not wait any longer. She had to know what the future held. At what she thought would be her last appointment she told Laura, "I just can't be pregnant any longer; you need to get me to the hospital right now. I need to have this baby now; I need to know now."

Laura, the wonderful midwife, gave her a wink and ordered a stress test, which showed Karen didn't have any placental fluid and needed to be induced. And with that the plan was established. Labor would be induced later the same day.

Once we were at the hospital all the customary steps were taken, and labor was induced. We knew most of the drill because this was our third, but we were also on our third obstetrician, and Laura was most definitely in charge. However, when Karen elected to use a midwife, she had to forgo the use of an epidural. Karen's labor went along rather routinely. My recollection is that labor lasted only a few hours. As the time drew near for Mitchell's grand entrance, Karen and I both noticed that there seemed to be a lot more nurses and doctors in the room.

When we asked why so many were present, Dr. Burns replied, "We're doing this for legal reasons."

It didn't take us long to figure out that the presence of numerous medical personnel were there at the end due to the risky nature of the pregnancy. Karen became more dilated and an instrument to monitor the baby's heartbeat was pressed gently against his little skull. Karen seemed more nervous than scared, having been through the birthing process twice before. I remained calm and confident that everything would be fine. At this point, there's no time to worry; all of the tough decisions had been made and there was no going back.

The cards had all been dealt.

It was time to push, but only at Laura's direction. Karen pushed several times, and it seemed as if we were getting close. Suddenly there was a panic in the room; Mitchell's pulse had dropped quickly.

Laura moved up close to Karen's face and said, "You need to bear down and really push; this child needs to come out now, or we'll have to take you off to surgery for an emergency caesarean section."

Karen pursed her lips, took in her breath, and at Laura's next command mustered all her energy to push out the long-awaited child. It was one of the most, if not the most, amazingly heroic things I had ever seen.

The customary spanking on the butt and the audible sound of the baby crying let Karen and I know the baby was alive and breathing. I turned my attention to Karen while the doctors inspected the newborn, Mitchell. She was exhausted and at that point I was more concerned about Karen's immediate condition than with Mitchell's. Besides, there was a congregation of doctors, nurses and technicians surrounding the child, so I wasn't about to fight my way through the crowded room. Karen seemed to be okay, but still very anxious to know our fate on this date: the 22nd of May in the year 1995.

I said an Our Father to myself, praying that our son would be fine. Days later Karen told me her super-human effort had nothing to do with the prospects of a C-section. Her efforts were totally out of concern for her little Mitchell. We had come so far through the entire ordeal, the 13 weeks of bed rest, more than 20 ultrasounds, the extraordinary efforts of our entire family—she was not about to allow for anything bad to happen that she had the power to control.

This experience was unlike the births of our first two children where once the baby was cleaned up and checked out, the child was handed over to the mother for the first time. Moments earlier there were numerous people checking out Mitchell, and at one point he may have even been taken out of the birthing room while Karen was birthing the placenta that generally follows moments after the baby is out. In the past, this was a part of the process where I didn't do much looking, but this time, given that the health of the placenta was at the core of this challenging and risky pregnancy, I couldn't help but look.

Once the bluish, gray mass was out, Dr. Burns probed at it and examined the tissue on a tray for a few minutes and then placed it in a plastic case. From there she asked whether it was okay with us for the placenta to be sent off to a lab in Dallas for further analysis. We both nodded in agreement.

We were more concerned as to the whereabouts of our new son. At least 15 minutes had passed since Mitchell's grand entrance and we still knew nothing of his condition, other than to know that he was crying and breathing just fine seconds after his arrival.

The door pushed open and Mitchell was finally brought in to meet his parents. The first thing I looked at was his forehead and his little face peeking out of the white linen wrap, and I couldn't see much. As they handed him over to Karen, I peered very closely at his forehead to see if there were any signs of a larger, more elongated forehead indicative of a mongoloid child, and from my vantage Mitchell looked just like Will.

Dr. Burns came in and said there were no signs of any problems that could be readily ascertained. In fact, Mitchell's APGAR scores were even higher than William's. His weight was 7 pounds, 11 ounces and he seemed in every way to be a perfectly normal, healthy baby boy.

Karen and I were elated!

We understood that there was always the possibility that Mitchell could have some other type of problem that we would not know about until later, such as a slow learner or some other sort of physical problem. We said a Hail Mary together, just to thank the Lord and the Blessed Mother for our good fortune.

He looked perfect!

We now knew we had done the right thing and felt we had been vindicated, given the events at the same hospital seven months earlier when Dr. Marino had so strongly suggested that we terminate the pregnancy. To me, this was one of our more challenging life decisions and if we had chosen to not proceed with the risky pregnancy, we would have had to answer to the Lord for this decision. We didn't know at this point in time that seven years later Mitchell would score five goals in a soccer game and get straight A's on his report card. We only knew at this moment in time that he was fine, and it was normal to cry tears of joy.

Two days later we brought Mitchell home from the hospital. Karen's father, Tom, his girlfriend, Peggy, and her daughter, Morgan, were there to greet us when we arrived back home at Crystal Cove with our new bundle of joy. When we arrived, Karen lay Mitchell down in the middle of our bed. The first-floor master bedroom was at the end of the house and a long hallway led through the foyer to the kitchen. As we all sat down to eat, Mitchell could be heard yelping from the bedroom.

Peggy went down to check on him a couple of times and finally, I said, "Bring him to the table." Upon arriving at the table Mitchell calmed down and was fine.

Then it dawned on me: from inside the womb they say a baby can hear just about everything that's going on, and for months Mitchell had been hearing all the commotion going on in the house created by his two-year-old sister, Samantha, and almost five-year-old brother, William.

I said to everyone at the table, "See, he just wanted to be a part of the party."

Karen referred to Mitchell as her "Miracle Baby" and she soon gave Mitchell a couple of interesting little nicknames: "Snig" and "Smelley." We had our healthy third child, even though the placenta was slightly detached from the uterine wall. Thank God there was a functional placenta that obviously provided sufficient nourishment and oxygen to Mitchell, otherwise Karen would have either miscarried or maybe we would have had a stillborn child. Anyhow, we had our "Miracle Baby" and a few months later he was baptized as Mitchell Joseph Volpe, with Karen's youngest brother, Tommy, and my sister, Lynn, serving in the important and honorable role as godparents. Karen, at age 34, and I had just had our last child.

Meanwhile, on areas of much lesser importance, the entire city of Cleveland would be shocked to find out late in the 1995 season that long-time owner Art Modell, had agreed to move the Browns to Baltimore.

When asked by my father-in-law what I thought about the transaction, I replied in jest, "I think my family will like the inner-harbor area and living in Baltimore."

Mr. Modell set the fan base in the Cleveland area on fire when he announced that the name, colors and records were all moving to Maryland. They would become the Baltimore Browns.

However, Mayor White and the lawyers in Cleveland found a "silver bullet" clause in the lease Mr. Modell had executed with the city for use of the old Municipal Stadium up on the lake. The lease called for the Browns to remain at the stadium through 1996 and the city told Art Modell and the NFL that the team would be required to fulfill the terms of the lease. They would play their 1996 games in front of friends and family if a deal weren't cut that would ensure that Cleveland would get either an existing NFL team or an expansion team by a certain date. In the end, the Browns were assured of retaining the Browns name, colors and records. A loan for a new stadium was part of the deal, and in 1999 a new expansion team would be born in Cleveland. I was taken aback by this turn of events. Art Modell had always been a horrible businessman, having accumulated loads of debt while residing in one the NFL's best markets.

I really didn't care. We had our healthy Mitchell and two other beautiful children, and it was about time I got a life other than the emotional ups and downs of being a Browns fan. Our family settled into some semblance of normality. Karen's Kurtains soon resumed business as usual, and for me things at Centerior Energy picked up in intensity.

At Centerior, we had been hearing through the grapevine about the potential for deregulation in the electric utility industry, similar to what had happened with banking, natural gas and telecommunications. Historically, providers of electricity served customers in a certified service territory where their rates were approved by state utility commissions. The rates were derived on a bundled basis and included the costs of generating facilities, high voltage transmission lines and distribution facilities. Congress had decided that wholesale competition was required in order to bring down prices for wholesale consumers, given that the U.S. economy was becoming more and more dependent on electricity. Continued dependency on fossil fuels for energy and the constant crisis in the Middle East required more domestic solutions to meet the country's energy needs, and electricity showed the most promise. The country has an abundance of coal, and small combustion turbine fire plants can be built quickly in order to meet the demand. The major problem is transportation or, as it is called in the electric utility industry, transmission. These are the high voltage lines used to transport power great distances from the power plants in bulk at a wholesale level, well before the end-use customer actually consumes the electricity.

The forecasted demand for electricity was increasing at an astronomical rate. In order for Congress to advance this goal of fostering wholesale electric competition, they gave the Federal Energy Regulatory Commission, or FERC as it is more commonly referred to, the authority to open up the use of the transmission system to third parties. It had been customary for the owners of the transmission system to leverage ownership of these high voltage lines, which are the functional equivalent of the interstate highway system, for their own use. In other words, these lines were generally used to transport their own energy from electric generating plants, but comparable access to a third party was seldom the case and usually only the result of protracted litigation. This anti-competitive behavior by the electric utilities was stifling competition. This was bad for consumers and Congress had seen open markets for electricity work in other parts of the world, so why not here?

In developing Centerior's 1996 budget Stan Szwed, who was the Director of Systems Planning, had me add $150,000 to the budget for consulting services in connection with what he termed "functional unbundling." I remember thinking to myself that this sounded rather complicated. I was glad I wasn't going to be involved in this complex and ominous endeavor. Little did I know that Stan would soon put me on a temporary assignment in the rates department to work with Gwen Luciano on Centerior's required filing of an open-access transmission tariff. This was part of the functional unbundling process that was required by the law and subject to the FERC's jurisdiction. There was a notice of proposed rule-making on this new tariff which allowed third parties comparable use of Centerior's transmission system.

Suddenly, I found myself engulfed in a strange, yet new and exciting part of an industry that had historically been rather dull and boring. I spent some time at the FERC in Washington D.C. learning about this new era of electric competition. I hadn't traveled much during the first 15 years of my career and was now away a few nights each month. Karen was very supportive and excited that my career had taken this turn for the better, even though it involved me being away from our young family more often.

This process had actually started prior to Mitchell's arrival. I remember a very pregnant Karen coming to the airport to pick me up. Gwen Luciano, who was my supervisor, was traveling with me from Washington D.C., and Karen said to me on the way home, "Gwen's so pretty and professional in her business suit and there I was pregnant out to here, not looking my best." This trip, which happened just after Timothy McVeigh had bombed the Federal Building in Oklahoma City, ended up being very fruitful for my career.

Gwen and I had dinner at this quaint little Italian restaurant in Georgetown. She had told me that both she and Stan were impressed with the work I had been doing, and she wondered whether I was interested in a permanent position in the federal rates area within her unit that dealt with Federal Regulatory Affairs. Of course, I was excited and accepted the change in career direction.

I was now totally out of the information technology side of the business. This type of climate was more conducive to my personality, and I finally felt as though I was using my MBA. It was only the second promotion of my career. I did receive one promotion while at Marathon, but at Centerior the only real change was the move from Davis-Besse to Independence, which was a lateral move. It was nice to finally get recognized and be promoted. It was long overdue and Karen always felt that I needed a break to prove that my career could be better than average. Usually, to move up you had to move out, as in find another employer who was willing to offer some upward mobility and the compensation commensurate with such a position.

The FERC had issued Order No. 888, which required all public utilities to file open-access transmission tariffs. Assembling the tariff and doing a full-fledged cost of service to file the rates was challenging, but it sparked my enthusiasm. It was very cutting-edge stuff, and a number of my peers were intrigued with the changes going on in the industry. Many neighboring utilities were merging, given the open-access era that was taking shape in the industry.

Part of Order No. 888 encouraged utilities to form independent system operators or ISOs. These ISOs would take over the functional control of the transmission facilities of several regional electric utilities in order to provide non-discriminatory open-access to the transmission system over a significant geographic region. My initial reaction was that on a voluntary basis, these utilities that were so entrenched in maintaining control of their own facilities would not be inclined to relinquish this authority to a third party that had been deemed an independent entity.

A few months later a handful of utilities in the Midwest region were discussing the possibility of forming a new company called the Midwest ISO. Centerior assigned me to represent them on the pricing work group that was exploring alternatives on how the rates for transmission service on a regionalized basis would work. Every two weeks a number of Midwestern utilities contemplating participation in the Midwest ISO would meet at the Skybird Meeting Center, which was located behind security at Chicago O'Hare, to talk about transmission pricing for the fledgling Midwest ISO. This process began in April 1996 and went on for more than a year.

On the home front, the children were growing up wonderfully. Will was in kindergarten at Holy Family, the same school I had attended, and Samantha was in preschool, having taken on the very outgoing and gregarious personality of her mother. Sam ruled the roost!

The dysfunctional Derringer family next door had moved to South Carolina. Once they sold their home and the long-awaited moving truck pushed off, Karen and I celebrated with glee. We had no way of knowing that a bad situation could get worse. Crystal Cove Circle only had 10 homes, and other than the Greens and the Pollacks, it was not a very family-friendly place to live. Ruth and Bill Glause, who lived two houses away, were nice to us, but some of the other people living on the Cape Code themed cul-de-sac were far from what we thought was ideal. There was a preacher who was trying to start his own following of churchgoers in Russia. The people who lived on one side of our house had a daughter who watched our kids a few times. We generally paid her with a check, but several times the check came back with "No More Checks" penned in the memo line. We thought this was a bit odd.

The people who bought the Derringers' home were from Yugoslavia. One of their parents, who spoke no English, lived with them, along with an adopted daughter. They were very friendly, and initially we got along with them fine. Then things began to change. First they took on a boarder, a mentally disabled adult recovering from surgery. We were told when he moved in, late in 1995, that he would only be there a few months and that there was nothing to worry about—he was not a sexual predator and we had no reason to be alarmed. He was still there a year later, plus there was some serious remodeling going on in the basement. In their lower level, which was also a walkout like ours, they were adding numerous catacomb-like rooms in order to take on more boarders. Somehow our neighbors had managed to change the zoning for their home to allow the house to become a group home for mentally retarded adults.

Bill Glause, who lived next door to the new group home, found out that the local zoning requirements had been changed at the state capital in Columbus without the consent of the other residents in the development. He was mostly concerned with the property values; my concern was not only with our property value, but also the safety and well-being of our children. Every day a bus would drop off daytime boarders, and slowly more permanent, full-time boarders were added. The State of Ohio paid the owners $1,500 a month per boarder. They had also managed to bypass the stringent zoning requirements that called for a sprinkler system and other food-related facilities to be installed at their residence. The house had become a full-fledged group home for the mentally and physically disabled.

Karen and I are not lacking in charity and understanding for people who are born less fortunate. Had it not been for the grace of God, we too, could have been parents of a less-than-perfect child, given our challenging pregnancy with Mitchell. It was as though the Lord was reminding us that He had spared us this cross by putting this home right next to ours. Even though I loved the lake setting and the view, I knew deep down that something had to change.

Karen was becoming more and more disenchanted with the neighborhood and in the summer of 1997, at dinner with my parents while on vacation at their recently purchased condo in Virginia Beach, she made it clear that she was unhappy and wanted to move. I was concerned mostly with the transaction costs for moving our household goods, closing costs and commissions. We began to look for another place to live.

I continued working on the pricing work group for the formation of the Midwest ISO and in July 1997, I made a proposal for the pricing mechanism in Cincinnati at the home offices for Cinergy Corporation, a large utility that had resulted from the merger of Cincinnati Gas and Electric and Public Service of Indiana. Several companies participating in the discussions did not like the Centerior proposal, and Stan Szwed called me from the road the next day to let me know what a good job I had done in spite of opposition from the other companies. One of the representatives from Indianapolis Power & Light Company referred to my proposal as "a pig wearing a tutu—underneath it all, it's still a big fat pig."

A few weeks later Centerior Energy announced that is was merging with Ohio Edison Company to form a new utility called FirstEnergy. In the wake of deregulation, many utilities were now uniting forces. For me, another merger did not seem to be a big deal. However, the new company would be based in Akron, not Cleveland. Most of Centerior's senior management staff were taking an early retirement package or, in some cases, being demoted. Many of my friends in administrative positions would be getting severance packages.

I was told not to worry because of my expertise in the new world of open-access transmission and because I was representing Centerior in the early discussions contemplating the Midwest ISO. I retained my job after the merger was announced, and still reported to Gwen. Stan Szwed fared pretty well. He had been promoted to Vice President of Transmission at Centerior and was retaining similar responsibilities at FirstEnergy. I was skeptical about my future with FirstEnergy. For the short term, I seemed to be in good shape. But I knew that over the long haul, given the fact that I had roots with Centerior, which was the firm being acquired, despite the use of the term "merger," my days were likely numbered. This was an acquisition and Centerior Energy was history. Coupled with our unhappiness on Crystal Cove Circle, I started looking for a change of venue.

One day I was on the phone with John Procario, a man at the forefront of restructuring the electric utility industry and the Vice President of Electric Systems Operations at the Cincinnati based electric utility called Cinergy. When we had finished talking about Midwest ISO business, I asked him whether it would be appropriate for me to forward him a copy of my resumé for consideration, if and when the Midwest ISO were to actually form. I went on to tell John that I was concerned about my future, given the merger. John was the chairman of the transmission owners committee, which was the primary group of senior management representing the numerous electric utilities that were conducting the negotiations on the Midwest ISO's formation.

After I explained my dilemma, John paused for a moment and then asked me a few more questions about my background and experience. John had seen me in front of the semi-hostile crowd of transmission owners months earlier when I made the Centerior pricing proposal and I guess he was impressed at how I held my ground.

John asked me what kind of money I made at Centerior, so I told him, wondering where the conversation was going.

"I can offer you much better compensation if you're willing to relocate to Cincinnati and work for me," John said.

"Of course, I'll have to talk to my wife first, but I would like to come down to check it out," I said.

"Great, we'll be in touch," John said and he hung up.

Although there was no written offer at that point, the interview was really a formality. I called Karen and talked with her briefly about the possibility, but one thing seemed clear to me—we had to get outta Dodge.

Northeastern Ohio was home and both of our families lived in the vicinity. Thanks to a career opportunity, we were moving to Cincinnati. This was a region of Ohio I had always loved. As a kid I had listened to Johnny Bench and the Big Red Machine teams of the '70s on WLW. Even though the Cleveland Indians had just made a major resurgence, losing to the Atlanta Braves in the 1995 World Series, and even though the Indians were contending for the American League pennant again in 1997, I knew we could all love the land of the Big Red Machine. Cincinnati had a lot to offer a growing, young family.

And besides, the weather had to be better than Cleveland, averaging six to eight degrees warmer than northern Ohio, with much less snow.

CHAPTER 9

Kings Island

After I interviewed with Cinergy in August 1997 and received the formal offer, which I immediately accepted, Karen and I took a long weekend to look at houses and communities. I had done some research and the northeast suburbs near I-71 seemed to be a fit. Most of our house-hunting focused on the cities of Mason, Loveland and West Chester. Our first visit, after locating the realtor, was to a new development called Crooked Tree, with a large regional residential builder named Zaring. When we walked into the model, Karen looked at the overall floor plan of the Edinburgh and we were impressed. When Karen saw the large upstairs bathroom, her eyes filled with tears and she said, "This is where we'll give our babies baths!" Will was entering the first grade, but he was still a baby to us. Beautiful Samantha had just turned four and Mitchell was only a year and a half.

Later on I told Karen the price and she cried again because she knew it was within a range we could afford. We looked at several other houses that day, but our minds were made up as we picked out a lot at the top of a crest on a street named Larkspur Lane in rapidly growing Mason. One of the perks I liked about Crooked Tree was the wonderful golf course by the same name within walking distance of the house. Even though our home wasn't on a golf course lot, living in a golf course community was still very nice. Later that evening while visiting nearby with

Karen's nieces, the Repass girls, we found out Princess Diana had been killed in a car wreck in Paris.

On our next trip we did all of our selections and made a deposit. Construction started in September 1997. Initially, we tried to sell our home in northeastern Ohio ourselves, but after a few weeks we decided to go with a realtor. In October, I resigned my position with FirstEnergy and took up residency at the Days Inn at the southern end of Mason.

Once again I had thrust Karen into the role of being a single mom, entrepreneur and realtor all at the same time. She was very supportive and understanding, but it was far from fair. My ultimate goal was to make her life easier, because I knew the demands on her time from the children would only increase as they grew older. The more money I made took pressure off Karen. While we were in Cleveland, Karen had to work in order for us to put groceries on the table and make a car payment. As my compensation increased, the new plan was that I would be able to give Karen a check every 10 days so she could establish a budget for the household and be at home for the kids.

Living out of a hotel can be a real low light. I kept tabs on the construction of our new home, but overall it was pretty boring. There was one nice diversion that kept me occupied. The Cleveland Indians were playing the Baltimore Orioles in the American League Championship Series. Paul stopped in for the deciding game versus the Orioles, and after a long pitchers' duel, the Indians light-hitting second basemen, Tony Fernandez, hit a solo shot in the seventh that proved to be the game winner. We had a case of beer and some cigars, and we were actually sitting in chairs in the parking lot so we could catch some sun while we watched the game on the hotel TV that we had pulled out near the door. We were pretty trashed by the end of the game, so we walked over to Applebee's to celebrate, drink more beer and get some ribs. It was a blast and one of those times Paul and I will always cherish. We were the only people in Cincinnati who cared. The Reds were playing golf and as for the Bengals, well, as usual they just plain sucked.

So the Tribe won the ALCS and went on to lose to the fledgling Florida Marlins in seven games in the 1997 World Series. Manager Mike Hargrove blew game seven when he allowed the Indians' semi-reliable closer, Jose Mesa, to come in for the bottom of the ninth where Mesa allowed the Marlins to tie up the game. Hargrove should have allowed the set-up man, Mike Jackson, who had just pitched a perfect eighth inning, to at least start the ninth. If Jackson had allowed the leadoff hitter to get on, then going to Mesa would have been warranted. In the end, Cleveland again remained the "Land of Almost." Cleveland had not won a world championship in a major sport since the Browns 27-0 victory over the Baltimore Colts in 1964.

I really liked my new position as a Senior Contract Analyst, even though most of my time was spent not on administering contracts, but helping Mr. Procario with the formation of the Midwest ISO. I was his caddy and we traveled around the Midwest to great places like Detroit, Chicago, St. Louis, Indianapolis, Milwaukee and even historic Green Bay, home of the Packers. I had taken on the responsibilities as the recording secretary for the transmission owners' committee, and in these meetings I really got an education from these men, most of whom were electrical engineers and had been in senior positions in the industry for years. I was a sponge and I soaked up a basic understanding on the technical aspects of a remarkably complex industry.

I came home on the weekends and it was very hectic. Open houses are a real pain and finding quality time with the children was difficult. Karen was also trying to close her business, fulfilling the orders of her last few customers in the pipeline. On the way north up I-71 for Thanksgiving, I ran into some major snow around Mansfield, Ohio, that made the final 80 miles very slow-going and treacherous. The last part of the trip, which usually takes just over an hour, took around three. I thought to myself we wouldn't miss all this snow while living in southwestern Ohio. Things had gone pretty slow as far as finding a buyer for our home on the lake, but finally on Christmas Eve we received an offer for a few thousand less than we had hoped to get. We accepted the offer. Sometimes you just take the lumps and move on.

Meanwhile, our new home in Mason was coming along nicely. There were no problems during construction and one of the owner's sons, Mark Zaring, was in charge of construction for our Georgian-styled home. Our lot lacked the lake view, and in fact, did not have even a single tree. It was almost perfectly flat and well suited for football. In early January 1998, Karen and the children came down to see the progress on the new house and to check on the transfer of Will and Samantha to new schools once they moved down in February. Will would be in the Mason Public School district, attending Western Row Elementary as a first grader, and Samantha would be in a new preschool program near our house. We were unable to get them into St. Susanna's, where there was a very long waiting list. In retrospect, Karen and I both felt that we had made a mistake not building in a community where our children could attend parochial school.

Finally, in February, the new house was ready. On a cold, cold evening, with all of our worldly belongings packed in a moving van, Karen and the three children made their way south to Mason, Ohio. However, there was one problem. An ice storm had just hit southern Ohio and when Karen got to the south side of Columbus, everything slowed to a snail's pace. In retrospect,

I should have told her to pull off and get a hotel room. The moving van was due to arrive early the next day, and she called a few times by cell phone to let me know that they were okay even though they were only moving at about 40 mph. We were going to have a slumber party. I had the sleeping bags all rolled out in front of the fireplace.

About 11:00 p.m., Karen and the beautiful Volpe children finally arrived at the new house, cold, but safe and sound. The risky adventure was all for naught. The driver of the moving van explained to us the next morning that there was no way his guys could get all of our furniture into our house, given the ice. We made do for a day until the movers were able to get our goods inside.

The next day was the ultimate in boredom and frustration. It reminded me of a rainy day at the beach. We ventured out on the icy roads searching for food and found a Boston Market on the verge of closing. They felt sorry for us, so they fed us before closing their doors in the middle of the afternoon, because only fools were out. Karen always had a way of charming people and she managed to use her wonderful people skills to get her children food when the hourly workers wanted to get home. Every business and school in Cincinnati was closed due to the ice.

The poor guys working for the man who owned the moving van had it rough. Karen had befriended them while they were packing up our things in Stow. One of the young men had apparently fathered a child with the daughter of the man in charge of the move. He didn't treat these three guys very well. They had to pay for their own meals, and when they couldn't move us in, the man in charge slept in a hotel while the boys were out in the cold of the moving van with only dingy moving blankets to sleep on. Karen made sure the guys were fed, and when they arrived in Mason on the day of the move she noticed they were only wearing sweatshirts, no gloves and thin socks. While they were bringing in the first few items, Karen drove out to Big Lots and bought stocking hats, gloves and wool socks for the movers. She was always looking out for the other guy. Eventually, all of our material goods were moved into our new home.

William and Samantha settled into their new schools without any major incidents. I'll never forget Samantha's teacher at her graduation months later in May.

"Samantha came to us in February and immediately took complete control of the class," she said.

I thought to myself, "That's my girl. Her mom was right—she's certainly not one to tiptoe through life."

We made many friends in the neighborhood right away. The Smiths lived a few houses down the street—Phil and Sandy with their daughter Samantha, who would become known as "Big Sam," and their son D.J. I really enjoyed Sandy's cooking. She was brought up in a traditional Italian home in suburban Cleveland and she used lots of garlic in her recipes. She made some wonderful spaghetti sauce. Directly across the street from the Smiths lived the Kuzner family. Jennifer and Bob were high school sweethearts from Detroit. Their oldest son Bobby and our Will became friends, even though Bobby was a year older than Will. Their other son, Ryan, cracked me up. Let's just say Ryan could get a little out of control and sometimes he would tend to overuse the phrase, "That sucks!" Just down the street was the Mitchell family. Keith and Lori had met at Purdue, and they had two very cute kids, even though their daughter had a knack for spilling grape juice all over our carpet, and one night she dumped an entire cup on me.

I continued to work on the development of the Midwest ISO at Cinergy and spent a good deal of time on the road negotiating the details for what we all hoped would eventually become a real company. We really enjoyed living in Mason. We had season passes to the local amusement park, Kings Island, and on weeknights we would head over during off-peak hours to hit a few rides and see the fireworks. It is really a neat place to live. We were only three hours from Cleveland, and thanks to inter-league play, the Indians even played a few games at Cinergy Field while we lived there.

William played little league and Samantha took some classes in hip-hop dancing. Mitchell was his mother's pride and joy. They were thick as thieves. When I would come home at the end of the day, I'd always ask Mitchell what he did that day and he'd say, "Chopping with Mommy." Karen had restarted Karen's Kurtains and had developed a nice client base near our home. This was one of the great things about her business, especially living in a new development. Everybody had a new house and Karen's services were in big demand. She was also a manufacturer's representative for Hunter Douglas blinds.

I loved my job at Cinergy. John Procario had given me tons of autonomy in helping him develop the Midwest ISO. In January 1998, we filed the tariff and the owners' agreement, the foundation documents for forming the Midwest ISO, with FERC. We knew it would be months for the regulatory process to take shape before the federal agency would issue an order regarding whether we could proceed with the new, non-profit entity.

After a conference call one afternoon, Procario said to me half smiling, "You know, when this thing gets up and running, you'll end up leaving when they offer to double your salary."

I just smiled and said right back, "You'd match that to keep me, wouldn't you!"

Karen's cousin Kyle Captain, who was the son of her mother's sister Ellen, had taken a job in downtown Cincinnati. We grew to be good friends and I always enjoyed our chats. Will and I helped Kyle move into his apartment in the trendy Hyde Park area. Kyle and I had lunch regularly at some of the area's casual lunch spots, such as the Red Squirrel and the well-known Skyline Chili. Kyle didn't have a girlfriend while he lived in Cincinnati, because his big love was hunting. He had an off-road four-wheeler that he used to chase deer through the mountains of West Virginia on weekends.

One day Karen hung up the phone after talking with her mom. Karen told me her Uncle Dick had a growth down his throat that was causing him some trouble and he was going to see some doctors in Huntington, West Virginia, to have it checked out. We both thought it sounded pretty serious and hoped he would consult with doctors at a larger hospital in either Columbus or Cincinnati. It turned out that they decided to radiate what was already a large cancerous growth. Radiation only made matters worse. The growth turned to mush and the cancer quickly spread.

Dick was in his early fifties and to say he was a character would be an understatement. At the family reunion a few years earlier, I was in a foursome with Dick in the annual golf scramble. He was hurting during the round due to Friday night's activities, and on one green he managed to hit a putt at a perfect 45-degree angle from the hole. It was probably the worst putt I had ever seen. None of the girls on some of my cheap dates in high school ever hit a putt this bad. Dick's son, Shannon, and Kyle grew up together in Huntington. Shannon had joined the Army and was in a Special Forces unit. Kyle had numerous stories about Dick that could fill a book. Dick passed away after a long two-year battle. My parents came down to Mason and watched the kids while Karen and I attended the funeral. We had prayed for Dick just about every night at dinner and in a way having someone to pray for was very fulfilling for our family.

On some nights we would ramble through grace and start to eat and Samantha would say, "Hey, we forgot to ask God to watch over our Uncle Dick."

Karen and I would just look at each other with a sense of satisfaction because we knew we were doing at least one thing right. It was the first person my children had ever known who had died. This was something that you know is going to happen some day, but you think that it's going to be a great grandmother or another elderly person who has moved on, not a vibrant man in the prime of his life.

I don't know for sure, but I suspect that Dick's troubles were caused by habitual use of tobacco-related products. He had smoked cigarettes earlier in life and never went anywhere without his pipe during the years I knew him. His death was an opportunity to instill in our children the dangers of smoking. Karen and I don't smoke, however I will occasionally fire up a traditional cigar to celebrate the birth of a child.

There was another major family episode that occurred while we lived in Cincinnati. As a teenager, attending a large, all-men's high school run by the Jesuits, the art of fundraising was always an interesting challenge. At Walsh an annual dinner-auction gala event called POW WOW, which stands for Promotion of the Winning Warriors of Walsh, was an event to look forward to each April. This endeavor depends on volunteerism in order to make it happen. I waited on tables as a freshman, ran auction items for a couple of years, and helped with the valet parking as a senior. In college, I tended bar one year when I was home on break. It was always a festive event with an open bar, a gourmet dinner and a variety of ways to spend money in either the oral or silent auctions.

Once my siblings had all married, my mom and dad, who had attended every POWWOW since its inauguration in 1973, would reserve a table, and for at least 10 years we would all be there together for an evening of family fun. When Karen and I moved to Cincinnati we knew that we would be traveling north to attend this annual tradition. Both of my brothers had also graduated from Walsh. My sister's husband, who I refuse to refer to by name, had graduated in 1979 in the same class as my brother, D.J., and Karen's brother, Kenny. Tommy also graduated from Walsh. He and Kenny were both great soccer players during their days there.

The POWWOW in 1998 was extra special!

This gathering would be part of a family celebration because it was also the weekend of my parents' 40th wedding anniversary. We would have a private Mass at Walsh on Sunday. There was one hitch, though. My sister, Lynn, called me to inform me that she and her husband had to miss POWWOW that year because of a "family" wedding on her husband's side in Canada. She was seeking advice as to how to break the news to our parents.

I remember telling her they'd understand and that, "After a 10-year run, there was bound to eventually be a scheduling conflict."

A wedding seemed to be a good enough reason to not make this "can't miss" event.

You know how they say there are always two sides to every story. A few days later my dad called me very upset over Lynn and her husband missing POWWOW and the celebration of their 40th wedding anniversary. "What's the big deal dad," I said. "They have this family wedding, and certainly you understood that this was bound to happen sooner or later?"

Well, as it turns out, my sister told my parents she didn't even know the name of the third cousin who was getting married in Canada. The previous year my brother-in-law had quietly announced when leaving POWWOW that it would be his last one. He had a problem with the public recognition given to my parents that evening. My parents were recognized that night for being the only couple to have never missed the event in the school's history. He found a plausible rationale, the wedding of a distant family member whose name Lynn didn't even know, as being of more importance in their lives than his wife's parents.

My dad called me at Cinergy one afternoon and pressed me a little regarding the situation. I remember sitting at my desk, sweating the situation, and I finally decided that it was about time someone told him the truth about my brother-in-law. I had gotten along fine with my brother-in-law, but he had grown to resent my father's success in the business world that now included my brothers. They are all dedicated and had worked very hard to grow their new business. I guess my brothers and dad made it look easy.

A few years prior, with only the benefit of a high school diploma and little to no small business experience, my brother-in-law embarked on a business venture with his brother and sister. Evidently there was something missing, maybe dedication, hard work and trying to work with his brother and sister, as they had their own complications and other priorities. I'm not saying one can't make it without higher education. I know a few self-made millionaires who had no education beyond high school. The difference is they worked hard to make it; nothing was ever handed to them.

His lack of business acumen, compounded by his propensity for over extension, ultimately proved to be his undoing. The problem began a long time ago, having failed to prepare for the living standard to which he believed he was entitled. He thought he was leading a charmed life after high school, as he left the mailroom for a position hosting special events that the major tire manufacturer sponsored. They paid him very well given his lack of real work experience. There was no need for more education.

Who cares about education and experience?

He started a business of his own with his brother and sister when the tire company finally figured out they could save some money by cutting him loose. So, his resentment of the success around him was understandable, in spite of all the things my parents did for him, including meeting his company payroll when the cash flow wasn't there.

This even extended to his inability to pay his mortgage.

A few months earlier, one morning, Lynn stopped by my parents' house on her way home from the hospital after a night's work in the intensive care unit. She was sweating her second missed house payment and a letter from the bank.

My dad had pledged they would not lose their home and he replied to my mom, "Marilyn, just make out a check!" as he left for work, not even asking about the amount.

What I felt compelled to reveal to my father wasn't mere resentment on my brother-in-law's part, but the particulars of his sentiment. He seemed to think that because my brothers were owners of the family business, they were getting more than they deserved from the business they were working so hard to build.

"They're getting theirs now," he had said. "How about ours, Mark?" referencing my sister's supposed inheritance. "I want mine now. I can't wait."

These weren't slips of the tongue, but a deep-seeded posture. It was these sentiments that I was painfully considering relaying to my father, of which he was totally oblivious. I never felt this way because I was handed an opportunity to receive a fine education, all thanks to my parents. Karen and I did not feel we were owed anything. We both had our education and career experiences, a solid foundation to build a family around.

Karen and I had worked very hard to dispel my brother-in-law's feelings. We hoped that once he got squared away financially, his adamant resentfulness would subside. But the hurt was there and I knew I had to finally give my father the facts.

I sat at my desk trying to decide whether to come clean and relay my brother-in-law's growing resentment of his in-laws' success. I decided to spill the beans. There's always something to be said for the truth. It beats being a coward and a fraud. To this day I don't know if I did the right thing or not, however, this much I know for sure: I told the truth!

Reluctantly, I told my dad his son-in-law had said, "I don't need it 30 years from now," referring to what he saw as his entitlement program, a significant inheritance given his marriage to Lynn. "I need it now!"

The next few weeks Karen and I spent hours on the phone trying to convince my parents that Lynn did not share the same resentment toward them that their son-in-law did. He didn't want to be a part of the family, but what he did want was an infusion of more capital. Blowing off POWWOW and my parents' wedding anniversary in 1998 was his way of showing his disdain for his in-laws. Lynn insists that her husband is "not that way" and has hung with him to protect her children. But despite Karen's and my efforts to mitigate the situation, it had grown to the point where the differences were not able to be reconciled. In the end, I had an estranged sister whom I would not talk to for years.

This was a situation where one must take a side, and I took up firmly with my parents. They were clearly the ones who had been wronged. Lynn asked that my parents, my brothers and I keep our distance in order to allow her to maintain some semblance of a marriage. We have abided by her wishes. It's difficult to explain to our children why they don't see their beautiful cousins anymore. Even sending birthday presents was frowned upon. Lynn's husband forced her to make a very difficult choice.

"It's either them or me!" he emphatically stated on more than one occasion to Karen.

This whole situation and the premise surrounding this set of circumstances are nothing short of incredulous.

For the greater good of her children, Lynn made the proper choice and chose to remain loyal to her husband. This was to be expected and was the right decision, consistent with the manner in which she was raised: upholding the sanctity of marriage and to maintain the family unit at virtually all costs.

Lynn was Mitchell's godmother at his baptism; however, Kathy quickly volunteered to assume this honored responsibility. She has been a wonderful godmother ever since, and if there was a way to change the name on his baptismal certificate, we would. Later on I would find out that Karen had pleaded with my brother-in-law on many occasions to reconsider his demand that Lynn separate from her parents. Karen had fully supported Lynn in the many ways a family member should.

Lynn worked full-time as an ICU nurse to keep the family afloat after their business went down the tubes, and my parents graciously helped them out. Karen had always gone out of her way to help Lynn. On numerous occasions, Karen was there for her as she labored to overcome her husband's failure to provide. She supported Lynn when her nursing responsibilities had her up all night. Karen, in her immense dedication to family, did everything she could to make life easier for Lynn. As Lynn's role as the main family provider increased, Karen occasionally helped with everything working mothers do: running errands, transporting children and watching Lynn's children.

Karen was steadfast in attempting to build a bridge between my parents and their daughter. Karen could not contemplate a daughter not having a relationship with her mother. She worked very hard in her role as the peacemaker, while we attempted to help reconcile this unfortunate situation. We could have easily decided to stay distant and not get involved, but in the end, Karen and I simply had a different definition of the true essence of family. This situation is sad and very difficult to come to terms with. We couldn't imagine a situation in which our Samantha would be married with children, living just seven miles away, and Karen and I would not be permitted to see our grandchildren. Imagine being forced to watch your grandchildren through binoculars as they frolicked on the playground.

Five years later when Lynn learned that Karen's darkest moments were looking even darker, as Karen battled leukemia, Lynn displayed total indifference and a lack of feeling. As things would turn for Karen, she could have used Lynn's professional experience when she faced what would be life's ultimate challenge. But Lynn would be AWOL. Maybe with her Bachelor of Science in Nursing and years of ICU experience, she could have contributed to some form of medical enlightenment and comfort given Karen's grave predicament.

This is shameful!

Karen, the consummate family champion, was shown no regard or consideration. Lynn demonstrated nothing, but cold indifference, to a sister-in-law who had supported her and tried to salvage this family situation.

I often pray there can somehow be a reconciliation of this episode, because life is too short. There is always hope for forgiveness and moving on as long as there is a willingness to talk.

For the duration of 1998, we settled into a fast-paced routine. We carted our children to little league games and other activities. All sorts of family visited from Akron on a regular basis, and we went to tons of Reds games, particularly because inter-league play allowed our Cleveland Indians to venture down to Cinergy Field. One weekend Karen's brother Kenny brought down about a dozen couples to party and see the Tribe pound the Reds. After the game we got into a little scuffle at the Ogden Bar. I remember somebody throwing a bowl of popcorn at Kenny. Well, at least nobody tried to wipe a booger on my wife. Way too much alcohol!

Karen had a cousin named Greg who had coincidentally built a new house in Mason about a quarter of a mile from our house. He and his lovely wife Cindy had two children, Tyler and Valerie. Naturally, we became really close with Cindy and Greg. We celebrated children's birthdays and hosted numerous cookouts at each other's homes.

I would spend numerous hours evaluating my options for seat selection at the new Cleveland Browns Stadium in conjunction with their return to the NFL in 1999. When the package arrived informing me of my seat location, I was practically trembling. I had really missed professional football during my three-year abstinence from the Browns. It was hard to have a life. I still watched the Steelers and hoped that they would lose each and every week. Some things just don't change. I was elated to open the package and find that I had received my first choice, in the corner of the end zone at the Club Level, and I almost cried when I was placed in Section 343, Row 2 seats 1-4. Being on an aisle is always a plus!

In September 1998, the FERC gave conditional approval for the Midwest ISO to begin operations and the odyssey I call a career continued. The fun was just beginning. There were more filings that needed to be made, plus issues that required discussion and settlement. This would keep me pretty busy at Cinergy. A site selection group from the transmission owners was examining where to locate the new organization. Numerous cities in the region were under consideration: Chicago, Detroit, Louisville, Indianapolis, Milwaukee and St. Louis. Cleveland wasn't in the mix.

I silently hoped for somewhere near greater Cincinnati as the site for Midwest ISO's headquarters.

CHAPTER 10

County Clonbur, Ireland

Some time early in 1999, Karen's father started into motion plans for all of his children and their spouses to venture over to Ireland to visit the land of his ancestors. He had been there several times, and Karen and I were always game for an adventure abroad. Karen had been to Ireland once, in 1982, at the outset of her backpacking adventure with Nora and Margot. I was intrigued with two aspects of the trip: the golf courses and the beer. Later on, the dates were set. We would travel over in early August. For the bulk of 1999, we had settled into a familiar routine with the children in school, my daily bus rides back and forth on I-71 to work, and Karen's Kurtains providing beauty and warmth, mostly to new homes in Crooked Tree without an outrageous expense to the happy homeowner.

In May 1999, Karen's Kurtains financed a long-awaited family trip to Orlando. It was a most memorable Mother's Day when Karen, along with all the other mommies, was presented flowers at the gate. We saw it all: Disney, EPCOT and MGM Studios. The kids had only seen Kings Island and had no idea about rides like Space Mountain and the new Buzz Lightyear interactive ride, which we went on at least 10 times. Our hotel room at the Ramada in Kissimmee really sucked. The toilet only flushed when we filled it up with water using the wastebasket, but we didn't care. We just slept there, showered and left for the day. Samantha lost her first tooth at Reagan National Airport on the way down.

The kids' first trip by air was a scream to watch as parents. "Mom, we're really above the clouds," chimed Sam.

Later on into the summer in July, we made our annual journey as a family over to Virginia Beach. Over the course of the summer, I had a lot of meetings related to the formation of the Midwest ISO in Indianapolis. In anticipation of the trip to Ireland, I would practice singing "My Wild Rose," with the hope of potentially singing the old Irish song to Karen at some point during the trip, but only if I had enough liquid courage, of course. One of the highlights of the summer was Samantha's participation in her hip-hop dance team at a competition at Mount Saint Joseph's College near downtown Cincinnati.

This summer was unique. Karen and I went on not one, but three vacations: Orlando, Virginia Beach and then her dad's big trip with her siblings to Ireland. In early August, we would fly into Shannon, Ireland, and stay in Gort. We all met at Cleveland Hopkins, except for Karen's brother, Kevin, and his wife, Colleen, who were unable to get away. We tossed down several beers and a couple of plates of appetizers before heading over to JFK to board our transoceanic flight to Shannon.

JFK was mayhem, even on a Sunday afternoon. We traversed our way through customs—it was a zoo and made domestic travel seem like kindergarten. The six-hour flight on AerLingus was wonderful; the plane was crowded, yet comfortable. We were well fed and I did my best to sleep as much as possible, because when we arrived in Ireland it would already be early in the morning local time. Everyone looked forward to getting to our hotel and getting a change of clothes and a nap. After we landed in Shannon and cleared customs we were told our luggage was not on the plane, apparently not making it through the zoo at JFK in time for an international flight. We were slightly upset because we knew that AerLingus knew our luggage was not going to make it over with us.

We were exhausted that first day and didn't do much. We got our bearings and went out to dinner, and I made some calls to set up some tee times. Karen was in her glory with her whole family there together, even though this trip was without our children. Karen tends to miss them much more than I do when we go on vacations without them. At dinner that evening we were still all wearing the same clothes with which we had started the trip, and Tommy informed us not worry because he had turned his underwear inside out. The next morning at breakfast he informed us that he had solved the problem again by going "commando."

"What's that mean?" Karen asked, and Tommy said, "I'm not wearing any underwear at all!"

Karen was laughing pretty hard and said, "That's just too much information."

Later that morning our luggage finally arrived, and everyone took great joy in getting a fresh change of clothes. A shower only takes you so far if you have to put on the same smelly clothes.

Much to my surprise the food in Ireland was much better than I had anticipated, primarily because of the varieties of whitefish they served. The sausage with the eggs in the morning was not the greatest, but that dried cow's blood junk, I forget its name, was so awful looking that I wouldn't even try it. Karen and the rest of the crew were content to tour the countryside and go into the quaint little shops. I could deal with this for about an hour. Tommy, Tom and I played three wonderful rounds of golf. The courses are tough and when the wind blew, it was hard to do anything that resembled the great game of golf.

On one hole, I hit a lousy tee shot, hitting the ball very thin, only about 180 yards out. I still had 200 yards to the green, but at least I was in the fairway. I pulled out my four-iron, even though we were hitting into the wind, thinking I could get the ball up somewhere near the green. I hit what felt like a perfect shot. After my follow-through, I looked up and saw the ball was very high, heading like an arrow straight toward the pin. I thought I'd hit a solid shot, but much to my disappointment, the ball fell about 40 yards short of the green. "Damn wind!" I muttered as I walked up to my ball. I think I took a double bogey six and for the three rounds I only broke a hundred once.

Another day, I hit a beautiful drive that was about two feet off the fairway about 250 yards out and slightly left. When I got to where the ball landed, it was hidden in the slightly dense rough. We couldn't find it in the time allotted, and I took a one-stroke penalty for a lost ball just a few feet from the fairway. The game can be frustrating, and in Ireland the level of frustration can definitely increase, especially on the two links-style courses we played. Tom, Tommy and I had a great time. For our last round we played with a man from the area. He added a certain amount of local charm and helped us with the unfamiliar course. He joined us for lunch and a beer after we completed our round.

While abroad we spent a significant amount of time in Galway City, shopping and stopping in at about every tavern we could find. There's an "O'Brien's Pub" in just about every town. We watched the local teams play in the curling championship on TV in one of the bars. Everyone flew the flag of their favorite team on their porches just about everywhere you looked as we traversed the countryside.

One of the highlights of the trip was our visit to Karen's father's cousin to see the Varley family. They had us to lunch and we visited the local church, where we said some prayers. I couldn't help but notice that many members of the Coyne family had donated stained glass windows a long time ago. Then John Varley escorted us all to the cemetery where his family members are buried. John, who was a strong classic-looking Irishman, told us with tears in his eyes the story about losing his daughter to illness years earlier.

For me personally, besides the golfing, the highlight of the trip was that afternoon when we ventured high into the hills where the view of Galway Bay was simply breathtaking. A thousand little islands dotted the bay. It was one of the most beautiful places I had ever seen.

We also ventured down to the remnants of a dock where Karen's grandfather had fled from a soccer game after finding out there were people after him. He eventually boarded a steamer and made it to the United States, settling in Wheeling, West Virginia.

By then it was time for dinner, so we went to a local bar in Clonbur for a few beers and a bite to eat. Karen and I sat at one of the tables as we all laughed and drank while waiting for our food. It was here that I decided to sing the song to my bride that I had practiced so many times in the comfort of my car as I drove along I-74 back and forth from Mason to Indianapolis. My mom had researched the lyrics, and she forwarded them so I could at least sing the right words, even if I was unable to stay on key.

A radio station was playing music softly in the background, but I was concerned that the music on top of my singing might be such a distraction that I would fall flat on my face in my attempt to serenade Karen in the very city where her ancestors still resided. I would never live it down. Finally, a commercial came on the radio and I decided to go for it. I just turned to her and belted it out in my low and lousy tenor voice.

> *My Wild Irish Rose, the sweetest flower that grows*
> *She'll bloom everywhere, no one can compare to my Wild Irish Rose*
> *My Wild Irish Rose, the sweetest flower that grows*
> *And someday for my sake, she just may let me take*
> *The bloom from My Wild Irish Rose*

Karen just smiled at me as I sang and said, "You're a nut!"

And her entire family cheered and applauded as I finished the final note.

One of the locals came over and said to Karen's dad, "If the Yank starts singing again he'll be singing alone because we're all leaving."

I was finally able to sing to my wife and had done so without making a complete fool of myself. This was a very special trip and I'll always be grateful to my father-in-law, Tom, for taking us to Ireland.

When the week was over we ventured back to Cleveland after doing some frantic last minute shopping. This time we arrived with our luggage and my parents, who had been watching our children, met us at the airport with our car so we could cruise back down to Mason right away. I needed to get back to work.

The ride down I-71 was exciting for me. It was early August, and the new edition of the Cleveland Browns was playing the Dallas Cowboys in the annual Hall of Fame game in Canton, Ohio. The Browns won their first exhibition game, and a month or so later, I would attend the first regular season game in the new stadium on Sunday night, September 12, 1999, versus the hated Pittsburgh Steelers. I invited Karen's cousin, Greg Smith, who lived just around the corner even though he was an avid Steelers fan, having grown up in Pittsburgh during their heyday of the '70s. He couldn't believe that I'd invite him, but I knew he would really appreciate the historical significance of the event. The game itself wasn't much as the Steelers blew out the expansion Browns 43-0 in a game televised on ESPN. This didn't matter because the pre-game tailgate in the Flats, west of the new stadium, was one of the best parties and wildest celebrations in the parking lots surrounding the stadium that I have ever seen. We had jumbo shrimp cocktail, filet mignon, fine cigars and champagne. Fireworks lit up the sky and live bands screamed rock-n-roll throughout the throng of gleeful football fans.

As we walked to the stadium from our traditional spot in the Flats where we had partied for a whole decade prior to Art Modell's decision to move our beloved Browns to Baltimore, the unified chant was, "PITTSBURGH SUCKS! PITTSBURGH SUCKS! PITTSBURGH SUCKS! PITTSBURGH SUCKS!"

At one point, Greg turned to me as we walked toward the new stadium, chugging down our final pre-game beers and shouted, "The little hairs on the back of my neck are standing up. This is incredible!"

CHAPTER 11

St. Louis de Montfort

Once we settled back down with our activities in Mason, a problem was emerging with regard to mold in the houses near us. At a new Zaring development called Lakeside, the original bricks on several of the homes were torn off and redone because the TYVEX covering that was put over the siding did not allow moisture to escape through the sub-wall. Our home was inspected and given a clean bill of health, although Karen was suspicious of the blackish substance on the floor that we could see when the carpet was pulled back. They sprayed a mold killing substance on these spots and I was sure we were okay given the thorough inspection.

Other area families were not as fortunate and several children were experiencing respiratory problems that were attributed to the mold. Zaring's insurance company was not covering the expenses associated with the brick replacement, and soon it became apparent that Zaring was having financial problems. Hundreds of homes needed $30,000 to $50,000 in brick replacement. Our neighbors were upset, but I didn't lose a whole lot of sleep over the situation. The real problem was the stigma attached to a Zaring home, resulting in lower market prices.

In December, the first-ever meeting of the Board of Directors for the newly formed Midwest ISO was held in Cincinnati. FERC had granted approval for the company to form a few months earlier in September. I helped John Procario prepare the presentation to the board. It would introduce them to the new organization and give them an overview of the industry, although several of the board members had significant electric utility experience. Indianapolis had been selected as the site for the new company's headquarters, and several suburban locations for the control center and corporate headquarters, mostly in the vicinity of Carmel, Indiana, were under consideration. The new board moved quickly to hire Dr. Matthew Cordaro as the CEO, and Jim Torgerson was named the CFO. A few weeks later Jim called me to ask me some basic questions about the Midwest ISO tariff and how the company would recover its operating costs, given that it was a non-profit company.

John Procario had referred Jim to me to help answer questions because of my familiarity with the founding documents and the underlying intent of the transmission-owning companies forming the Midwest ISO. I had played a small role in founding the new company. I knew if I answered competently, there might be a career opportunity with Jim at the Midwest ISO, or MISO, as many people in the industry had started calling it. I was always deliberate and yet thorough in responding to Jim's inquires. However, we had just settled in Mason, and Karen's Kurtains had taken hold, with numerous families taking advantage of Karen's creative services. I knew the prospects of another move would not be popular.

We had a special New Year's Eve for the turn-of-the-century celebration, spending the evening at a Holidome with an indoor pool just up I-75, outside of Dayton. The kids had a blast in the pool and Karen and I had a portable TV, away from the water, as we watched ABC's coverage from around the world prior to the clock striking 12:00 midnight at Times Square. There were no problems with Y2K, as everyone had predicted. The lights stayed on and computers continued to function. All the precautionary measures appeared to have worked and the paranoid people who bought electric generators didn't end up needing the expensive devices.

I spent a considerable amount of time in Indianapolis over the next few months during the first quarter of 2000 attending transmission owner meetings as MISO continued to unfold. Most of our meetings were held at the offices of the Wabash Valley Power Association near the airport on the west side of town. Dr. Cordaro and Jim Torgerson had executed a lease for temporary office space nearby, while the final plans and construction for the permanent control center in Carmel proceeded. Groundbreaking was set for May 2000. One day when I was on the phone with Jim, he asked me if I would be interested in interviewing for a position reporting to him at the MISO. At first, I tried to politely get out of interviewing because I was fearful of making my young family move again. We had only been in Mason for a little more than two years.

Eventually, Jim said to me a few days later, "It never hurts to listen." On an afternoon in March I dropped by, dressed in my best suit, to talk about an opportunity to become a part of this exciting new organization.

Karen had her misgivings, but true to form she said, "I'll follow you anywhere, but at some point we need to put a stake in the ground and have some semblance of stability for these beautiful children."

I told her even if I get the job I could commute the two hours each way. And I remember telling our good friend Sandy Smith that if I get the job, "We're not moving!"

The interview with Jim went very well. I learned that he had been the CFO at Dayton Power & Light, and prior to that he was at Puget Sound Energy in Seattle. He had a picture on the wall of his office of where he had lived on Mercer Island in Washington State. Jim is very intelligent, soft spoken, and I was intrigued with the idea of reporting directly to a CFO. During the interview I told him that the only way I would move my family to Carmel would be for an opportunity that would be a major jump from my current position as a Senior Contract Analyst at Cinergy, a company with a set of working relationships that I truly enjoyed. I would need a position at either the manager or director level, with a compensation package that was significantly greater than what I had in Cincinnati.

At the close of the interview Jim told me, "I'm going to make you an offer. I'll call you in a couple of days."

When I called Karen and told her about an offer being imminent she said, "I'll support whatever you decide."

I certainly picked a wonderful, understanding and totally supportive woman to be my wife and mother of our children. I assured her that moving was not part of the plan and besides, Zaring homes were not selling well. I was genuinely ready to treat the job as if I were a consultant, content to live out of a suitcase. Many close friends told me that a long two-hour commute each way would be detrimental to the overall welfare of our young family.

A few days later, Jim called to tell me about the offer he had put together and would send it to me in writing the same day. The offer, including a signing bonus, was well above the compensation level I had mentioned seeking during the interview. The position was Director of Regulatory Affairs and I would report directly to him, the Chief Financial Officer. I was ecstatic and upfront about the opportunity when I spoke with Mr. Procario, who had been so good to me at Cinergy. As I thought about the offer and the possibilities, I was saddened because I knew in my heart that Cinergy wasn't going to be able to come close to matching the handsome offer Jim Torgerson had made.

It was bittersweet as I thought about leaving Cinergy, because John Procario was such a great guy. He is also Italian.

"Us *paisanos* have to stick together," he said as he smiled, and then he added, "I can't believe you're leaving me for money."

The most important aspect about the offer was that Karen didn't have to work anymore to make a car payment, buy groceries, buy shoes, haircuts and pay the dry cleaning tab. Instead, she could buy things on the "want list" instead of the "must list" like she had back in May 1999 when Karen's Kurtains financed the family trip to Orlando to see Mickey Mouse. Taking this job was, as Kyle put it, "a stupid test." He couldn't believe I'd even consider not taking it. I just felt a certain amount of loyalty to Cinergy. By taking this job, even though I knew deep down moving was probably inevitable, it meant that, number one, I was assured that my children could go to college, and second, we could afford to travel. Karen loved to hit the road and always seemed to be the happiest when she knew there was an adventure to look forward to. The idea of traveling to exciting places with her husband and children was most exciting.

As word of my resignation spread through the halls in Electric System Operations at Cinergy, a younger guy named Dave Espling came up to me and said, "I hear you're going to MISO. Congratulations." He then told me that he was from the Indianapolis area and a graduate of Brebeuf Jesuit Preparatory School.

"I think they're building a new Catholic grade school in Fishers, which is the town right next to Carmel," he said. "It seems like the name of the parish is St. Louis de Montfort. I'll check it out on the Internet and get back to you."

I ran to my computer and did a search. He was right on and then I called Karen immediately to tell her the news.

After working the new job for a couple of weeks, it became obvious that my initial thinking of not moving the family was totally impractical. So while Samantha and Will were at school one day, we drove to the Fishers and Carmel, Indiana, to check out the possibilities. This time, finding the right church and school was our top priority.

When we arrived at St. Louis de Montfort, or SLDM, as we would come to call it, in May 2000, we found a busy and dusty construction site behind the church, and only four months remained until the start of the inaugural school year. One of the parishioners who worked at the rectory greeted us warmly and made us feel welcomed right out of the gate. They were accepting applications and there were openings for Samantha and William in the second and fourth grades, respectively, but there was a waiting list for Mitchell's kindergarten class.

We were slightly disheartened, but we filled out the applications and made a deposit for two of our three children. "You'll just have to wait on an opening," the principal told us. I think we were third on the waiting list.

After our visit to SLDM, we drove west into Carmel and came to the intersection of 116th Street and Hazel Dell Parkway. I immediately took a right turn and remarked to Karen that Zaring had a new development underway called The Lakes of Hazel Dell. We went into the model home, looked around, introduced ourselves and grabbed some floor plans. We had to drive like hell back to Mason if we were going to beat Sam and Will home from school. The convenience of the school, home and work in a span of eight miles was too good to be true.

A few weeks later, Ursula, the principal at SLDM, called Karen to tell her there was an opening for Mitchell, but we only had until four o'clock to give them an answer and a check for $500. I raced back to SLDM and out of shear luck had one check remaining in my checkbook. So now all three Volpe children were enrolled at St. Louis de Montfort Catholic School. Karen and I were elated.

Now, one might wonder why we would invest in another home built by Zaring, given the mold problems in Mason. We knew that we might have problems getting a fair price for our wonderful home in Mason, but we had a strategy that in retrospect turned out to be a smart move. Here's why we decided to build another Zaring home in spite of the mold issue. First of all, we liked the quality of the home and the layouts. We settled on the Franklin II, a slightly larger version of the home we owned in Mason. We signed a contract with Zaring to build the house in Carmel and put down a non-refundable deposit of $10,000.

The catch was that when construction completed, we had better be ready to close. Otherwise, Zaring kept the down payment and was free to sell the home to whomever they wanted. My goal was to tie the sale of the home in Mason to Zaring being able to get its profit out of a significantly more expensive home in Carmel. The most we could lose was the $10,000, so this was a calculated risk that Karen and I deemed worth the gamble. This strategy forced Zaring to work with us and our realtor to get our home in Ohio sold for a reasonable price. Otherwise, they had one more home in their inventory with all the associated carrying costs. Besides, Karen picked out a beautiful wooded lot adjacent to the tree preserve in the middle of the development. We finally had some trees!

The first realtor we had in Cincinnati stunk, so when her contract was up we hired Dave McDonald, one of the best. Dave worked his butt off to put on open houses and get us some showings. We finally got an offer in August, but it was $30,000 below our asking price. I then started to use some of my negotiating skills on Zaring. We had met Zaring's CFO at a grand opening party for the Lakes of Hazel Dell. We took the opportunity to explain our dilemma.

"Look, I'm taking a beating if I take this offer and there's nothing wrong with my house. The buyer has all the leverage, and isn't willing to pay a fair price given the problems with mold in the other homes. I need a $20,000 credit toward the contract price on the house in Carmel, otherwise I'll walk," I said.

"I'll give you 10," he said.

"We have a deal," I replied. "Please put it in writing and thank you."

I had lost a lot of sleep over this move, but things eventually worked out.

One of the last big events we enjoyed before moving to Indiana was to see Jimmy Buffett at Riverbend with all of our neighbors in Mason. What a blast! We packed the party bus and cruised down to the concert. I had not seen Buffett since he warmed up for the Eagles' *Hotel California* tour more than 20 years earlier. The show was awesome! "Fins to the left, Fins to the right," "Cheeseburgers in Paradise" and "Margaritaville" in front of a packed house of loyal, hardcore, partying parrot heads.

Karen's final big project in Cincinnati was having a local photographer take some really cute black and white pictures of the kids near a little stream down by an abandoned railroad station. Karen was thrilled with the results and was happy to have these cherished pictures of her three beautiful works of art.

In August, at Zaring's Lakes of Hazel Dell grand opening party, we met many of our new neighbors. We got to know Amy and Joel Jackson, who had just completed the home next door. They had a house of their own in Carmel that they had on the market as well. They had two children the same ages as Will and Samantha. They were named after state capitals, Austin and Madison. Actually, Madison goes by "Maddie." Samantha and Maddie really hit it off.

We also met Bill and Leslie Grace, huge LSU Tiger fans, whose twin daughters, Courtney and Lindsey, were about to be seniors at Carmel High School. Their oldest daughter, Ashley, lived with them just five houses down from ours. After the party, our kids wrote their names in the garage floor concrete that was curing. We went to Sahm's for dinner and then back to the Residence Inn for some sleep.

Later in the summer, after our annual journey to Virginia Beach, the Volpe kids checked into the Residence Inn in Fishers, Indiana, just down the road from SLDM. School started in the middle of August in Indiana, and the new house was still three weeks from completion. The first day of school was exciting. The kids were really pumped up, and another guest at the Residence Inn in the suite below us was upset with all the early morning commotion. For the first time ever, Samantha put on her green plaid uniform.

The first week of all this "togetherness" was fine, but our nerves and patience were wearing thin by the middle of week two. We had closed on the sale of our home in Mason, and once again Karen was dispatched back to Larkspur Lane to supervise the packing of our belongings that would remain in storage until the new house was ready. Karen worked all day on her birthday with the movers. She took it in stride and was most understanding, given such rotten circumstances.

The move went smoothly in early September, except that one of our TV sets, including the remote, had been stolen while our things were in storage. The movers' insurance covered the loss, but a few weeks later I discovered that Karen's engagement and wedding rings had also been stolen from my top dresser drawer. Not one of my brighter moves, leaving the valuables in such an obvious hiding place. Karen had been wearing the 10-year anniversary ring that we purchased on a whim at a Zales store at a mall in Virginia Beach in 1998. The movers' insurance company wrote us a check that covered replacement of the rings at wholesale cost, which was approximately what I had paid for her rings 10 years earlier. The man from the insurance company had said he would come to the house with a box of rings and Karen could "just pick out a new one!" She was upset at his audacity. There was no way she was going to pick out a new ring on our kitchen island.

Nothing could replace the moment or the ring I had given her out on the ski slope in the Canadian Rockies where she said, "Yes!"

CHAPTER 12

Harpo Studios

In late fall 2000; I devised a plan to put together a unique Christmas present for my wife. She had always mentioned that it would be so cool to actually sit in the audience during the taping of one of Oprah Winfrey's shows in downtown Chicago. I was lucky to be able to work with and become casual friends with a handful of consultants from Arthur Anderson's Chicago office. They were helping the Midwest ISO develop the settlements system software. As a result they interfaced with me directly because the system had to be consistent with rates, terms and conditions of the tariff. In many cases we would decide on policy and work to make sure the business practices, the tariff, and the systems were all in sync. Ed Lennox, Darlene Tolbert and Mollie Titler worked tirelessly to implement these systems, and eventually the Midwest ISO hired a manager of settlements. In the meantime, I was their go-to guy for answers on interpretation of the tariff, so they could build the right set of functionality into the software.

My idea, given that Ed, Darlene and Mollie had all sorts of connections in Chicago, was to get tickets for Karen, her mom and her sister to see the taping of one of Oprah's shows. As Christmas drew near, the trio was unable to actually procure the tickets, but they assured me that it would be child's play once everyone at the studio returned from the holidays. Darlene had a friend who knew Oprah's producer, so I just trusted that it would all come to pass.

I put together a card with pictures of Oprah on it, and I presented it to Karen, Pat and Kathy at the annual Coyne Christmas party. They were absolutely giddy with joy. Karen's brother, Kevin, noticed that I didn't actually have the tickets for the show in hand, but I had all the confidence in the world that Darlene and Mollie would come through.

Kevin said, smartly, "Oh, I understand this is more of a concept present than a real present."

Early in the first quarter of 2001, I think it was in March, Darlene and Mollie came through and the tickets were in hand. Karen took a cheap flight up to Midway from Indianapolis on ATA and met up with Kathy and Pat at the hotel. They had a great time, did a little shopping, and ate fine seafood. While they waited in line to get into the studio they socialized and made friends with other Oprah fans outside Harpo Studios. Karen was a little disappointed in the show because it was the taping of the "Book of the Month Show." The featured book was *The House of Sand and Fog*, so there were no Brad Pitt, Mel Gibson or Tom Hanks sightings. Karen said that during one of the commercial breaks Oprah was talking with the audience and Karen said to Oprah, once she got her attention, "You're just stunning!" Even though it looked a little iffy at first, my friends, Darlene and Mollie, came through and I was able to score some major points when this unique little trip actually became reality.

Pressure at work had intensified over the previous months, and for the most part, I had not been home for six straight weeks during February and into March 2001. Three of the large companies that had helped form the Midwest ISO, two of which were essential to our survival, announced that they were withdrawing to join our chief rival organization, The Alliance. The fiasco had begun in December 2000, when one of our smaller companies, Illinois Power, gave formal notice of their intent to leave. All by itself this event was not that devastating, but when Chicago-based Commonwealth Edison, our largest transmission-owning member, also announced their intent to leave, we knew we were in big trouble. Citing closely interconnected operations with Commonwealth Edison, the third company to file with FERC to withdraw was Ameren, the large St. Louis-based utility that also had operations in Illinois. If FERC granted approval for these three companies to withdraw—and all indications from the FERC chairman indicated that this was likely—the Midwest ISO would not survive. Commonwealth Edison and Ameren formed the heart of the Midwest ISO. FERC consolidated the three cases into what became known as the Illinois Power Case, but to the executive management of the Midwest ISO, this was really about our continued viability.

Imagine the 1927 Yankees without Ruth and Gehrig.

We knew our organization would not survive if we could not work out some sort of financial and operational settlement. The Alliance was not willing to merge because their for-profit business model was at odds with the Midwest ISO's non-profit setup. As a company that provided transmission service over a large geographic region, the departure of these two companies would have been devastating. Many industry observers thought we were on life support.

After six weeks of intensive negotiations in Washington D.C., we managed to come to a settlement in which the departing companies would pay us a total of $60 million in order to honor their financial obligations. We also agreed to implement an agreement that would allow the Midwest ISO and the Alliance to coordinate their operations at the seams between our regions; otherwise things would become operationally untenable.

This was a stressful time for our household. We had just moved to Carmel, and then it looked as if the new company was going to take a dive. I was feeling guilty about having just moved my family, and now the whole plan was about to backfire. But thanks to the superb negotiating skills of Jim Torgerson, who had just been named CEO, we were able to settle the case after countless hours of closed-door negotiations. We knew we would fare much better if we could work out a settlement, especially on the financial aspects, without the case going to hearing. And I was grateful for having helped play a small role in those arduous negotiations.

But we still needed to issue additional bonds before we could finish our systems and recruit the skilled people necessary to run our day-to-day operations. Finding investors for the bonds was the difficult part. News of the Illinois Power Case caused a downgrade in our credit rating.

Wall Street does not like risk.

In the end it worked out, but at times I thought I had moved my family out into the middle of a cornfield for nothing. Karen grew weary of my calls; it was a real roller coaster ride. On some days things went great, and on other days I considered sending out my resumé because we were never in the driver's seat.

After the settlement, the company was on a roll. I helped manage a major filing that was very successful, as it resulted in the Midwest ISO being named the country's first Regional Transmission Organization compliant with FERC's Order No. 2000. The company proceeded with its plans to move into its brand new control center in Carmel in April 2001. This was a great achievement and a real team effort.

There was another time when Karen went the extra mile involving her cousin, Ricky Coyne, who lived an hour north of us in Rossville, Indiana, not far from Purdue University. Ricky had not been dealt the best hand in life. Karen had become concerned about his job and the people he was hanging around. She visited his trailer and found the living conditions to be far from ideal. Ricky was nowhere to be found, and the owner of the trailer park told Karen that Ricky owed him some money. He had not paid his bills. The power was turned off, and after asking around she finally found him living on the front porch at his girlfriend's house not far away. Karen immediately called Ricky's brother Marty. Tom also drove across the turnpike from Ohio to see what he could do to help out his nephew.

Ricky eventually received some much-needed medical attention for a chronic neurological problem and finally was placed on full disability. Ricky was back on his feet, but without Karen's actions he could have died. He was living like a homeless person and being taken advantage of by people he thought were his friends. They took his money and were not very nice to a guy who couldn't fend for himself. Karen got him help, and now he had some direction. Despite his problems, we were always amazed by Ricky's extraordinary memory and his ability to recall the tiniest of details.

Samantha made her First Communion in early April. It was our first opportunity to have a big family party in Carmel. We did it up right and both sides of the family came to Carmel for the big event. A bizarre accident happened the night of the party. Our new neighbor, Joel Jackson, slipped on the garage floor with a Molson beer in his right hand. In order to break his fall he dropped the beer bottle, breaking the glass, and then lacerated his right hand on the glass. I remembered that a new neighbor,

Dr. Todd Arnold, had just moved in that day a few houses up from ours. Even though he had spent the day unpacking, he was willing to come down and take a look.

"I can sew this up right here on the kitchen island," Dr. Arnold said, and Joel said, "Fine with me, I'd rather not go into the emergency room and have them ask 64 questions."

Besides, none of us were in good enough shape to drive, except for Joel's wife, Amy, whom we promptly dispatched to get us another case of Molson. So Todd sewed up Joel's hand in our kitchen surrounded by all sorts of helpful onlookers.

In late April things were going well, and we were on our way to northeastern Ohio for POW WOW. Karen was browsing through the catalog of auction items when something caught her eye. It was a trip to New York City that included airfare for two, three nights accommodations at the Edison Hotel on Times Square, a Sherwin-Williams gift certificate for $250 and a tour of Martha Stewart's enterprise, including a taping of her television show.

"What do you think this will go for?" she said.

"Probably four or five thousand dollars that we don't have," I said.

"What if it's a really good deal and it doesn't go that high, what can I bid to?" Karen persisted.

"If you can steal it for $1,500 then it's ours, but don't get your hopes up too high," I said.

The next evening, while we were at the big night, the oral auction started after dinner. I was talking to Lewie Seikel, one of my classmates, when he noticed Karen had her paddle up in the air. "Watch out, I think your wife is spending some money!" Lewie said.

As I walked toward the table she was grinning from ear to ear. "How much did it go for?" I said.

"I stole it just like you said for $1,300!"

Karen was very excited with her bargain and was trying to decide whom to take on the trip because she knew I wouldn't be interested in seeing Martha Stewart's trappings. I would only be interested in going if the Browns happened to be playing the Jets at the Meadowlands that weekend.

For the rest of 2001 we slowly settled into our new surroundings in Indiana, finally finding some semblance of normality, except for the events of 9/11. This shook up everyone, and of course, made us all take a step back and look at ourselves from a totally different perspective. Karen called me right after I arrived at work on September 11th and said that a plane had just crashed into the World Trade Center. I didn't know it was a jet. I just took it as some stupid guy flying his Cessna over Manhattan who had lost control and somehow smashed into the building while trying to fly between the massive skyscrapers. Moments later Ed Lennox came down to my office and said that the Pentagon was on fire. Then I learned that a second plane had crashed into the other building at the World Trade Center. I think it was right then when we all realized the world would never be the same. Karen went to SLDM to pick up the kids, but the school was in lockdown and the children were not allowed to leave.

She called me very upset with the situation and I tried to reassure her by saying, "The state obviously has a well-thought-out set of procedures for this type of situation. Our children are safe; these animals are not going to target a small Catholic school in the middle of Indiana."

"You're right, they're safe," she said.

As Karen and I watched the endless hours of television coverage over the following week, there were times when Karen would sit and sob, unable to understand how people could hate so much and do it all in the name of their alleged god. At one point I thought to myself, she is such an amazing, caring and loving person. I would understand if the Lord decided that this world, with all of the hate and evil, was no longer the right place for her, that one day before her time, he might call her home.

Then I thought to myself, "Shame on you for having such an awful thought," but in the back of my mind I knew all things were possible. I never assumed anything and these tragic events reminded us that life is precious and way too short.

Karen is a patriot and she loves this great country of ours. She had software installed on the PC that allowed her to embroider sweatshirts. Like most Americans, the tragedy of September 11, 2001 motivated Karen to rally around the flag. She ordered red, white, and blue hooded sweatshirts in assorted sizes and embroidered PROUD TO BE AMERICAN on them. She sold them to friends and family and gave all the proceeds to the Carmel Fire Department to help them defray some of their costs of going to New York City to help with the cleanup. At the Carmel Firemen's Fire and Ice Ball a couple of months later, Karen was recognized with a plaque from the department in appreciation for her efforts.

On a cold and rainy morning in late October, Karen was at home talking to her Uncle John on the phone when she looked out the window and noticed that our little four-year old neighbor, Brady Arnold, was walking in his pajamas from the Jackson's house to our front porch.

She hung up on her uncle and as Brady rang the doorbell Karen opened our front door and asked, "What's wrong, honey?"

Brady grabbed her hand and said, "Come, it's my Dad!"

They ran in the rain together to Brady's house. When Karen walked in the front door she found Dr. Todd lying on the floor, partially in shock, having fallen 17 feet through the drywall ceiling in their hallway foyer. Insulation and drywall were scattered everywhere. Todd had been hunting in the crawl space for a leak in his roof when he fell through the ceiling and hit the hall railing at the top of the steps. He broke his pelvis, several ribs and his wrist. Karen immediately called 911, made sure the children could stay with Miss Kimmie, located Todd's wife, and then followed Todd in the ambulance to the emergency room. Dr. Todd underwent surgery and after a long rehab was able to fully recover from his injuries. Later, Dr. Todd would tell me that 45 percent of all people falling from such a height do not live to talk about it.

It was a bonding experience for Karen and Dr. Arnold.

In May, Karen and Grace Hineman, her good friend from SLDM, held the first-ever Teacher Appreciation Party at Craig Willy Hall. Karen and Grace, along with the help of several other ladies, called on local merchants in order to put together a nice array of gifts for the reverse raffle. We were amazed to find out how many people in Hoosierville had never heard of a reverse raffle. Here's how it works: instead of the first number selected, being designated as the winner, it's the last number pulled out that takes home the grand prize. Each ticket costs $25. About every third number pulled wins some sort of prize, saving the grand prize of cash for last. There was a nice buffet dinner and a DJ played music so everyone could dance throughout the evening. Karen served as master of ceremonies. She was downright funny, often saying, "So sorry, you're just another big fat loser!" as the numbers were dwindling down.

Karen is a visionary and she started what has become an annual "thank you" event at the school. The goal of the event wasn't to raise money, but to recognize the faculty, staff and their spouses for their hours of dedication throughout the year.

The Volpe family closed out 2001 on a happy note with a road trip to Nashville, Tennessee, for New Year's Eve. We went into a few of the country music bars where children were welcome if they hung out in the back and took in the sights. After we walked out of one of these fine establishments Samantha spotted a limousine. Our "shy" young lady walked up to the driver and asked whether she could see inside. Much to our delight, the driver offered to take us on a quick tour of the city and then drop us off at our hotel.

The next day was the last day of the NFL regular season and Will and I went to see the Browns battle the Titans in a meaningless game. Tim Couch and company were down by 14 points in the fourth quarter and the hometown faithful headed for the exits. The Browns rallied with two touchdowns in the final five minutes and won on a Phil Dawson field goal as time expired.

"What a bunch of wimpy fans, they don't know what it's like to be really cold," Will said, "Thirty degrees is downright warm for December."

The next day we visited the beautiful Opryland hotel and headed back north to Carmel to start 2002.

CHAPTER 13

The Ministry Center

Throughout 2002 Karen was very involved at SLDM. The Midwest ISO had begun commercial operations as the regional provider of transmission service over a 15-state region on February 1st and I was working long hours. Karen's activities at SLDM centered on coordinating the hot lunch program, teaching sewing classes as part of the after-school enrichment program, and decorating the church as the liturgical seasons changed. The biggest project Karen worked on was the school's first dinner/auction fundraiser. Karen and Fr. Dave Hellmann sold the idea to the pastor, Fr. Tim Kroeger, and they were given the go ahead.

The inaugural edition of this event would be in early February 2003. Karen had been to POWWOW many times, so she had the vision and the organizational skills to get in motion the necessary committees that would prove to be the backbone of the event. Staging an event like this requires hundreds of hours of planning, if it is to be successful. The name of the event would be Mardi de Montfort, of course.

One Sunday morning at Mass in January, Scott Zigmond went up to the pulpit after Communion and invited the men of the parish to participate in a two-day retreat called Christ Renews His Parish, or CRHP (pronounced "chirp"). I have always admired Scott; he was the first friend I made at St. Louis de Montfort. As he spoke, his selling points amazed me. He said he first heard about CRHP one Sunday morning six months earlier as he was zoning out before Mass came to a close. Then he recited a litany of reasons why one would not make it to CRHP. One reason in particular made a big impression on me, "I don't have time!"

Scott went through the math and one weekend takes up only 0.4 percent of the year. I am not what I would call a religious zealot, but I stay true to my convictions. I believe what I believe. I consider myself very traditional and am conservative in a Catholic sense, but I would not call myself hardcore. I was instantly sold on the CRHP invitation. After Mass I told Karen that I wanted to attend and went to the Narthex to sign up right away. Normally, I wouldn't consider doing something like this, but for some reason I felt that it was something I needed to do for myself. Karen was very supportive and said it was fine with her.

A few weeks later Jay Feller picked me up at 7:30 a.m., along with two other guys. I had my duffle bag with a change of clothes and my sleeping bag. When we arrived at the Ministry Center, CRHP Team #15 welcomed us. Breakfast consisted of Sausage McMuffins from McDonald's and lots of coffee. I saw a lot of new faces and it didn't seem like this was going to be one of those religious retreats that was way over the top.

Once the day started we heard several men give testimony about their personal journey with Christ.

I heard it all.

Scott Zigmond, the witness on Christian Community, talked about losing several good friends and comrades from West Point during Desert Storm. I saw this man, whom I considered to be the pillar of strength, get teary-eyed, swallow hard and continue to discuss his journey with Christ, his family and his country.

I was genuinely moved.

After the weekend is over, there is no commitment to continue on with the program over the next six months, although one is encouraged to continue. When I initially walked in I had an open mind, but I really didn't think my busy work schedule at the Midwest ISO would allow me to take a night a week for about three hours to continue participating in the program. I remembered thinking that if the meetings were on Sunday nights, I might be able to make a go of it. The weekend had been well organized and was well run. It was a long day and one of the first things we did when we walked in was take off our watches. No clock watching is permitted.

After dinner we had the opportunity to go to confession, then a Mass at which we heard a teenager speak about her love for the Lord. I had the privilege of speaking about my shortcomings and the evils of temptation with the new associate pastor, Fr. Dave Hellmann. He knew Karen well, given her involvement at the school and church. Once confession was over we had some free time, and several of the guys went over to the gym to play basketball. I could have used a few beers at this point, not to get drunk but just to help me sleep. By my estimation, it was well after 11:00 and I was beat. It had been a long day after an even longer week at work.

I rolled out my sleeping bag in one of the meeting rooms at the Ministry Center that we were using as a dorm room. Eight guys had staked out their spots, and everyone was trying to get some rest. I wasn't comfortable at all. Some of the guys had already fallen asleep; there was a chorus of snoring and lots of miscellaneous farts flying around as a result of the lasagna dinner we had eaten earlier in the evening.

The room was hot as hell.

After about 45 minutes of tossing and turning I decided to see if there was another place that might work out better for me, so I grabbed my sleeping bag and pillow and headed toward the door. I staggered down the hall and took a right into the big meeting room where we had eaten. A couple of guys were still awake, working on their witness presentations for Sunday.

The room was dimly lit, and I looked to my right and saw a dark corner where a portable chalkboard sat on a diagonal. I thought to myself, if I tip the chalkboard forward I could shield myself from the light. My plan worked great; it was quiet and I had my own private tent in the corner.

I lied there awake for some time. In spite of the serenity, I was still on a floor in my sleeping bag and far from comfortable. I was lying on my left side facing the room. My left butt cheek was growing numb, and I was starting to feel as if I was on the verge of drifting off to sleep. Then my left elbow and shoulder were also a bit numb, so I decided it was time to flip over to my right side, without waking up, because I was finally relaxed.

As I went to roll over I found that my entire body was totally petrified and I became scared that I had inexplicably become paralyzed.

I could not move.

My heart began to pound in my chest. As I tried to open my eyes all I could see was a very bright light. Then my body felt very warm, as if I were experiencing a low-level, full body orgasm. It was a feeling I had never experienced before. I was no longer scared and wasn't worried about being permanently paralyzed.

I heard a voice that sounded very much like the deep, graveled tenor of my father's voice.

"Don't worry! I've got you," the voice said, "I've got you and you're going to be fine."

I still felt the orgasmic glow all over my body and then it felt more like I was a little baby, after a warm bath, all wrapped up in a nice warm blanket. The next sensation I felt was like I was rocking and being cradled, gently by a pair of hugely powerful and reassuring arms. All this time I still couldn't see anything but the bright white light, which had become less blinding and intense.

I heard my dad's voice once more. "I've got you," he said.

The feeling that I was being rocked back and forth gently continued for a few more seconds. Suddenly, I was able to see the tables and chairs in the Ministry Center again. I curled my knees up toward my chest, just to make sure I wasn't paralyzed anymore. I remembered thinking, "What the hell was that?" I knew it certainly wasn't a dream. In a matter of seconds, I was sound asleep and I didn't wake again until the next morning.

When I woke up I took a shower and joined the men in the Ministry Center for some coffee and donuts. As I chomped down on a donut I looked back over at my makeshift hut, with the chalkboard still tilted, and I thought briefly about my mysterious experience. It would be several months until I would realize the depth of my experience

I had just been touched by the power of the Holy Spirit. I just didn't know it at this point in time.

Several members of my wonderful family had sent me encouraging letters. Many of them brought tears to my eyes as I realized how blessed I was to have such a beautiful family and such a great wife. We had a late afternoon Mass in the school's new chapel. It was the first Mass in this new facility, which had just been completed, with pews salvaged from an old country church. After Communion we were instructed to tell Father Hellmann of our intention to continue. I told him I wanted to continue, but I was concerned about the timing and the demands of my job.

When I arrived home, I was in a great mood and felt totally rejuvenated. I thanked Karen for allowing me to take the time to do something for myself. She was curious about the weekend and pressed me for details. I told her that many of the witnesses had requested that we keep what was said in confidence.

Two weeks later my new CRHP #16 team met for the first time and we started on our own six-month journey in preparation for our turn to put on the weekend for what would be CRHP #17 team, in August.

We met on Thursday evenings for about three hours. At the beginning of every meeting we said a prayer and sang "Here I Am Lord." For the first few weeks we went through a process called faith sharing, in which each of us talked about our life's journey and our faith. After listening to the other men talk for about three weeks, I decided it was my turn to talk about where life had taken me.

These men were like brothers, and most of us were in similar situations. All but one of us, David Gregg, was married. Some of the guys were going through some pretty tough times. As I started to talk I spoke initially of my youth. I said that the first day I truly remembered was November 22, 1963, the day President Kennedy was shot. I spoke about how I remembered the Vietnam War era as being a time of political unrest with the assassinations of JFK, RFK and Martin Luther King Jr., and the attempt on George Wallace's life as he campaigned for the presidency. I mentioned being a big fan of the space program, following all of the Apollo missions. I spoke about my parents, how my dad worked so hard and drove all over the Midwest selling auto advertising specialty items to car dealers, especially license plate frames. He was a great dad, and in spite of all the time he spent on the road, he was a wonderful provider and a great man. We never experienced any financial difficulties and I was very grateful to him because his sacrifices made it possible for me to have great educational opportunities.

I talked about what I did as a kid: altar boy, my days as a catcher behind the plate, family vacations to the beach. I also talked about my very smart mom. She had a 4.0 grade point average in college, majoring in chemistry, and about how she taught me to respect women and have good manners. I mentioned my high school days at Walsh, my early drinking days and the time I got spiked in the face during an intra-squad game, putting an end to my modest baseball career. I spoke about the responsibilities inherent in being the oldest child. Then I went on to discuss my days at Ohio Northern; how I studied hard during the day and then had college fun in the evenings at Sigma Pi fraternity, yet was always able to maintain good grades.

I talked about my career, my frustration at Marathon, and how I found my niche in the electric utility industry. I talked about the women I chased, but never caught, and the beer I drank. I spoke further about the numerous innings of softball, and the work I did on my MBA at Ashland University while I lived in Findlay. Then onto the summer of 1985, when I separated my shoulder on a bang-bang play at second base, the victim of a cheap shot, and that was when I decided to follow Bruce Springsteen and the E Street Band's *Born in the U.S.A.* tour around the Midwest.

I talked about meeting Karen, how she had saved me from myself, the birth of our children, my blown-out Achilles, and my career moves that brought us to Indianapolis. Then I relayed the major test of faith we had with our problem-plagued pregnancy with Mitchell.

I closed my faith sharing with the following words:

"So far my life has been a bed of roses; nothing really bad or major has happened to me. I know there will come a day when

I will have to bury my parents, but that's a part of life. I have this feeling that there's something lurking behind me. Every once in awhile I take a look in the rearview mirror because I just feel that God has something else, maybe something out of the ordinary and challenging in mind for me, while I'm still here."

CHAPTER 14

Indiana University Medical Center

It was now a couple of months after being touched by the power of the Holy Spirit, and I was facing a real life or death situation. I finally realized what had happened under the chalkboard; it all made sense and I knew the Lord was with us. I was unusually calm.

My wife had leukemia.

Karen had been diagnosed with the disease after five frightful days at St. Vincent Hospital in Carmel. When we arrived at the ER, one couldn't help but to be impressed with the speed and efficiency with which Karen was admitted. The first thing they did was transfer Karen's entire medical file from St. Vincent's onto a computer outside her ultra-modern, brand new, state-of-the-art room in the ICU. A team of at least four oncology residents plowed through the files, entering all sorts of data onto the computer.

Moments later a small doctor of Asian descent began preparing to conduct a bone marrow biopsy. We were introduced to Karen's oncology nurse, Katie Hincher, who explained to us what would happen over the next few days. The first step was to perform a bone marrow biopsy. A small piece of bone would be extracted from within Karen's lower hip and then the marrow would be drawn from within the bone marrow cavity. The extract would be put on slides and sent off to the laboratory for analysis. The initial diagnosis, based on the blood work from

St. Vincent's, indicated that Karen had acute myelogenous leukemia

Dr. Li put Karen on her side, and then gave her a series of local numbing agents that really stung Karen's behind. I crouched down close to Karen's face and tried to help her get through the pain. She was so strong and brave. Then the doctor took a long hollow stem or cylinder that was about five inches long and slowly worked it into her upper buttocks, twisting it back and forth in a manner that reminded me of a struggle I often had extracting a stubborn cork from a bottle of mediocre wine. Karen was still in some pain despite the local, and I think she could feel a lot of what was going on. Once the piece of bone was pulled, the doctor attached a syringe to the deeply inserted stem and pulled back on the trigger.

Nothing came back into the syringe, except for maybe a minor trace of a reddish liquid that looked like blood.

Looking at just Dr. Li's eyes—the rest of his face was covered with a surgical mask—I could tell he was perplexed. He pulled back the cylinder and attempted to work it into a different area in order to extract the bone marrow.

Again the well was dry.

This went on at least two or three more times, although it was probably more like five or six. Karen was in severe pain.

Her pain was excruciating.

It was hard on me too. All I could do was watch and help coach Karen through the procedure. She began doing the same breathing techniques learned during Lamaze. I was about to go over the table after the doctor, figuring he was just another incompetent doctor, otherwise the procedure would have been done by now. I was very wrong; he knew exactly what he was doing. Katie Hincher stayed with us even though it was well into the early evening. She rubbed Karen's leg and told her to relax. I was still on the verge of going ballistic as Dr. Li hunted around for a bone cavity where the marrow might reside. In my mind I questioned his competence, but later I realized his inability to find the liquid was a basic manifestation of the underlying cancer. Finally, after an agonizingly long 10 minutes, he hit a spot, yielding just barely a sputter of the marrow. It was enough for the laboratory analysis.

Karen rested as comfortably as possible the rest of the evening. It had been one of the toughest days of her life. She finds out she has cancer; she's transported to a new hospital and is immediately put through a painful bone marrow biopsy that literally drills a whole through her hind end, well into the bone. Then there was the digging around until a splattering of marrow could be found. All of this on top of a seven-inch cut in her lower abdomen, coupled with the lingering effects of what appeared to be pneumonia in both lungs.

The oncology team Dr. Cripe had assembled to deal with Karen's case informed us that, based on the initial review of the blood chemical analysis from St. Vincent's, Karen had acute myelogenous leukemia, or AML. Dr. Li informed us that there was a good possibility that Karen had contracted a subtype of AML called M3 or APL, which stands for acute promyelocytic leukemia, and if the biopsy confirmed M3, this was a very good outcome, given the circumstances. Subtype M3, although it was a rare form of AML, was curable in many instances.

Karen had somehow acquired a chromosome defect. This disease was not inherited. We did our research from the simple booklets the hospital provided, which read as follows:

> Cells that accumulate in the marrow could be identified as promyelocytes, the next step in blood cell formation after myeloblast or blasts. AML, subtype M3 patients have a

specific chromosome abnormality that involves chromosome 15, usually in conjunction with a translocation with chromosome 17. With APL, the cells are stalled at this stage of production. A derivative of vitamin A, all-trans retinoic acid, often abbreviated as ATRA, is administered with chemotherapy and is capable of inducing the leukemic promyelocytes to develop into mature cells called neutrophils. ATRA decreases the concentration of leukemic blast cells in the marrow and remission frequently ensues.

The last sentence gave us hope.
I liked the sound of the word "frequently."
We would later find out that only 1,200 Americans are diagnosed with APL each year. Katie told us that chemotherapy would begin the next evening. Karen's white blood count had gone through the roof, escalating to 77,000, an extraordinarily high number. The chemo had to take hold and reduce the white count quickly, so the plan was to hit her hard with chemo. This would be the first of three rounds of chemotherapy. The goal was to take her white blood count to zero, wipe everything out, good cells as well as bad, and then she would be given injections of Neupogen, a growth hormone that would jumpstart her bone marrow into producing new, healthy white blood cells, red blood cells and platelets. This was the path to remission Katie sketched out for us.

It seemed a million miles away.

The path to recovery was long. Karen would be in isolation for 30 days and then the other two rounds of chemotherapy would be administered in the fall. We had barely scratched the surface.

Next, I had to perform a task that no parent should ever have to do. I headed home to assemble my children and inform them their mother had cancer.

Fr. Dave Hellmann had arrived at the hospital, and he drove me home. We talked in the car about my unenviable task of informing the children that their mother had cancer and might die. Earlier in the afternoon, after consultation with Kevin and my dad, we had decided the best thing to do was to send all three children to Kevin's home in Hudson, Ohio. Kevin referred to this as "Camp Coyne." Each one of Kevin's three children corresponded in age with our three. Cousin Sean was born 12 hours before Will; Katie was just a few months older than Samantha, and the same was true for their Timothy and our Mitchell. Besides, Kevin had a large house that could easily accommodate the additional three Volpe children for an extended period. Kevin had also just acquired a GMC Yukon XL, so there was plenty of room for the kids and even their bikes.

When I arrived at home Pat, Kathy, Tommy and my dad went for a long walk in the neighborhood, allowing me to have private time with my children. I sat the three of them down on the big blue leather couch in the family room. I told them the truth. I told them their mother was very ill, she had leukemia and it was very serious. This was the hardest thing I ever had to do in my entire life.

Will piped up immediately, saying, "Mom just helped me with this subject with my homework last week in school. We just studied leukemia in school. This is when your white blood cells aren't able to fend off diseases and act as your defense system."

How ironic, I thought. The two of them had talked about leukemia just a few weeks earlier.

"Right now Mom has to be the number one focus. There's no way I can be a good dad and a good husband at the same time so even though I don't want to, the best thing to do is for us to send all three of you to Uncle Kevin's house so I can concentrate on Mommy," I continued.

"We're doing everything we can do to make sure that she'll be okay," I added, trying to be strong for all of us.

"Could she die?" Will asked.

And I said, "Yes, there's a chance that she might die, but we're going to do everything possible to make sure that she lives. That's part of the reason why I have to send you to Uncle Kevin's for awhile."

By now both Samantha and Mitchell were in tears. William was just taking in the whole situation. He internalized his feelings, just like a man. I told them I was sorry, but their baseball, soccer and gymnastics activities were over. Will wasn't too upset by this news because his baseball team, the Diamondbacks, really sucked. He referred to several of the players as "The Bedwetters."

"MaMaw's mommy got breast cancer and died from cancer, and now my mom has cancer. Does this mean that I'm going to get it, too?" Samantha reasoned.

I couldn't hug my Samantha fast enough and I quickly reassured her that leukemia is not inherited and passed on from our parents; somehow, Mommy had acquired this disease. We just didn't know how.

I found this question and insight from a second grader rather remarkable. Mitchell, the youngest, tried to be brave, not saying much, and crying ever so softly. It was amazing that, at his age, he took this news so well. He's sensitive, but he hung tough. Samantha mothered her little brother and kept her arm wrapped tightly around him constantly. By now I could see that Pat, Kathy, Tommy and my father had returned from their walk, and I knew they could help comfort my shell-shocked children. I told them we would spend the rest of the evening packing their things, and they would head over to Ohio with Kevin in the morning. I felt terrible, but I knew it was the only logical thing we could do under the circumstances.

I then headed across the street to the Wetzel house and told Amy Jackson, Kimmie Wetzel and Melinda Bruggemann, our wonderful neighbors, of our horrific news. All three of them cried while I asked them for their help over the next few weeks, if not months. Marty Wetzel offered me a stiff glass of scotch.

"I know you will do whatever I ask to help save my wife's life," I said.

Melinda looked at me and said, "You're amazing! Do you hear what you're saying?

"I don't have much of a choice to do anything else, do I? We are going to win, because there is no other alternative. I know I can count on all of you to help save her life," I said.

A commotion at the Wetzels' front door caught our attention. Mitchell and Sam were wearing hula skirts and acting pretty silly, and I thought this was cool. Acting goofy and cutting loose a little had to be much healthier behavior than crying or anger. I gulped down the rest of my scotch and left. We spent a good part of the evening organizing the kids so we could get up early the next morning and pack up the Yukon.

As the Yukon backed out of the driveway on Thursday morning, it was very hard for me to fight back the tears. Once they had gone out of sight it dawned on me that it was time to put up the Ohio State Buckeye flag. While I hoisted it up, I sang the "Buckeye Battle Cry" quietly to myself. And when I finished the song, I said out loud, "Come on, my Buckeye Girl, it's time to fight. I know you can do it." Then I burst into tears for the first time, but somehow managed to wipe them away as I jumped into my dad's white minivan to go to IUMC to help Karen fight the fight.

My dad drove downtown, and we spent the first of what would be many long days at IUMC. Karen's nurses were superb, and one nurse in particular, Marcie, was very diligent and compassionate. Upon our arrival, Karen had already undergone minor surgery to install a Hickman catheter line or port under the skin and directly into her jugular vein. The port would make it easier to administer intravenous transfusions and drugs she would be receiving over the upcoming months.

We were very impressed with the IUMC staff's level of care and attention to detail. Dr. Cripe remained a mystery man because we never saw him. Katie Hincher assured us that even though we didn't know him at this point in time, he was very involved in Karen's case and was working hard to map out a strategy that would lead to remission.

When we met with Dr. Li, the lead resident oncologist assigned to Karen, he explained to us again that they were reasonably sure Karen had a form of AML called M3, or APL, but that this could not be confirmed until the results of the bone marrow biopsy had come back. He further explained again that even though this was a rare form of leukemia, there was a silver lining in that it was curable. In recent years, great strides had been made in the survival rates for people who had acquired the M3 subtype of AML. Dr. Li also told us that Karen's chemotherapy would begin later that evening even though the definitive results of the biopsy had not come back from the lab.

"Shouldn't we wait a few days for Karen to recover from the female surgery and the effects of the pneumonia-like symptoms she's experiencing?" I asked.

Dr. Li and Katie replied that Dr. Cripe was very concerned about Karen's rapidly accelerating white blood count and that waiting for her condition to improve was not an option. Katie went on to explain that the same protocol for the chemotherapy would be prescribed for the first five days regardless of which type of AML she had. If the test results showed that Karen had contracted a form of AML other than M3, then we would go down a different chemo track starting on Day 6.

In other words, we didn't have any time to waste. If Karen's white blood cell count continued on its spiral climb, we might not be able to achieve remission, and her days on this planet were numbered.

It was one of those damned-if-you-do, damned-if-you-don't situations.

Katie explained the side effects associated with the two forms of chemotherapy Karen would receive, idarubicin and duanorubicin. Katie said that in most cases, patients experience a lot of nausea and vomiting. She also mentioned that Karen's hair would fall out and probably grow back in a different color, and that the texture would likely be different, usually curlier.

Finding this out, Karen said, "Fine with me. I never liked my hair anyhow. Let's get this show on the road. I need to get home to my babies."

"Does this mean that her hair could come back blonde, and I'd have a blonde for a wife without having to switch wives like some guys do?" I said.

Katie just smiled and said, "No, Mark, it will probably come in darker, not blonde."

Meanwhile, something else was going on in Stow, Ohio, that we didn't have the heart to tell Karen at this point in time. Her good friend Nora Wilson, formerly Nora Haas, was burying her mother the same day Karen was beginning her chemo. It was Nora who had planned the awesome ski trip to Kitzbuhel, Austria, that ultimately brought Karen and I together. Karen had always sworn that she would be there for Nora whenever she needed her. But we knew we couldn't tell her about Mrs. Haas' passing. My mom attended the funeral, having known Mrs. Haas as a fellow parishioner at Holy Family for years. Mom found it impossible not to cry when she gave Nora a hug outside of church. Nora probably suspected something was wrong when Karen wasn't able to be there, but we knew this was not the time to tell her about Karen's leukemia. This would be too cruel a blow on the same day Nora buried her mother.

Life can be so bizarre at times. I remember thinking to myself, "Wow, who writes scripts like this? Oh, yeah, how could I forget? God wrote this script and He's known we would be facing this turn of fate our whole lives."

Karen started her first round of chemo at 7:00, exactly when Dr. Li had had said she would. It was hard for me to imagine that the contents of two IV bags clearly marked "HAZARDOUS," with the skull and crossbones that we usually associate with poison, would be my wife's salvation. The fluids took a few hours to flow through to completion. My dad and I left about an hour after the chemo started and went to a nice restaurant specializing in fine seafood called the Keystone Grille. I tried to relax and enjoy the meal, but I felt horribly guilty that my wife was downtown fighting for her life and I was sitting at a nice table in one of the area's finest eating establishments dining on exquisite seafood. I went home, and my dad headed over to his hotel room.

I had a very restless night and tried to use Coors Light as a sedative, but I couldn't stop my mind from wandering from good thoughts to bad thoughts and then back again. I had all the faith in the world that she would beat this thing and would survive, but in my mind I was a realist, and I was reluctantly forced to think about the possibility that "Thy Will Be Done" might mean Karen would be prematurely called home to be with the Lord, despite our efforts to keep her here with us on Earth. I hated that I was even thinking things like:

"Would I ever date or remarry?"

"Who would serve as pallbearers?"

"Would I be able to handle life as a single parent?"

"What were the amounts of coverage on those life insurance policies we took out several years ago?"

"How could I do an adequate job of parenting these beautiful children she had given me?"

"What would I say during her eulogy? How could I do this wonderful woman's life justice in 20 minutes?"

"What about our trip to Rome? I can't go without her."

We're only human and you can't help where your mind goes even if you're trying to stay positive. I've always been a planner and my mind churned through the permutations of what may, could or would happen. Other thoughts shot through my mind as I vividly recalled her telling me one thing in particular during dinner out at the Reserve Inn in Hudson. It was October 1993, long before we had our Mitchell. We were celebrating our fifth anniversary. That night Karen gave me three very strict instructions.

Her tone was emphatic. I couldn't forget what she had said that evening. I don't know how we got on the subject, but here's what my wife said:

"If I die before you and you leave the casket open, I'll come back and haunt you the rest of your days. Secondly, don't waste money on any expensive casket. A cheap pine box will work just fine, and third, there will be no crying. I want it to be a party with lots of alcohol. Don't cry! Celebrate my life. No moping will be tolerated!"

As I lied there in bed totally awake, I decided that even though we lived in Indiana, Karen was pure Buckeye, and I would let her mom pick out her final resting place in the rich soil of Ohio if she died. Not that I had anything against the spectacular Hoosiers who had welcomed us so warmly. In fact, I was counting on the expertise at the Indiana University Medical Center to save her life. But if she were to die, this proud graduate of The Ohio State University and member of Alpha Phi sorority would go back to Ohio. Even if I left the casket closed, I figured she would still figure out a way to come back and haunt me if I put her in the ground in Indiana. The last thing I needed was to suffer the scorn of my wife from the hereafter.

I probably got all of an hour and 45 minutes of sleep that night before heading back to IUMC at 7:00 the next morning. I remember at some point talking on the phone with Scott Zigmond, when he called to check on the situation, about my wandering thoughts. I was concerned because it seemed to me that even though we were doing everything we could for Karen I had almost accepted the fact that she was not going to make it. Scott told me this was normal. We're human and we can't help but think that the worse thing might happen.

The hospital bombarded us with informational brochures. One of the most helpful brochures was about a website called Caringbridge. This site allowed us to keep family and friends posted on Karen's progress. Readers could send Karen words of encouragement, advice and prayer through a customized guestbook that resembled a one-way e-mail. Late in the day Friday, I sat down at a computer in the library on the sixth floor at IUMC and typed out the first journal entry and posted it to Karen's web page. Friends could enter the guestbook dedicated to her by typing in "karenvolpe" under name and "IN" under directory. Tommy set up the header:

Karen Volpe

Welcome to the <u>Web Site</u> we have created to keep the friends and family of Karen Volpe updated on her progress as she beats leukemia.

My initial journal entry attempted to capture what had happened during the previous six days. Word of the website spread through hundreds of emails and distribution lists of our broad network of family and friends who knew and loved Karen.

Friday, June 14, 2002 at 03:38 PM

Many of the questions and concerns regarding Karen focus on how this happened, so rapidly. This initial entry is intended to be a chronology of the events leading up to this point in time.

During the week of June 2, 2002 Karen was here in Carmel carrying on with her active schedule of summer activities. Will, Samantha and Mitchell keep her on the move—school is out. She was slightly fatigued and had trouble getting a good night's rest all week. She complained of lower back pain on occasion. On Friday evening the 7th, we went to dinner and a play with friends.

Saturday morning she awoke with an upset stomach and minor pain under her left rib cage. She described it as stomachache. We went to the Urgent Care center near our home. While being examined her pain increased and her vitals deteriorated. EMT transported her to the ER at St. Vincent Hospital in Carmel.

The ultrasound revealed an immense volume of blood in her lower abdomen; a ruptured ovarian cyst was the suspected cause. She had surgery to remove the left ovary and tube. In recovery clotting was of major concern; many units of blood were required to get her hemoglobin levels up. Several blood products were administered over Sunday and her CAT scan revealed cloudiness in her left lung. Sunday was spent stabilizing her in the ICU. Throughout Monday her breathing was very shallow and labored, but the clotting issue seemed resolved. Her platelet count remained mysteriously low. No progress was being made and the hospital staff was noticeably puzzled with her lack of improvement.

Early Tuesday the family made their lack of satisfaction with Karen's treatment known to the hierarchy at St. V, and the level of treatment, especially addressing her respiratory system was noticeably increased. We had also switched her pain medication from morphine to percocet at her mother's suggestion. Later in the day Karen seemed out of the woods and was able to joke and talk with her family. She had a restful evening in spite of her shallow breathing, all other vitals looked well.

At 6:00 a.m. Wednesday morning the critical care specialist, after consultation with a hematology-oncologist, informed her brother, Tommy, and her husband, Mark, that her blood chemicals indicated a 99.9 % probability that she had leukemia or cancer of the white blood cells.

The next hours were spent determining where to transport Karen to verify the theory. After a thorough analysis of the available options, it was determined that Dr. Cripe, at Indiana University Medical Center in Indianapolis, was the place where Karen would be treated. A bone marrow extract was performed for lab analysis. The family was immediately told that the numerous blood draws at St V. revealed a very high likelihood that Karen had acute myelogenous leukemia, or AML, which is a curable disease that must be attacked aggressively with chemotherapy. Thursday was spent preparing Karen for chemo and the focus remained with verifying the suspicion that it was pneumonia that had developed in both lungs. Her white blood cell count raced out of control, with 92-95% being deemed as bad cells. Lots of antibiotics had been consistently administered to deal with infection. Chemo began at 7:00 p.m. on Thursday and Karen remains in good sprits and rests most of the time. The white blood cells are in the process of being destroyed and thus far everything is going as planned.

In the early morning hours of Saturday, still unable to sleep, I updated the website again. I had spent many hours Friday evening calling several of Karen's closest out-of-town friends. I had talked with Mary Kay Kibler, a good friend we had met in Mason who moved to Atlanta right before we moved to Indianapolis. I also had talked at length with Margaret Evans in Portland, Oregon. I felt bad after I hung up with Margot because I knew the news about Karen had to be hard on her. Margot was miles away, out on the West Coast; she had never married and lived alone. Her best friend had cancer; she must have felt as if she were on an island, a feeling of total helplessness.

"What can I do?" she asked.

All I could say was, "Pray!"

In the early morning hours of Saturday, sleepless and still wrestling with the same tormented thoughts from the night before, I updated the website. It was another night of very thin sleep as I tossed back and forth. Just prior to trying to get some rest I wrote:

Saturday, June 15, 2002 at 01:25 AM

Karen is now 32 hours into chemo and is resting comfortably. All signs are positive as the white blood count continues to decline. There are no current problems with any side effects—minor sore throat and her hair follicles hurt a little. She has received more units of blood.

Yesterday when she was informed that her hair would fall out in 2-3 weeks Karen replied, "Fine, I never really liked my hair anyway." Her attitude remains very upbeat, and we are all encouraged, as the race to beat this disease begins. Her brother, Kenny, is on his way.

Continue to pray!

Hope and courage will prevail. We love you all for everything that is being done, the prayers, the cards, the rosaries and the novenas. Please continue to pray.

Time for another Our Father.

On Saturday, my CRHP brothers and a group of neighbors arrived at the house at the same time. Both groups of men were set on mowing, edging and doing whatever else needed to be done. I think my CRHP brothers ended up washing the windows. Our yard looked great. Karen was stressing about everything with her house. I tried hard to reassure her that the house wasn't that important and in fact had never looked better. Well, at least the outside was well groomed.

We finally started to make some progress resolving Karen's breathing problems and her stamina was improving. She was able to converse freely with her friend Gretchen Koch, a sorority sister from OSU, and her husband Steve, who had come over from Columbus. Karen and Gretchen visited for hours. Pat and I were concerned that Karen was overdoing it and that we would end up going backward if she didn't take an occasional break to rest. The high drama for the day occurred when Steve fainted while wearing the mask that was required while visiting with Karen. He ended up in the ER so they could check his vitals. There were times when I had trouble with the mask myself, especially if her room was warm.

Karen's dad, Tom, had gone back to Akron for the weekend. Returning home for a few days greatly helped his mental outlook because he had been struggling to accept the fact that his daughter had cancer. Later in the afternoon I had my only really challenging moment with my mother-in-law, whom I love dearly. She had pushed one of my buttons on an issue I just couldn't let slide. The details do not matter, and in the end she agreed with me and apologized. It was the one and only time during this ordeal that I got upset with Pat. I'm sure there were situations where she wasn't happy with me, but all in all we worked well together and generally agreed on the major aspects of Karen's care.

Pat takes copious notes, while I rely on my memory and take only a few notes. Most of my back-of-the-envelope notes were taken during morning rounds and consultations with the doctors. I'd use these notes to help me update the website. Pat kept a journal, which was always helpful and served as a reminder for us to keep track of some details that the hospital staff might lose track of, especially the nursing staff due to shift changes.

In the middle of the afternoon on Saturday I updated the website again.

Saturday, June 15, 2002 at 02:02 PM

Contrary to earlier reports, Karen will not be sleeping most of the day. The cardio-pulmonary specialist is very pleased with her breathing pattern and her ability to communicate with ease. He indicated that, "If it's not broke, why fix it?" As she tires, she will rest and visitor time will be restricted as appropriate. Father Dave brought Karen and other family members the Holy Eucharist.

The white blood cell count continues to decline and is currently at 17,000. The chemo is doing its job as planned without any drastic side effects thus far. She looks great. Her latest bed configuration is much more comfortable, having her much more vertical than horizontal (like a dentist chair), which helps her breathe.

The facility is a truly magnificent, state-of-the-art medical center. Karen is a graduate of The Ohio State University; however, we are currently big fans of the Indiana University Medical Center. Go Hoosiers!

The medical staff's management style would be likened to a semi-military regiment with compassion and care toward the patient and family. The terms "strict discipline" and "tough love" both come to mind.

Keep praying and sending messages to this web site. Karen will see them ASAP. My laptop is here. She is strong and we are here every step of the way. Our Holy Father is hearing the name Karen Patricia Volpe over and over and over…This is only one battle. The war is on. We shall persevere.

Karen's Aunt Patty and Uncle Bob visited IUMC. While they were visiting, I recall Pat getting visibly upset with the reality that her daughter had been stricken with cancer. I told her we had to be strong. It wasn't as if she were a victim of 9/11: dead with nothing we could do to change it. Karen had hope and plenty of courage.

"She'll beat this thing," I told Pat.

I asked Kimmie, Amy, Dad, Pat, Aunt Patty and Uncle Bob to join me in saying the Lord's Prayer. We formed a circle in the family waiting area of the ICU, holding hands, and saying the Lord's Prayer. I'll never forget the beauty of that prayerful moment.

The level of stress I was dealing with was starting to take its toll. On Saturday night one of my neighbors invited me to join in on a little get-together they were having over at Stan's to continue rallying the troops for Karen. I had quite a few drinks and my neighbor, Stan Crisci, a local investments and banking executive with whom I had recently entrusted the management of a large chunk of our 401(k) savings, warned me, saying, "Volpe, take good care of yourself. Play some golf, get good sleep and eat good. Otherwise you'll end up being a patient yourself."

He had a sister who had died years earlier from breast cancer, so I knew Stan had been down this road before. I scoffed at his suggestion and continued to drink. I think I remember giving up on Coors Light and switching to Bacardi and Sprite, with a twist of lime. I drank the better part of a fifth.

One of our neighbors, Amy Jackson, visited Karen on Friday and had also met Dr. Li. At the party she told everyone his accent didn't allow him to say "chemotherapy." Instead, it sounded like "chemosarapy." Amy recounted how she found it hard not to giggle out loud every time the adorable Dr. Li said "chemosarapy" instead of "chemotherapy." She said, "I was trying so hard to be serious, but every time he said chemosarapy, I just started cracking up."

When I returned home, I made another journal entry that seemed semi-coherent, in spite of the level of alcohol racing around in my system. Thanks to exhaustion and the better part of a bottle of rum I actually slept a little. It was probably not the most restful type of sleep. At least I was out cold for a few hours, with my mind unable to wander over the endless myriad of dark potential outcomes that had been taunting at me.

Sunday, June 16, 2002 at 12:27 AM

Karen's brother Kenny, long-time OSU friend Gretchen Koch and her husband Steve (a brilliant and well-accomplished professional graduating from Ohio Northern University back in the early '80s) made it in from out of town. Dave Helle of CRHP 16 also visited with Mark for a while. Kenny's plane landed in the middle of the 6:00 p.m. storm and he had no problems getting to the hospital from the airport, even though John Bird encountered numerous backups and traffic mishaps along the way none of which involved him directly.

The arrival of these family members lifted Karen even higher as she spent the day talking and napping. Day 3 of chemo began at 7:00 p.m. The congestion in the lungs is diminishing with minor audible grumbles being heard through the stethoscope. The 4:00 p.m. blood labs continue to provide encouragement as the WBC is now down to 10,500 from the morning's 17,000 figure. Hemoglobin is at a 9.0, indicating a French judge is obviously on the take. Karen is a 10! This is also most encouraging because the more recent numbers have congregated in the range of 7.6 to 8.8. Platelets are still low, but these get fixed later as I understand.

Since coming to IUMC, we feel that we're on a three-game winning streak to open the season, but there still are 159 regular season games to go. The World Series ring will be won. Speaking of sports, Karen and Gretchen turned on the U.S. Open today to watch Tiger's swing.

They say to take it a day at a time day, but it feels more like minute to minute.

Karen did get to read a few of her guestbook messages and these pumped her up big-time as visiting hours wound down. Paper copies of everything sent as of this entry will be there tomorrow morning for her to read.

Last evening she called at 2:30 a.m. with a long "honey-and mommy-do" list, giving her mother and me an additional jolt of joy, even though we were supposed to be sleeping. Right!

No real flowers today good job!!!

For the second evening in a row I had the pleasure of having dinner with my father, John Volpe. We can't help but to replay old stories involving Karen, plan for future fun in the sun, and discuss and philosophize on the day's events. His advice is most helpful. Despite the circumstances I will treasure these two simple meals forever. He's my mentor, my rock and a superb logician. One last thing: I'm very glad his boss gave him the time off to be here.

Lisa Roach, Samantha's second grade teacher was right on with her recording of the SLDM classic hit. "Our God Is An Awesome God" and he does reign with power above.

Our Karen is an Awesome Woman! She feels the power of prayer and her family does as well.

I know the pews will be crowded tomorrow, so be cordial in the parking lots or, better yet, come early and stay for two. Bring two envelopes as well because SLDM needs a boost to fix the AC. Congrats to Father Dave on 29 years in the priesthood.

As you can tell by this entry we're all in a very good mood, but we know how fragile the situation remains. Change is inevitable; the key is to keep the train on the tracks.

Happy Father's Day to All!! Our yard and home look great thanks to a team of men headed by Bill Grace and Gary Dufek.

Love one another as I have loved you.

Be peaceful.

Amen.

CHAPTER 15

Camp Coyne

It was Father's Day, but I really didn't give it a second thought. I woke up slightly hung over from the previous evening's activities. I finally got to spend some one-on-one time, almost alone, with my wife for awhile early Sunday morning. I put Bruce Springsteen's *The River* album on the sound system in Karen's room in the ICU. While Karen lay back, with me listening to Bruce, she had her hair shampooed. She was totally relaxed and enjoying the pampering from Emma.

"Emma, you're an artist," she purred.

I sat back and enjoyed the simplicity of the moment. Karen was comfortable and relaxed compared with the state she was in exactly one week earlier back at St. Vincent's in Carmel. Sometime earlier in the day Dr. Li had said, "Time was on our side."

I was beginning to believe him.

As long as she kept progressing, the treatments would have a chance to get Karen into remission. Sometimes I'd just sit there with her and pray and watch the second hand slowly move its way around the clock. Five minutes seemed like an hour, but it didn't matter as long as the second hand continued to move and Karen continued to breathe.

During the day, Lori Spence, my friend from the Midwest ISO, came by and visited for at least an hour. She brought Karen a huge care package of goodies, a journal, a little camera, some lotion and all sorts of fun stuff. It meant a lot to me personally that Lori had taken so much time out of the day to spend time with us, especially considering that it was Father's Day. She had three children of her own and a husband at home.

Father Dave Hellmann stopped in later and visited with Karen. At this point, Pat had returned to Akron because her husband, John Bird, had his own medical issues and she needed to be there. Only my dad and I were left to hold down the fort at the hospital that Sunday. After visiting with Karen, I talked with Father Dave for a bit and I replayed for him Dr. Cripe's overall game plan and strategy to get Karen into remission. My dad and I both received Holy Communion. I felt as if I were receiving the Eucharist for the first time.

As Father Dave went toward the elevator door to leave, I said to him, "Father, I feel kind of guilty because I've missed church now for two straight weeks."

"Don't worry about it," he said. "You're living the Word of the Lord right now as we speak."

I got a feeling in my gut that I'll never forget; it reminded me of how I felt on the Sunday of the first Super Bowl back in 1967, when my dad told his children, "Grandpa died last night." He was so very strong when he broke the news to us, and as the oldest, I knew he had to feel terrible inside. But he was strong and didn't show any weakness in front of his children. Now it was time for me to do the same.

Later on my dad told me that during the day he had been on the phone with Kevin, coordinating a time when it would be good for me to call and talk with my kids. I had forgotten that it was Father's Day. I was so focused on my wife that I had hardly given my children a second thought. They had been down at Kevin's in-laws' summer home on Lake Mohawk, which is about an hour and a half south of Akron, Ohio, not far from New Philadelphia. Fishing, water skiing and other fun adventures had filled their day. "Camp Coyne," as Kevin called it, was a wonderful diversion. Our three children were happy, healthy and well-loved. Colleen's brother, Chris, and her sister, Tricia, were also there, along with the rest of the family, and they were showing my kids the time of their lives. This was great for our children, and I was glad they were having so much fun. This was the closest they would get to Virginia Beach—the shores of Lake Mohawk in the middle of Ohio would have to suffice because there would be no big family vacation in 2002.

I made the following update on the website, and then went back to make the call to my kids that my dad had coordinated with Kevin. As you read it, you can tell the ordeal is starting to wear me down.

Sunday, June 16, 2002 at 07:25 PM

Today began with Kenny's second visit, then home and off to Montreal—he'll be back soon. Fr. Tim was here for a wonderful visit and lots of catch-up conversation. Fr. Dave also peaked in for a quick visit. My colleague from the Midwest ISO, Lori Spence, brought in wonderful gifts: a journal, a camera, stationery and much more. Her experience with a friend's AML battle was most inspirational.

Karen was concerned about naming the people in this story by name. I believe the friends and family need to be identified by name. If this bothers anyone, please let me know, as I am aware of your right to confidentiality. In the meantime, I believe the Constitution's 1st Amendment rules the day. Freedom of Speech. Gotta love it!

Pat Bird, Karen's beautiful mother, gives me strength, and I hope that I do the same for her. She is an amazing woman, resilient, strong and unbelievably courageous. Today she returned to Akron for just a day and will be back Tuesday. She knows I love her too; she helps with Karen and everyone whose life she has touched.

On to Karen's condition—two oncologists stopped by to review her progress and the Big Picture looks good. The prime concern focuses on bleeding, and this remote possibility remains, but we have minimized all risks by keeping her in bed. By the end of the day on Monday or Tuesday, the minimal risks will diminish; however, the clotting issues will still be monitored on an ongoing basis. A unit of blood is dispensed to keep the hemoglobin levels up, we're at 8.8. The lungs continue to clear up significantly, and although the presumed pneumonia continues to lurk, her breathing is perfectly fine. The antibiotics, historically a Karen favorite for fending off strep throat and the like, are also working wonders on her lungs. She receives pain medication for the lungs, at her request. Her present heart rate is 64! She has been so relaxed, it's a beautiful thing. Most importantly of all, the white blood count is continuing down to 4,400 as of 4:00 a.m. and is now down to 2,500 as of mid-afternoon. Those numbers on a simple piece of paper are the only presents this father, who majored in accounting, needs. Zero is the only correct answer that can be accepted, as one is one too many. The physicians said time is everything, every second counts.

Now, get out your Kleenex.

For me personally, this morning was an awesome spiritual and totally romantic experience with my bride of 14 years. I know that this will sound somewhat strange, but here goes.

Karen's nurse, Emma, was washing Karen's hair and applying conditioner. She was so laid back, and Karen complimented Emma in a relaxed mumble, uttering, "You're an artist." Selections from Springsteen's *The River* album played softly in the background as I quietly said three decades of the rosary.

Bruce feels free to visit us here in Indy—we've got the fastest cars in the world.

The peacefulness and calm was overwhelming as I fought back the mist emerging from my eyes. Karen's good friend Nora Wilson (formerly Haas) gave me the advice with respect to saying the decades of the rosary—it's all about a feeling of total inner peace. Nora recently lost her mom, and she is a special friend having played an instrumental role in bringing Karen and I together in 1987 with the ski trip to Austria that Nora had organized.

This one precious hour will never exceed the joy of our wedding day and the birth of our children, but this one hour on Father's Day 2002, ranks way up there on the flagpole, at least for me. My faith and hope is that there will be many more moments like these.

Picture this one: It's June 2017—Karen and I together walking Samantha up the aisle at St. Louis de Montfort.

I warned you to get out the tissue.

We Are One Bread—One Body in Christ

This is only the Beginning.

During the week, the popularity of Karen's website grew immensely. There was constant activity in the Caringbridge guestbook, and as a matter of routine, I would print out the most recent entries and take them to Karen for her to read. Here are just a few of the entries that Karen found most interesting. She appreciated all the words of encouragement. From my perspective the website allowed friends and family to vent while also staying connected with her progress. This was tough on everyone. The website was under constant surveillance.

Hey Sis,

Lil T Calling. We seem to talk every few days, so I'll put a call into you now and then it's up to you to get better and call me the next time. As I look back on our conversations, we tend to ramble a lot; we discuss many miscellaneous issues, and get interrupted too…. so let's talk.

I know we don't generally talk at 4:43, but this is kind of different. You have leukemia—what's up with that, Karen? That wasn't part of the plan. But the cool thing about having AML is that, at least, it sounds cool. When I found out that you had this type of cancer, among many thoughts that ran through my head, I was hoping that you didn't have "Hairy Cell Leukemia." That just sounds bad. I mean come on, Hairy Cell Leukemia? When I was researching this stuff on the internet at St.V's Hospital and that came up as a possibility, I was thinking that it is bad enough my sister has leukemia, but how am I going to tell my friends that it's called Hairy Cell…. so at least AML (the M3 version, I hope) sounds cool. And to boot, you are doing great. Keep getting better, Sis.

Karen, can you sense that? I know it's like other people are listening in on our conversation. Maybe it's just my imagination or perhaps the government.

Why in the h*** am I up at almost 5 in the morning? I'm not sure if the chicken or the egg came first. Let me explain—you are always on my mind (even while sleeping), but I did have to get up because I had to pee really badly. So to recap, did I have to pee or was I thinking of you? To be honest, I guess we will never know.

This is a great conversation Sis. Although you must be preoccupied, you haven't interrupted me, taken a swig of beer, or burped in my ear.

Some more miscellaneous thoughts from your Baby Brother: Riley is cool as cool gets. She totally gets "Da-Da." She can say it, kind of give what may resemble a High 5, and that smile of hers—she is so proud of herself. Which takes us to another topic.... it's Father's Day! I actually got a card this year! As John Scanlon puts it, I have considered Kelsey and John my kids from Day 1, but this time, I should get a "Happy Biological Father's Day" card. I'll call Hallmark.

Hold on, I have to pee again.... I'm back. Wow, that new soap Diana bought is great on the hands. You know, it's probably best you weren't on the phone to hear this call.

What else, Sis? You are in great hands. I am glad I was able to get to you during this time of transition. You had me scared there for a bit, but I have all the confidence in the world in you...and the chemotherapy is helping a bit too. You want to know something else that scared me too?

I roomed with Kevin for a few nights while we were in Indianapolis…Please don't tell anyone this…he'd probably get upset. But Kevin wears a thong to bed! Oh, My God! A thong! One time, he was prancing around in the hotel room in a pink one with rhinestones. I know everyone deals with stress differently…but what would the textbooks say about that? That's the real reason I was at your bedside that night at St.V.

Honestly though Karen, Kevin and I weathered the beginning of this storm together—thank God for Kevin and humor because we used a lot of the humor part to cope.

Seriously, though Karen…I am sorry that you have to fight this battle. But fighting you are. You are an inspiration. You have brought the Coyne and Volpe families closer together. As a result, I am looking inward at my life, my job, my wife and my children. If you can make room for leukemia on your plate, then I can work on being a better person. Don't get me wrong; the really odd, rude, suffocating humor will stay, but I am looking inwards. Thanks.

Lil Kare, I don't want to run up your nickel. I love you. Mark loves you. Family and friends will take care of everything outside of Room A1 in the ICU—you continue to take care of everything inside of A1.

My plan is to get back to you this Thursday or Friday night at the absolute latest.

I'm going to go back to bed now. This conversation is way too much one-sided…and I really do sense that someone is listening in on us. Next time we talk—remind me to call Nextel to check it out.

Love,

Tommy

Tommy
Akron, OH USA—Sunday, June 16, 2002 at 04:29 AM

My darling Karen O'Coyne O'Volpe, Leave it to your wonderful family to hook up this great way of talking to you. I am thinking and praying for you every minute of every day. According to Mark's notes, our prayers are being answered. I doubt if God has ever heard so many prayer requests for one person. He knows he is dealing with a very special angel here on earth. I can't wait to see you and hug you. I know you are fighting this thing with everything you have and we all know you have more fighting power than most. Keep it up, girlfriend. I am visiting my brother Rob in California right now, and my folks and Mark are here too. They all send their love. Carla, Rob's wife, who you met and shared your Oprah bond at my parents' anniversary party, told me that she emailed Oprah about you and asked Oprah to pray for you too!!!!

I am coming to see you soon. I love you more than you will ever know.

Your little sister,
Margaret Jane
Margaret Evans
Portland, OR USA—Monday, June 17, 2002 at 11:15 PM

Dear Karen,

It may surprise you to know that I have suffered severe withdrawal symptoms since last seeing you Saturday night. But I am heartened by the progress Mark is reporting. Yours is an amazing comeback, but you are an amazing woman, so that's to be expected. I fully anticipate your visiting us in July and disrupting our home with some major project you feel necessary. Karen, we do not need to do any more painting for the next 10 years. Judging by the number of messages, half the world is pulling for you. If there is strength in numbers then you are well on your way.

I have held you in high regard since 8th grade at St. Hilary. I know you have the moxie to beat this scourge.

And so does everyone else who knows you.

All my love,

Your favorite stepfather.

PS Mom misses you so much that she called your home phone and

TALKED TO YOU ON THE ANSWERING MACHINE. Do you believe that???? I certainly do. Mom will be there Wednesday afternoon. Tuesday she will be seeing your precious children.

John Bird
Akron, OH USA—Monday, June 17, 2002 at 09:05 PM

HOW KAREN CONQUERED CANCER

Karen and Mark,

I just arrived in Ohio at my Mom and Dad's and was able to get onto the website for the first time. From Mark's messages, it sounds like you are fighting this just as I knew you would. Karen, you are one of the strongest, funniest, most beautiful and caring people I know. This illness doesn't stand a chance!!!

Just so you know, I always tell you how much I love all the 50,000 wonderful pillows you have made for our house; we want to hug them just a little harder now. We can't wait until it's you we're hugging. And, that will be as soon as I know you can have me there!!! Not only are you in my prayers all day long, but Katey, Jillian and Chris are praying for you, too. I miss you and your infectious laugh and cannot wait until I hear you soon!!!

Much love and prayers,

Mary Kay Kibler
Alpharetta, GA USA—Monday, June 17, 2002 at 10:48 PM

Hey Ya-ya sista—Remember what we told you today: I CAN, I CAN, I CAN! Look at that picture of those three beautiful children and fight your way up!!! You are gonna get out of there, You're gonna fight and YOU are gonna win. REMEMBER: GO, FIGHT, WIN!! OK—now read these inspirational notes and KICK BUTT!! WE love you with everything we have, Kimmie and Amy

Amy Jackson
Carmel, IN USA—Monday, June 17, 2002 at 11:31 PM

Hello Karen!

I am not at all surprised by the number of e-mails you are getting—probably as many web site hits as Britney Spears, and you are more beautiful!!!! Cindy, Tyler, Valerie and I are praying for you every day. God has a wonderful plan for you and your family. You will beat this, Karen—you are a very strong woman...We love you...

Cindy, Greg (Zak), Tyler, Valerie

Greg Smith
Mason, OH—Tuesday, June 18, 2002 at 03:36 PM

Hey momma how are you i know u hate being in that poopie hospital...haha.. u will be out in no time...i love you so much...keep in touch

Samantha Volpe
hudson, ohio USA ROCKS—Tuesday, June 18, 2002 at 3:18 PM

Your friends at FirstEnergy just found out through an email from Joe Bambanek. We're here for you, Mark and Karen. Though miles away now and business paths take us different directions, you're still "family" to us in the Transmission Group. You have my prayers, my thoughts, my love. Mark, you really know how to make a gal weepy!! But still nothing for me beats the story you have engraved in your wedding band—"The adventure continues." Right?

Gwen Luciano
Akron, OH USA—Wednesday, June 19, 2002 at 04:08 PM

HOW KAREN CONQUERED CANCER

Yea………….

"God's in his heaven all's right with the world"

You go girl!

I knew if anyone could do it, it would be you!!!!

Just talked to your BIG SISTER and I got the scoop from her. Kathy had just finished writing her e-mail below when I called her; she is still floating on cloud nine. What great news to have heard, and of course that is what sisters are for!!!!!

I know your Mom (my BIG SISTER for those of you that do not know me) is chomping at the bit to get back to you tomorrow, I sure am glad John is driving :)

What a support group you have, we ALL love you,

your aunt ellen :) :) :)

aunt ellen
Myrtle Beach, SC—Wednesday, June 26, 2002 at 11:39 AM

Hi Karen,

As I went about my day, my last day with your beautiful treasures, Will, Sam & Mitch, I kept singing and humming to myself that old '70s-something song by maybe The Who…Oh, The mother and child reunion is only a (motion? / moment?) away!…And I got a big smile in my heart each time! I can only imagine how excited you must be to hug your babies tomorrow, but they too, are SO

EXCITED!! Kevin and I have enjoyed each moment with them; they are such a joy to be around! We are actually looking forward to spending 5 hours in the car with them tomorrow—something I'm not sure I would say about my own three children!! But think of us speeding away along that road to Columbus and through those Indiana cornfields tomorrow—we're on a mission to reunite mother and child!!!

I have to share with you a Kodak moment from this past week when we were at Lake Mohawk with all the kids and my parents. Actually, it was much more like a MasterCard commercial than a Kodak moment. I have to preface this story with telling you I can't remember if you have ever been to the house at the lake, but there is a rather large, steep hill between the house and the yard and the lake. Also, we had talked all day about the kids camping out in tents. They were so excited to do that. My story begins with a cookout on the deck, followed by s'mores.

Graham crackers, Hershey candy bars, stale marshmallows...$3.79

One lone birthday candle to stick in a marshmallow so we could sing Happy Birthday to Uncle Kevin...$0.20

Time spent pitching two tents, complete with rain guards (no rain in forecast, but just for the full effect!)...1 hour, 40 minutes (we do not do this regularly, obviously!)

Trips spent up and down the hill to get kids settled with blankets, sleeping bags, just the right pillow, cups of ice, water bottles, flashlights...Trips by kids—2; Trips by me—about 10 (I never said I was a bright woman!) (And let me remind you that this is a BIG, STEEP hill!!)

Sitting on the deck after "settling" (very loose definition) the kids and making bets on the number of children that would last the night outside…Papa and me—3; Nana and Kevin—2 (Unanimous agreement that Will would be a "survivor")

Time actually spent in tent…anywhere from 20 minutes (Timmy) to 1 hour and 30 minutes (Sam) (With the exception of Will who did in fact make it till about 6 a.m.!!)

Smiles on sleeping children's faces while in comfy beds with lifetime memories in tact…PRICELESS

I love you Karen and Mark; can't wait to see your beautiful faces tomorrow afternoon!! Love, Hugs, and Prayers, Colleen

Colleen Coyne
Hudson, OH—Saturday, June 29, 2002 at 10:50 PM

Meanwhile back at the ICU, Karen had just been given some pain medication. She was somewhat uncomfortable and edema had set into her feet because of all the fluids she had been taking on, making them look like huge overstuffed sausages. I had massaged her feet several times during the day, but in spite of the progress she had recently made breathing, she still had assorted pain, mostly in her back.

It was about 8:00 p.m. and I was beat. The phone in Karen's room rang, and I was able to spend a little time talking with each of my children as they drove north from Lake Mohawk in Kevin's big Yukon back to his home in Hudson. They all took turns, passing the cell phone around, except for Mitchell, who had fallen asleep. When I was done talking with William, I handed the phone to Karen and said, "Hey, Will wants to say hi." She just held the phone to her ear with a very puzzled look on her face the entire time, never speaking a word.

Then she hung up the phone and started to take off her hospital gown, pulling at all of the monitoring devices that were attached to various parts of her body.

"Why am I in the basement of Kroger's?" she said. "Go get the minivan right now. I've got to get out of here and get to my kids, they need me."

"No Karen, you're very sick," I said.

"You're at the IU Medical Center, not Kroger's grocery store. You have cancer and you can't go home yet."

At that she became more defiant, almost violent, and she continued to strip off her clothes and pull at her IV.

I yelled for Marcie, her nurse, who came on a dead run.

"She's having a reaction to the medication you just gave her! What was it?" I asked.

"Haldol," said Marcie.

"She's really out of it," I said. "She thinks she's at Kroger's and she's bound and determined to get out of here."

Marcie called the doctors to try and figure out what to give her to reverse the effects of the Haldol and its interaction with Ativan.

My dad had hit the lounge chair in the waiting area to try and get some shut-eye. I had told him that it looked like it was going to be a long night, so he needed to get some rest. Marcie and I battled with Karen for an hour and a half. Marcie did get an order to administer some medication to negate the effects of the Haldol. Karen kept insisting we leave at once. I tried to divert her attention to pleasant thoughts and happy times, but

Marcie told me it would take a long time for the Haldol to work its way through her system, maybe as long as eight hours.

I was exhausted, but I knew I had to dig in and help my wife get through this part of her ordeal. I tried to rest at the foot of her bed and could feel that my body was beginning to waiver. I had to press on; I had to try and say anything to get her to snap back into reality. I reminded Karen of the recent trip we had taken to Las Vegas and the fabulous singer-impersonator Dany Gans who put on an awesome show at the Mirage. I reminded her, the tickets cost $100 apiece. Karen's mind was off on a tangent. She mistrusted me because I wouldn't get the minivan and take her home to her three children.

At one point she said, "You spent all of our money on that stupid timeshare condo in Vegas, and now we don't have money for medical insurance. That's why I'm stuck here in this basement at Kroger's and not a real hospital."

A little later, she said something about not being able to trust Marcie.

"I've been doing my very best to help you and what you said just now really hurt my feelings," Marcie said to her.

Karen sat there with a blank stare, determined to rid herself of the monitoring devices. I was most concerned about the port that was sewn into her jugular and afraid that she might attempt to rip it out. If she did this, I was certain she would bleed to death, given her inability to clot due to the leukemia. Later, I'd find out that my preoccupation with the port was unfounded because it was able to withstand some 300 pounds of pressure. I wish I had known this in advance because I was consumed with preventing her from doing any physical harm.

At times, she would sit still and not say much, and then suddenly she would burst into bizarre talk having nothing to do with reality. She made me take down the pictures of the kids that we had put up. I did everything she asked, knowing eventually the Haldol would work its way out into the little plastic bag that held her urine. I remember looking down at the yellow liquid often wondering if the Haldol would ever work its way through her system.

At one point, I thought of Linda Blair in the movie *The Exorcist* and wondered if Karen's head would spin all the way around and she'd projectile vomit a large quantity of gross green liquid at me.

A little while later, I thought we had stemmed the tide. She had started to doze, and seemed to have calmed down. I rested my head and tried to close my eyes during these brief respites. Then I blew it all by somehow bringing up that my dad was sleeping in the lounge. Once Karen found out he was there, she started screaming at the top of her lungs, "John, John, John, John! Come here right now! John, John, John!"

One of the nurses went out to find him. It seemed like forever while Karen continued screaming for him. Eventually, I saw him outside the sliding door. It was taking what seemed like a long time for him to get in the room. I kept motioning for him to get inside. He did his best to wash and suit up quickly. This is not a simple process, as it required some time to scrub up to your elbows and then put on the gloves, gown and mask.

As soon as he arrived, Karen began to calm down.

The first thing she said was, "I'm so glad you're here. Go get your minivan and take me home to my babies; they need me."

My dad, who had been quickly clued-in by Marcie as he suited up, then responded, "Karen I can't take you home today. You're very, very sick, and right now, you have to stay here in the hospital."

"I don't trust your son Mark at all; he keeps everything

from me; he bought this stupid condo in Vegas, and now we don't have any money for insurance, and now he's got me stuck in this basement at Kroger's. Take me home to my babies right now, damn it. Go get the minivan," she demanded.

And then she made a motion toward her port as if she were going to rid herself of the contraption so she could head toward the door. I was on her right side, camped out near the foot of her bed. Out of the corner of her eye she caught me watching her and could read my apprehensions. My dad hugged and consoled her from the other side of the bed. Suddenly I was the bad guy, and he was the good guy.

She accused me of trying to sneak up on her.

"You sit down right now and do what you're told," my dad said to me sternly, just like when I was a little boy. Then Karen noticed that I hadn't taken down all the homey pictures we had hung in her room, so she ordered me to take them down, all of them. I complied, thinking it was only a matter of time before she would snap back into reality.

By now, it was about 3:00 in the morning. I was exhausted. I could hear my pillow calling me, and prayed that the effects of the Haldol would wear off soon and she would be back to normal.

For about an hour and a half Karen lied back and rested. Occasionally, she would catch my dad and I passing notes back and forth. We wanted to communicate without making any noise, but Karen was no dummy. A few times we were busted. Finally, she fell asleep and I was able to rest my forehead on top of the base of the bed as I sat in the same chair I had been ordered to occupy earlier. I was out of gas, but there was no way I could have moved from that spot! As the sun was coming up, she started to return to normal and seemed to realize where she was.

About 8:00 on Monday morning, she had stabilized—no more incoherent or outlandish demands. She was back to normal.

As we left, Marcie said, "She won't remember a thing!"

"Good!" I said, and I thanked her for hanging with us through a difficult evening.

While we were driving back to Carmel, the normal Monday morning traffic was moving into downtown Indianapolis. I remember thinking how much nicer it would be to be headed off to another week of work at the Midwest ISO. Finally, my head hit my own pillow at about 9:00, and I managed to rest until around 11:00. Even though I was beyond exhaustion, it was hard to sleep given the bizarre circumstances that had occurred just a few hours earlier. By 1:00 in the afternoon, I was back downtown. I was running purely on adrenaline at this point, and rapidly turning to toast. I could sense that my system was deteriorating, but I had to work through it because Karen's chemo treatments were to continue until the white blood count was down to zero.

I had to stay on the horse even if it killed me.

The rest of Monday went fairly well, and I didn't even attempt to explain to Karen what had happened. At around 11:00 on Tuesday morning, Karen was transferred from her room in the ICU to an isolation room in the Adult Cancer Care Unit.

As we loaded her up to make her way down to the fifth floor, I was somewhat upbeat because I saw this as a positive step. She was no longer in critical condition requiring the ICU level of care, and now she was transitioning to the area of the hospital where the nurses dealt with only cancer patients and understood the special needs of patients like Karen. To me, this meant we had survived the initial scare and were moving on to a unit that dealt strictly with cancer. But to Karen there was nothing to celebrate.

"I'm not looking forward to this," she said.

When we got to the isolation unit, I better understood her lack of enthusiasm. The room was very, very small consisting of a utility area near the entry separated by a wall with a large picture window. There was a bed, a lounge chair, a portable toilet, a TV and a little table on rollers. This was definitely much simpler than her room in the state-of-the-art ICU unit.

Reality had set in for Karen, and she had to be thinking, "Yes, it's true, I have cancer, and now I really am in a living hell."

Karen had been to the Jewish concentration camp called Dachau in 1982 when she backpacked throughout Europe. And now she was in her own little virtual Dachau. She was held hostage, imprisoned and was no doubt wondering whether she would make it out alive.

My dad headed back to Akron on Tuesday, while Tom, Pat, and Nora were slated to be in Indianapolis. He had been an invaluable mentor for me during the past several days. We had dined together; he had offered sound advice, and he complimented me several times on how I was handling this difficult situation. As he prepared to leave, he told me, "I think the Lord kept me around just for this one Father's Day." I think he was making reference to his own recent ordeal with his heart. It was a Father's Day we'll both never forget.

On Tuesday, I finally had the time to write the following journal entry. I had obviously decided to leave the details of Father's Day evening out of the public domain. I had relayed the details of the incident to her immediate family and reassured everyone that she was fine, except for the cancer.

I had no way of knowing the update written below would be the last one I'd make for a long time.

Tuesday, June 18, 2002 at 12:35 PM

Karen described her last night in the ICU as a little confusing. Early Monday she spoke with members of Dr. Cripe's Oncology Team assigned to her case. A group of three interns, resembling ER's Dr. Carter of five years ago, watched the briefing. The bottom line of the briefing was that Karen would be moved to a cozy unit in the isolation wing of the 5th floor.

Isolation means just what the word says: The visiting policy in this unit is very strict and will be followed to the letter. No exceptions, including Mark!

Her blood labs at that point were: WBC down to 1,360 and is NOW to 534. Hemoglobin is 8.4 and platelets at 24. The subtype strain of AML, with a 99% probability, is M3.

Respiratory therapy ended after she arrived in the isolation wing. Her lungs are clearing just fine and in a few days are expected to be near normal.

Miss Kimmie Wetzel and Amy Jackson, our wonderful neighbors, monitored her care. These ladies are wonderful as they immediately volunteered to staff Day One of the newly established Karebear Nursing Corps. Their mission will be headed by Karen's mother, Pat Bird, and is designed to help Karen as she recuperates while in the isolation unit. More details to follow. Mark worked on coordinating staffing and continued to monitor numerous fronts.

Rejoice—it's a beautiful day here in Indy. Her loving and devoted father, Tom, returned from Ohio for a visit, as did other family members. Pat Bird is in transit.

CHAPTER 16

Soldier Field

When I awoke on Wednesday morning at about 5:30, I had a stroke of genius. I called Scott Zigmond to see what he thought about my idea. I had remembered that Karen, when told almost a week earlier that she would receive the chemotherapy intravenously, had said, "Fine; as long as I don't have to do 100 pushups, I'm okay. If I had to do pushups I'd be dead, so if all I have to do is lie here, then let the chemo flow."

My idea was that I'd get all my CRHP brothers to do pushups for Karen; we'd tape them doing the pushups on her behalf and then play it back for her on the VCR. I thought it also would be cool if the guys on my CRHP team wore Cleveland Browns jerseys, sweatshirts or T-shirts to give the video that training camp look. I called Scott with my idea and caught him at the Louisville Airport traveling on business. His first response was, "You're crazy, but okay!"

He picked up all the Browns gear and talked my CRHP brothers into doing "Pushups for Karen." They must have thought this was nuts, but they did it anyway.

I arrived at the hospital a little later in the morning, and Karen's mom and dad were already there. One of things I was worried about was Karen's care for the month of June and into July while she was in isolation. My reference to KareBear Nursing Corps in Tuesday's Caringbridge journal entry was no mistake. My goal was to create an organized workforce consisting of female members of the family and friends who could coordinate with one another and make sure Karen had adequate coverage during her prolonged stay in the isolation unit. Also, Karen was feeling very vulnerable, and most men, other than immediate family and me, were not welcome in the isolation unit.

About one in the afternoon, David Gregg, one of my CRHP brothers, the lone bachelor in the group, had stopped by Karen's room looking for me. He cared about what was going on with Karen, but his major concern was with me, and eventually he tracked me down at Chancellor's, where I was eating lunch with Tom. Over lunch, I could tell Tom's overall attitude had changed. He was now totally on board and had accepted the fact that Karen had leukemia. His attitude was better and he was impressed with the level of care his daughter was receiving at IUMC. The effects of the morphine were gone and Karen was becoming more assertive and responsive. To me, it was a time where you had to be positive and play with the cards we were dealt, even though we didn't like them.

While we were at lunch, I mentioned to Tom that maybe we could play some golf later in the week given that Karen's situation had stabilized. Then I started to grow more and more agitated with how long it was taking to order, eat, get the bill and get out of there. David Gregg tried to calm me down and get me to relax. On the way back to the hospital, I decided to sit down in the grass and say an Our Father. David joined me, but Tom continued walking back toward the hospital. David sensed I was not acting like myself. He gave me a quick hug and said we were in his prayers, and then headed off to an appointment.

The hospital had strict rules on the number of visitors she could have each day and the number of times one could go in and out of her room. She could have a total of three visitors only and they were allowed to cross over into her living area six times total between the three visitors each day. This was a strict rule. I was bound and determined, given Karen's compromised immune system, that those rules would be followed to the letter.

I needed to get back to the office at the Midwest ISO to check on some paperwork for Karen and make sure my paychecks would continue. Lori Spence had also prepared a healthcare representative power of attorney that I needed to get Karen to sign. When I went to the parking deck and attempted to start the Bonneville, the battery was dead.

I decided to just lay down flat on the seat where I couldn't be seen.

My mind was starting to play tricks on me.

I had just seen a scene in some cop show where a guy got blown away in his car, a sitting duck trapped in a parking deck. At that moment, I was positive someone might try and do the same thing to me. After lying low in the car for about five minutes, I decided the best thing to do was to get away from the car. Once I got out of the parking deck, I made two calls. I called Jim Holsclaw, a new young attorney at the Midwest ISO with whom I had been working on a proposed merger, and told him I needed a ride from the hospital to the office and back. Then I called my Bill Grace, another one of our great neighbors on Garden Gate Way, and told him my car had massive electrical problems. I gave him the location and asked him to take it to the Pontiac dealer. I left the keys for Bill at the information desk at the hospital, and waited for Jim Holsclaw to drive me north to the office.

When I got to the office, I stopped by and saw Jim Torgerson, our CEO. I had only talked to Jim once over the phone right after Karen was admitted to IUMC. He was very supportive and reassuring. His instructions to me were clear: "Don't worry about your job. Your job is to take care of your wife."

I tried to relax; at one point I put my feet up on his desk, but only after asking Jim if it was okay first. This was all very out of character for me and for Jim, who is very professional and proper, but he cut me some slack and was tolerant of my request.

I was really trying to chill, but I just couldn't.

A little bit later, I saw many of my friends at the company. Donna Dare, Dorothy Shute, Kelli Williams and Anastasia Heinzelman stopped over to give me a hug and wish us their best. I took some time to show them the critical path Karen was on, and I charted the startling acceleration in Karen's white blood count that was at the core of our concern. This number had to be lowered if remission was ever going to be achieved. Lori Spence came in with the power of attorney documents I had requested, and then around five Jim Holsclaw drove me back south to the hospital. Lori could tell I wasn't right. Later she told tell me she had thought about calling my dad.

On the way back downtown, I was growing more paranoid, telling Jim of the hazards that lied ahead of us and how to drive around them. As we drove south on Meridian, I got a call from Katie Hincher, and she told me that my family was not following the rules regarding visitation in the isolation unit; that it was up to the family to follow the rules and act in the best interests of the patient.

"The family is on the honor system to follow the protocol," she said.

"I can't be there every damn minute. It's your hospital, you figure out how to maintain adherence to your policy. I can't be there 24 hours a day," I shouted back at her and hung up.

I know I used some bad language while I talked to Katie, which wasn't like me.

"Volpe, you've got to relax, man," Jim said.

He dropped me at the entry, and I ran into the hospital. Nora Wilson had arrived earlier in the day, and I vaguely remember telling Nora that I needed to get Karen to sign the healthcare power of attorney. I remember getting Karen to sign it, and then I stashed it in my black leather briefcase.

Next, I started roaming the halls. I ran up to the ICU waiting area on the sixth floor for some reason, and I ran into a set of little boys who were just adorable. They were black, and I remember hunching down to their level to just say hello and ask them their names.

It was a large family, and when I said to them, "Are you two twins?" they all smiled at each other as if to say, "Stupid white boy, of course we're twins. Ain't it obvious?"

I said, "I know what you two are thinking; you're thinking, stupid honky."

And then I stood up and was out of there, cruising back to the fifth floor. I could feel my pulse and heart starting to pump so rapidly that I could hear it. I stopped one of the nurses on the floor and made her take my pulse. I even flirted with her a little, which was very out of character for me. Then, as I was walking in front of the nurses' station, I remember saying, "Nonsense, I haven't any indigestion," which was my last line in a play back in high school when I played Mr. Kirby in *You Can't Take It With You*. This line had just popped into my brain.

I saw myself as an actor on a stage.

Then I heard a voice inside my head that sounded exactly like the voice I had heard months earlier in the Ministry Center on my CRHP weekend. "Don't worry, I've got you!" This time I recognized it as the voice of God, not my dad, and I heard him say to me, "Let it loose, you've got to make a point and take one for the team. I won't let anything bad happen to you, but it's time to go for it and say whatever is on your mind to make your point. Release your inner inhibitions and say whatever you need to say. Your father-in-law is out of control and you need to do whatever it takes to make him follow the rules."

I saw my father-in-law coming down the corridor from Karen's room and I let it fly. "Tom, you're such an asshole; it's time that you all start following the rules."

Next, I grabbed a diploma or something that was framed off the wall and I rifled it sidearm through the CRT that sat at the nurse's station. Pat was there too, and she just looked at me with a shocked and horrified look.

I loved her dearly, so I didn't say anything bad to her. But I let her ex-husband have it again, yelling, "Tom, you're so arrogant, I've had it with your attitude."

And then all of a sudden I was taken down very quickly, although gently, by two big black security guards. They were dressed in their brown security uniforms, having been called in to handle my tirade. There I was flat on my face, eating the carpet, as they slapped handcuffs on me. I remembered the words I had heard from the voice inside my head, and I wasn't scared at all of being hurt.

Then I heard the voice say, "Don't worry, you won't lose track of any of your things that are important to you."

The security guards slowly rubbed my back and tried to calm me down. We were in a small office just behind the nurse's station. The security guards were pretty cool to me. These guys had biceps four times as large as mine, and they had no trouble handling me. I had made my point, but now reality had set in and I had to pay the price.

I remembered the voice telling me again, "Just let it all hang out, say what's on your mind."

So I turned to one of the security guards and said, "What is it with you black guys? Is it true that just because you have bigger dicks than us white guys, you think you're better than us just 'cause of that?"

He kind of laughed as I pointed out all of my stuff that they were taking inventory of: my cell phone, cash and wallet. Then I saw a hockey puck on the floor, and I decided that it belonged to my William, who had just taken up ice hockey, even though I knew it wasn't his. I just laid there, face down and tried to gather myself.

Then I said to the security guy, who continued to rub my back, "So are you a Colts fan?" I figured he was from Indianapolis.

And he said, "No, I'm actually a Chicago Bears fan."

This simple reply made me go absolutely ballistic. Now I was screaming at the top of my lungs, "You are the luckiest bastards. I still can't believe that game. You lucky bastards!"

I was referring to the game I had seen at Soldier Field the prior season with Ed Lennox, Darlene Tolbert and her new boyfriend, Eric. The Browns led by two touchdowns with about four minutes left, and they let the Bears drive down the field and use up the clock, scoring a TD with inside of a minute left in the game. Then the Bears recovered the onside kick, ran a quick pass to get near midfield. As time expired, a deflected "Hail Mary" pass was caught out of the air on the rebound by the Bears running back trailing the play just before it hit the ground. The game was tied, and on the Browns first possession in overtime, Tim Couch had a third-down pass deflect off one his own offensive lineman's helmet out to Mike Brown of the Bears, who grabbed the floater, took it to the end zone, and then took a hard left straight to the Bears' locker room, having repeated the feat for the second week in a row—a miracle win in overtime. The Niners had been the victims a week prior. I walked out of that historic stadium feeling very dejected.

So now I had gone nuts a second time, and they knew it was time to get my ass out of there. They put me on a gurney, and as they wheeled me out of the hospital. I was screaming at the top of lungs the same words Al Michaels yelled into the microphone during the final seconds of the U.S. Olympic Hockey team 1980 upset of the Russians at Lake Placid:

"DO YOU BELIEVE IN MIRACLES? YES
DO YOU BELIEVE IN MIRACLES? YES
DO YOU BELIEVE IN MIRACLES? YES
DO YOU BELIEVE IN MIRACLES? YES!"

Rapid-fire thoughts consumed my mind. I was convinced that God had picked Karen to restore man's faith in the existence of God after 9/11. In my sleep-deprived mind, I had also contrived a theory that Karen had been chosen as God's vehicle to restore man's faith in God—she would be near death and miraculously recover from cancer against insurmountable odds and return home. She would restore the tarnished image of the Catholic Church, which had been in the news with so many allegations involving priests molesting young boys in Boston. Her recovery would quickly become a well-documented, modern-day miracle that would be in newspaper headlines all over the world, and Karen would become famous as the person who survived an incurable form of cancer and then returned to everyday life. I figured she would be on *Oprah*, *The Today Show* and even do her own speaking tour telling her fabulous story of faith and courage.

I pictured her leaving the hospital in her wedding gown with all of the news media present.

As they wheeled me out into the parking lot, I was screaming and half-singing like a jeering schoolboy over and over: "I broke the story, I broke the story, hah, hah, hah, hah, hah!" I was positive that I was a modern-day prophet and knew something the entire world would know in just a matter of days.

My wheels had come off, just as Stan Crisci had predicted. While they loaded me into the back of the paddy wagon, I noticed Aunt Patty and Uncle Bob had just arrived to visit Karen and they witnessed the end of the incident.

"Patty, I need a hug," I said when I saw her, and she obliged, reassuring me that everything would be okay. She had a calming effect on me, and Nora's husband, Barry, who also happened to be in the IUMC entryway, told me to just calm down and do what they said.

Then I saw an Indianapolis police officer whose nametag read "James Taylor." So I struck up a verse of "Sweet Baby James," singing away at the top of my lungs, *"Sweet greens and blues are the colors I choose; won't you let me go down in my dreams..."*

Reality set in again as the door to the paddy wagon was slammed shut and locked.

It was hot and dark inside.

I thought to myself, "I think I'm in big trouble now. My parents are really going to be so pissed when they find out."

I was in handcuffs for the first time in my life.

CHAPTER 17

Margaritaville

As the paddy wagon drove off, I sat there in the warmth of the darkness and tried to gather myself in this scene straight out of *Cops*. I thought that I was dreaming, or maybe even dead. Then it dawned on me: I'm in handcuffs. I had been a bad boy and now it was time to pay the price. I had taken one for the team. I had a big smile on my face because finally the incident on my CRHP weekend made sense to me. The voice I had heard moments earlier that evening before my outburst was God talking to me through the Holy Spirit. I was convinced I was actually touched by the power of the Holy Spirit and God was using me as his mouthpiece here on Earth. I believed deep down in my heart that this was the case.

I knew better than everyone else, they'd soon see.

What was I supposed to do now, I thought, as I muttered to myself, "Now you've done it!" The acoustics in the paddy wagon were superb, better than any shower.

I started to sing, *"Wasted away again in Margaritaville, searching for my lost shaker of salt. Some people say that there's a woman to blame, but I know it's my own damn fault."*

Okay, so I took some liberties with the lyrics. *"It's nobody's fault"* are the right words, but this predicament was definitely my own fault.

I'm sure the two guys driving thought I was totally out of my gourd—well, I was temporarily off my rocker. So I sang it again, just to entertain them. Actually I was only entertaining myself, but it sounded so good that I cut it loose again.

"Wasted away again in Margaritaville, searching for my lost shaker of salt. Some people say that there's a woman to blame, but I know it's my own damn fault." When you stop and think about it, the irony of the lyrics was most apropos.

We didn't drive too far from IUMC when the paddy wagon came to a stop. I heard the policemen outside talking a little, and then they swung the door open and I scooted out with my hands cuffed behind my back. I thought, if this isn't a dream, I might have to call Lori Spence and have her send me over an attorney. I could be in deep shit.

Then they tried to get me to sit on a gurney, and I said, "Officer, with all due respect, I'd love to cooperate, but if I sit down on that thing I'll be giving myself a handcuff enema and that won't feel so hot."

Finally, they let me lay on my side. I was in some sort of large indoor garage; the setting kind of reminded me of the arena where Ruby shot Oswald.

I eventually figured out that I was at another hospital as they wheeled me into a large room near the emergency room that looked like the drunk tank. I was in there for the longest time, and my mind continued to play tricks on me.

At one point I was convinced that I was able to ride on a magic carpet like Aladdin, and that my kids and I could glide through the air just like Aladdin. Everything was so colorful. I also thought that maybe I was dead.

Then a nurse came in to check on me, and I said, "What's your name?"

She said, "Nurse!" and she turned on her heel and left. She was a redhead with a beautiful face, and one big butt that reminded me of Matilda.

I was thinking, "Wow, a pretty Irish-looking redhead like my Karen and the rather large hips of my former girlfriend all built into one."

I wasn't sure if my mind was still playing more tricks on me. Moments later, I was sure that our old dog, Calgary, that I had put down years earlier on my birthday, would return to us as a puppy.

Then I yelled, "Nurse!" and eventually she came in.

"I have to pee."

She brought me a portable container like the one they gave me in the hospital with my Achilles surgery, which I filled to the brim while still restrained by the handcuffs. Then they wheeled me into the ER, and I finally got a clue as to where I was. It was Wishard Memorial Hospital, where they take the indigent.

This was not a pretty place!

An armed policeman roamed the room. Just behind the drape next to me sat a very crabby lady from a trailer park and her son. Her boyfriend had just beaten her up and her son was talking about getting revenge.

"I'm so pissed at that man I could do about anything right now, including killing that son of a bitch myself," he was saying.

I took off my shoes and held them near my head, afraid that someone might start some random shooting at any time.

By now I was genuinely scared, but I kept going back to the words I had heard in my head earlier. I knew God was not going to let anything bad happen to me, but I was still in a scary place. The mother and son next to me argued about their situation for an hour.

By now I had calmed down and kept promising the ER people I would not do any other stupid things. They relented and took off the handcuffs in favor of soft restraints. Then

I managed to get the attending physician to lend me his cell phone. I had trouble remembering phone numbers, but finally I got in touch with the Wetzels. I explained my situation, and asked Marty to come down and stay with me.

The folks at Wishard told me that I had to go over to Community North Hospital for a psychiatric evaluation. I was also informed that I was very lucky because they weren't going to press charges against me for disorderly conduct. Someone told me that my parents and brother were on their way. I couldn't figure out why no one from Karen's family had come to check on me; I was dismayed that they had abandoned me.

Later I found out that the social workers at IUMC had advised my in-laws to keep their distance because they were the objects of my anger at the time of my outburst. I want to make it crystal clear. My in-laws were not the reason I had lost it. It was my own damn fault. I had not taken care of myself, not slept enough, and probably drank too much even though I had been warned of the danger.

While I waited for Paul in the ER at Wishard, Marty Wetzel, Bill Grace and Gary Dufek eventually arrived. I could tell Marty was pissed. He had been trying to get with me to have a talk for a week, and I hadn't been able to find the time. I really admire and respect Marty. He had lost his second wife years earlier. He wanted to talk with me about my situation, and I knew he had a message for me.

Marty's a big guy and hard to miss. He played one year in the NFL, as a linebacker with the Jets in '82 after a great college career at Tulane, but a knee injury ended his pro career early. When he got a chance, he told me we were going to have the conversation I had been putting off. Marty told me that the neighbors were willing to dig ditches for my family, but I had grown to be very demanding. He told me some of the details regarding what happened with his wife and the events related to her death. He had tried to help the doctors figure out what was wrong, and had done a lot of his own research in an attempt to help.

Bill Grace, the self-designated Mayor of Hazel Dell, and Gary Dufek were very supportive and helpful. Paul heard about my trouble and drove in directly from Grand Rapids, Michigan, and was in Indianapolis in a record four hours. My parents and Kevin weren't far behind. Paul picked me up, and I was released to his custody, contingent on me seeing a psychiatrist at Community North immediately. I was so happy to get out of there. Paul took me to Community North, and my parents arrived soon thereafter, at about 3:00 in the morning.

I explained to the psychiatrist that I had been under a lot of stress with my wife's cancer, and I hadn't been sleeping well. I told him that I was mad at my father-in-law because he had been so negative 10 days earlier. I said my anger was directed at the old Tom and not the new Tom, who had returned with a totally different attitude and was now on the A-Team.

I purposely didn't mention anything about my recent revelation that I had been touched by the Holy Spirit at my CRHP retreat and had been hearing voices prior to and during my outburst even though it was the truth. I knew that if I spilled my guts they would admit me to my own rubber room, and I might never see the light of day again.

My parents both stuck up for me and my mom said, "Mark never had any problems growing up. He was the gem of consistency. He's a good dad with a successful career. This was an isolated incident."

Community North released me to my parents' supervision, and at about 5:00 in the morning, I got into bed, but my problems didn't go away.

Around 7:00 I awoke and I found some scratch paper. I drew out my mind's view of what was transpiring. The picture I drew was a rough rendition of the front cover of Mario Puzo's *The Godfather*. I drew hands and wrote a label above that said, "The Hands of God." Then, I drew puppet strings down to a man I labeled as Mark Volpe. This was how my mind was working. God had chosen Karen as the vehicle to prove to all mankind that he did exist, and I was the person who would break the story and announce to the world that the collective Coyne-Volpe Family was chosen to bring this message to all non-believers, including those Catholics who had strayed from their faith. All those who questioned whether a benevolent and loving God would allow so many innocent lives to be lost on 9/11 and then also allow priests, his representatives on Earth, to prey on young boys would see the light. Karen had been hand-picked to fix it—she was worthy of the miracle, and I believed this was all part of his "Grand Plan." I was not to question his commands, if I truly believed. I would do what he asked of me despite the fact that everyone would call me crazy.

I spent Thursday morning relaxing at home and lying on the hammock in the backyard. My dad found my drawings and other ranting and ravings that I had written and he tore them up. Many neighbors stopped by to see how I was doing. I just hung out on the hammock. At times I thought that if I fell asleep, I would accidentally fall through the hammock and strangle myself to death. Solid sleep had eluded me for days, and my mind was not sound.

Around noon I asked Paul to crawl into bed next to me to make sure I didn't do anything stupid. The suicide scene from *An Officer And A Gentleman* kept running through my severely compromised little brain.

Somehow, I had formed this theory that some people do not voluntarily commit suicide. God just takes them by the hand and makes them take their own lives, leaving us behind to question why this person took his or her own life, when they had so much to live for. I did not want to hurt or kill myself, but I knew I was not in total control of my own thought process. I was very paranoid and totally hyper.

Paul lay there next to me for several hours. At one point, about 3:00 p.m., I got up and my mom suggested I take a shower. While I was in the shower I thought I was Dany Gans from Vegas. I remember singing some Billy Joel songs, *"In the middle of the night I was walking in my sleep..."*

When I got out of the shower, I decided to totally blow my mom away. I was singing every word to "Born To Run" in perfect key, and I was strumming my air guitar like Bruce. The difference was Bruce wears black jeans, and I wasn't wearing anything at all as I left the master bath area and strolled out into the bedroom.

I told Paul, "The entire generation of Volpe men is going to die. We were all going down the toilet. It's our turn, and there is nothing we can do about it; my sons are toast and so are your little boys, Anthony and Matthew."

Paul just couldn't get through to me.

My mind was way out there.

I had some sort of vision of the names of all the saints and my mind flashed back to Grandma Schultz's funeral. Then I remembered Aunt Diane and Aunt Dorothy, my mom's twin sisters, who are 12 years younger than her, and how they seemed so calm and at peace at the funeral. I remembered Diane telling me that right before Grandma died, Grandma awoke one morning and said she had a vision of heaven and that it was so beautiful.

All the family and people she loved were there including her husband, Bill, who had been dead since 1963.

My mom handled my oddball behavior pretty well. Later I found out that she had called Amy Jackson and Kimmie Wetzel to tell them I had lost my mind and it was time to get me some real help. My mom tried to get me back into bed, and she attempted to get me to relax and visualize the sand between my toes, with the waves of the ocean running over my feet. She had given me a Valium, but it didn't help me at all. My mind was hypersensitive. The lack of sleep over the past two weeks had finally caught up with me.

I had officially lost it!

Meanwhile, Kevin was downtown with Karen and his family. The situation was ugly. Confusion reigned over who was in charge of Karen's care and who had access to her isolation room. Kevin was standing guard outside her door, limiting access to her room. He felt the situation was out of control and he made sure access to Karen's room was limited. Bear in mind that following the hospital's rules regarding visitation and access to Karen was critical at this point because Karen's immune system had been so heavily compromised. Even a common cold could kill her. Everybody was doing what he or she thought was best and were acting in the best interests for the both of us, but this situation was far from ideal.

Kevin had to do all of this without Karen even knowing he was there because he was supposed to be in Ohio taking care of my kids. Colleen was handling our children and theirs all by herself. Karen remembers my parents as the ones who were asserting control over the situation and restricting access to her room, while my parents insist the shots were all being called by the social workers at IUMC. I know that everybody did what he or she thought was best at the time.

It was my perception, based on the phone call I had received the previous day from Katie Hincher, that the visitation rules were not being followed, thus jeopardizing Karen's condition.

At the insistence of the hospital social workers, Karen was kept totally in the dark as to my condition. Without anyone having access to Karen's room, she was left alone for a long time when she needed her mother.

She was only told that I was relaxing on the hammock in the backyard and taking it easy. When my parents visited, Karen inquired as to my status, and my parents told her not to worry about her husband, that I was going to be fine, but that it was going to take some time.

This situation was entirely my fault, and I feel horrible about having created this set of circumstances when my wife was in what essentially amounted to solitary confinement. Right before my outburst, I had asked her to sign the health care power of attorney form. She said later that she had noticed I was very hyperactive, that I wouldn't sit down, and I kept wringing my hands. She was worried about me, but her mind was primarily on her battle with cancer.

So far, the chemo was slowly working its magic, and her white count was coming down. The goal was to strip her of all white blood cells and get her count down to zero.

Winning the war with cancer was what really mattered and whatever happened to me was of little consequence.

CHAPTER 18

Psychiatric Unit

Twenty-four hours after my outburst, my delirium got worse. I called Amy and Kimmie and asked them if they believed in miracles. They were very nice and told me everything was going to be okay. I remember sitting down at the PC and typing out some nonsensical gibberish on America Online that I had intended to send to everyone. I remember writing something to the effect that Mark and Karen were the "New Adam and Eve," sent here by God to restore man's faith in his existence, that he was omnipotent, and that despite all the evidence of prevailing evil that was going on in the world, "God still ruled and his love for us as his children would prevail." I predicted out loud that a magnificent and majestic cathedral would one day be built, before the turn of the century, on the site where St. Louis de Montfort Catholic Church now stood.

I never sent the e-mail.

I also recall looking at a set of numbers and colors, from a magazine, with my mom in the kitchen. Every number and color had meaning and symbolized something to me. I still look back at these events and wonder why it never dawned on anyone to give me something that would make me sleep. Hours later it was time for bed and I refused to lie down, so my mom called our neighbor, Gary Dufek, and turned me over to him because they were all exhausted after dealing with my antics for a day. I hadn't slept right for 12 days. No matter what I did, I could not get my mind to calm down.

I told Gary I wanted to go over to the fire department to see the trucks and maybe sleep there with his firemen buddies. It seemed like a safe place to me; besides, when I was a kid, I loved fire engines. Gary took me out for an ice cream cone, and while we ate the ice cream a couple of teenagers were driving in circles in the parking lot, making me very paranoid. They were far away from us, but I was certain they were going to turn and run us both down. Then Gary drove back to our subdivision, and as he drove I was having panic attacks at every intersection. I was sure that as we neared each intersection, the cars heading in the opposite direction would miss their stop sign or blow off the light and slam into my side of the truck, killing both of us instantly. There had been a recent accident in the news in which an area high school basketball star had died at an intersection when his car was hit broadside. I was sure the same thing was going to happen to Gary and me.

Then I noticed Gary was on his cell talking to someone, but I couldn't tell who it was; I thought it was one of the guys at the fire station. Later I found out that he was talking to Dr. Todd Arnold, our neighbor, and I remember Gary saying at one point, "No, he's not right. We're on our way."

As we approached the entry to the subdivision, I told Gary to hurry up. I was sure my dad had just had a heart attack. When we rounded the corner, I expected to see lots of emergency vehicles. It was probably midnight or 1:00 a.m., and there were no EMTs to be seen. I was still sure that my dad was dying from a heart attack and we had to go in the house and check on him. Stan Crisci, Todd Arnold, Bill Grace and Joel Jackson were there. I started screaming that we had to check on my dad right away, that I was sure his heart had given out, we needed to get him to the hospital stat and shock him with the paddles right away because he was going to die. The guys assured me he was okay, and that I needed to shut up because I was going to wake up everybody in the house. Then I asked Stan if I could autograph his Cubs T-shirt, and he kept telling me to get away because he liked the shirt. Next thing I knew, they had me back in Gary's Chevy Avalanche headed toward Community North Hospital.

When we got to the hospital they put me in a little room with a bed, and they started playing euchre.

"Volpe, lie down and get some sleep, you're a hurting unit," Stan said.

I stayed there for 40 minutes, still hypersensitive and paranoid that I would try to hang myself. Every time I would come out to check on the card game, which made zero sense because I absolutely hate to play cards, they would say get your butt back in there and sleep. It was like I was a little four-year old that refused to put his head down.

After about the fourth time, Stan said, "That's it, you need to check yourself in here and get your shit together. Billy Joel just did the same thing today at a substance abuse center; trust us buddy, we wouldn't steer you wrong; we're your friends and you've got to do this for at least 24 hours."

I reluctantly agreed, and they took me into the psychiatric ward where I signed myself in on a voluntary basis for at least 24 hours. They told me I was doing the right thing and everything would be fine. When the door slammed behind me I approached the desk, and this older lady wearing all sorts of jewelry made me fill out some forms. I could hardly fill out the forms and I was making no sense. She tried to ask me some questions. I could hardly talk or understand what she was saying. They put me in a room and told me to try and sleep, and explained that

I'd do better at my evaluation the next morning if I slept. I kept leaving my sleep room and going out to the main room, where there were tables and magazines. I tried to hide on the floor, but the staff knew I was roaming the place.

One of the attendants offered me an injection to help get me to sleep, but I refused. I remembered something my dad had told me earlier in life that didn't allow me to trust them.

"Once you let them stick that needle in your arm, you're not in control; they're the ones in control," he had said.

I think he was talking about what happens prior to surgery, but I just remembered not to trust anyone who would try to stick me with a needle, and in all honesty, this was all I needed. If I could be put down for 12 hours of sleep, then my brain would return to some semblance of normal functioning, but I was not going to fall for any tricks.

I thought the guy who insisted I get a shot to help me sleep told me to write a letter to my kids, but in actuality he gave me no such set of instructions. For hours, I sat there in my room and wrote out advice to each of my three children; parts of the letter read like a will. Then I noticed the sun was starting to come up, and I still hadn't slept. I had now been dealing with Karen's ordeal for 12 days without the benefit of any meaningful sleep. I tore up my written instructions to my kids, suddenly realizing that if these incoherent writings were discovered, I'd never get my ass out of there.

For a time, I thought about the horrors of the Holocaust, Hiroshima, 9/11 and all the wars and plagues that had happened during the course of recorded history. Somehow I concluded my own death would be the result of colon cancer, or maybe mental illness had set in, and I was destined to kill myself even though I had everything to live for.

When I came out of my room, there were all sorts of people wandering the halls and most of them looked like shit. I was convinced I had signed myself into some sort of insane asylum, and that I was one of those people who would be institutionalized for life like Dustin Hoffman in *Rainman*. I would become a lost case, forgotten for years. I screwed up and left my friends and was now in the hands of strangers.

Talk about totally delusional!

Dr. Seward came in and interviewed me. I made no sense as I explained what had recently transpired. He said I was definitely in a state of mania and that they could help me. As they escorted me off to my room, I was positive that someone was plotting to blow my head off like what had happened to JFK. I did manage to call Paul, and I told him to please come and get me, that I had figured everything out. To me this was a big joke, like an old episode of *Mission Impossible* that had accomplished its goal. I promised to be a good boy, but I was also wary of getting too close to windows for fear that I would throw myself out to my death. I was still very confused.

I was in the Community North Psychiatric Unit with the worst patients. After the first night, I finally slept for eight hours straight, thanks to the medications they had put me on. I was starting to feel like myself again. I did what I was told. I knew I had to toe the line to get back to my wife, so I really tried to follow all the rules.

There were no delusional behavior or bizarre thoughts happening after I got a solid night's sleep. My fellow patients in the ward had a broad spectrum of assorted problems. There were multiple personality types, substance abusers, schizophrenics, people who were suicidal and others suffering from depression in the ward. And then there was me, a successful aspiring executive, whose wife had cancer, and after 12 days of sleep deprivation, my mind had finally come apart. I had a manic episode and was delusional to the point of panic attacks. I played by all the rules, took my medications, ate all the meals, and went outside on cigarette breaks just to get some fresh air. I completed all the workshops on coping skills and stress management.

I even did some arts and crafts as part of the program, making a poster for Karen that had a *Born in the U.S.A.* theme with a guy in the Army from a recruiting ad in a magazine. I put my initials on his helmet, like a football helmet logo, and I added the caption, "I'm going in after Karen." Getting back to my sick wife was my primary concern.

Dr. Samuels was in charge of my case. He interviewed my parents for awhile in the hall after I was there a few days. I could barely hear them as I tried to eavesdrop on the conversation. My parents stuck up for me and explained that I had never been in any trouble, no substance abuse problems, no similar behavior previously, a successful career, a good husband and father.

A day later they visited me and brought along Jim Holsclaw, our new young attorney at the Midwest ISO. I signed a financial power of attorney that allowed my dad to make financial decisions on our behalf. Karen was concerned that we might lose our house, and she expressed this concern to my dad, so my parents and Stan Crisci took over our finances until we were back to normal. My dad assured Karen that there was no way we would lose our home.

While I was in the psych ward, I tried to help and befriend other patients in the ward. Many of them took a genuine interest in my circumstances, wished me the best and encouraged me to leave. The most interesting patient was a woman suffering from a split personality. In actuality, she had three different personas.

My roommate made me paranoid. His name was Michael Jamerson, and he confessed to me that in his younger days, when he dealt drugs on the streets of Chicago, he had popped a guy in a drug deal gone wrong. He said he had actually seen the gray matter pour from his head just above his ear.

He seemed to be a gentle and changed man, but I had to keep my guard up when I tried to sleep. Now, if you had heard this story from a roomie, wouldn't you also sleep with one eye open like a German shepherd?

By now I was back to reality even though the medication seemed to have dulled my brain and overall ability to react mentally. The meds did help me sleep. I felt as if I was in a prison—you had to wait your turn to use the phone. I always used my time to talk to Karen, and she said I sounded mysterious and weird. I felt like I was under the microscope and that my calls might be monitored in order for the shrinks to figure out where I really was as a psychiatric patient.

Karen was making great progress. Her white counts continued to plummet, and she was concerned more about me. She was convinced I would never work again because my once semi-smart mind had turned to mush. My parents told her that at some point during this general timeframe, although I'm not sure exactly when, that her husband had been diagnosed as suffering from bipolar disorder. They never told me anything. Karen was doing very well at this point and was thinking for herself just fine.

She found this alleged diagnosis to be totally absurd.

After three days of stellar behavior I thought it was time for me to get out, and I expressed a desire to sign the papers that would allow me to depart and get back to my wife. My parents had talked to Dr. Samuels a day or so earlier, and I figured my parents had been able to convince him that my troubles had been an isolated incident and that I just needed a couple of days to gather myself. When I informed the hospital staff I wished to sign the papers for my release, they ignored me. Then I started to show my displeasure with having to stay. I raised my voice and said loudly to the incompetent nurse, who visually reminded me of my estranged sister, and that I needed to get back to my wife. The brown-clad security guys showed up at the door moments later, so I just took a seat right in the middle of the floor so as to not threaten anyone. I decided to go with the flow and not create any more waves. My dad arrived in an hour, and he convinced me not to sign the papers, that it would be a mistake. He was very serious. I trusted him and did as he wished.

I trusted my key mentor in life, my dad. I guess dad had been informed about the incident earlier when I made a little bit of a stink about not being able to sign the papers that would allow me to get back to my wife. My doctor had advised against it, but I thought I was there voluntarily and could leave at my option. My dad advised me that it would be unwise to go leave. A guy who worked there named Mike had taken an interest in my case. Mike talked with me and convinced me that it would be a bad idea for me to leave so soon.

This was a tough time on my parents too; they were both somewhat distraught hearing the names of both Karen and Mark Volpe during the prayers of the faithful at Mass later that week. My dad and mom both teared up, not able to believe what was happening to this fine family.

While I was in the psych unit, several of my friends visited me: Bill Grace, Scott Zigmond and even Alvin Jones, our builder who was working on our lower level, stopped by to see me in the loony bin. Once I had finally gotten some solid sleep, I knew I was fine. So I just went with the program, played by all their stupid damn rules, took the meds and waited. Finally, after a week in the unit, I was allowed to leave for a short time. My dad brought by some nice clothes. I had been given a four-hour pass to see my wife downtown at IUMC. How ironic that both of us were incarcerated. Her fight was with cancer and me for what was allegedly being called mental illness.

It reminded me of the Eagles' "Hotel California."

"You can check out any time you like, but you can never leave!"

On Friday, following my fireworks, Tommy made the following update on the website. Only the people in Carmel and my immediate family knew my wheels had come off and that I had been hospitalized.

I'll always be thankful to Tommy for his outstanding contributions and personal sacrifice throughout this entire ordeal. I'd go to war with this man anyplace, anytime to battle any enemy with the sole purpose of winning no matter what the cause. In this case, it was his sister's life that hung in the balance, and Tommy was just like his strong sister. He refused to lose.

As Vince Lombardi once said, "When the going gets tough, the tough get going!"

Friday, June 21, 2002 at 03:51 PM

Wow. This web page is 1 week old and it has been hit 3,605 times. That is wonderful. Thanks for the support.

Things have been Busy...Busy...Busy. But, everything seems to be moving in the right direction now. I will also try to provide updates a bit more regular as well, but thanks for understanding.

A quote from the nurse who has primary care of Karen might be appropriate to start this off… "She just looks awesome!" Karen is really hanging in there and working hard. The nurses have hung the last bag of chemo…whoever it was who said, "Good to the last drop" WAS OBVIOUSLY NOT TALKING ABOUT CHEMO. She is trying to take a daily walk in the hallways to build her strength. You have never seen someone as motivated. Karen is an inspiration for making it thru this first week.

Her Platelets are up. The Hemoglobin is up. The White Blood Count is floating right around 250 to 300. The doctors are pleased with what they are seeing and how Karen is responding. They are ready for the next step.

This evening Karen will begin receiving hormones via IV that will last 2 weeks. It is designed to help her body begin to grow healthy cells. How cool is that?

Enduring chemo was bad enough, but the immediate fight is boredom. Although, Karen is not ready for visitors, one person can only take so many episodes of Jerry Springer.

Thank you for the love and support of our family as we drive over this speed bump. Will, Samantha, and Mitchell are loved and missed like no other child could be. Please keep them in your hearts and minds, as this is difficult on them too. Upbeat and silly cards to them certainly couldn't hurt.

Thank you once again. Love and Peace.

I continued to fight to get out of the psych ward, and finally Dr. Samuels allowed me to go home on June 26th, but only if I stayed on my meds, Depakote and Zyprexa. All this time, I never lost focus on Karen—helping save her life was all that mattered to me; my own battle was of little meaning because I knew I would live through it and get out. I shaved, showered and put on my best button-down shirt. I needed to get back to my bride. I had played the game, and it was finally time to get back to the woman who needed me. I felt terrible for having let my body fall apart at such a critical time when she needed me most.

I always knew in my heart it was all about sleep deprivation. Nobody had told me about the bipolar diagnosis while I was at Community North. I reviewed the circumstances leading up to my mania for Dr. Samuels, and he just listened. It didn't seem to matter to him, that I had been a straight arrow for 43 years, and under these extraordinary circumstances I had let my brain wear out.

Mike, on the hospital staff, explained to me that once the body doesn't get enough sleep, the chemicals in the brain start to come apart and the cells are unable to connect in a logical and coherent manner. What happened to me is very common among soldiers who are pinned down in a foxhole under mortar fire for days. After no sleep for multiple days, they literally go crazy. The mind can't handle the extreme stress coupled with a lack of sleep. The same thing can happen to adults as it does with little kids who don't get a nap: by late in the day, the child gets nasty. The same anger extends to adults, but can be much more pronounced.

Think about the times during the prior 12 days when my attempts to sleep were thwarted: First there was the incident at St. Vincent's where Karen's heart had stopped for 12 seconds; she had flat lined according to the monitor, when Marty woke me up at 3:00 a.m. to go to the hospital; then there were many nights when I was up late updating the website or consoling

Karen's good friends, who all lived far away, like Margaret Evans, Katie Kibler and Nora Wilson. Each of these wonderful friends felt so helpless being so far away unable to do anything but pray, although Nora was actually in the room with Karen on the evening of my little outburst. Nora did a great job of shielding the truth from Karen when my tirade occurred. Even Karen woke me up one night with a phone call, giving me a laundry list of things for me to accomplish.

The kicker was spending 42 out of 44 stressful hours awake on Father's Day evening and into Monday dealing with Karen's Haldol-related hallucinations. This was the pivotal event, and in my own mind, I know this was the straw that broke the camel's back. If I had gotten to bed that evening at a normal hour, even if it was with the help of a glass of Dewars on the rocks, I don't think I would have ended up in the psych ward. I'm mentally strong and most men would have collapsed from the physical demands much earlier.

My friend Stan Crisci's warning me that if I weren't cautious I would become a patient, too, had come true. It was never intended to become a self-fulfilling prophecy, but he was right. I had spent the longest week of my life in what might as well have been jail. Even though I wasn't free to go home, my mind was constantly on my wife. I read magazines and spent as much time as I could in the gym shooting baskets, dribbling the length of the court and taking long jumpers from three-point range. Then I'd chase down my errant shot and take off dribbling toward the other end. At times, I started to find the range and would occasionally make three or four in a row from long range, announcing out loud just like Joe Tait, the long-time voice of the Cleveland Cavaliers, "Price for 3—Got it?" I tried hard to work at sharpening both mind and body.

Over this general period of time, Karen was receiving literally hundreds of cards, letters and gifts. There are a handful of items she received from Ohio-based sports celebrities worth mentioning. She received several shirts and hats from the women's sports teams at Ohio State. The women's hockey and basketball teams both sent Karen get well soon wishes. We figure the Gans family from the neighborhood had something to do with these really cool items arriving at our house. Kari and Fred Gans are OSU graduates. Most of their wedding pictures with the bridal party were taken on campus, and some were done at the Horseshoe.

In late June, Karen received two separate packages from Cleveland. Her favorite Cleveland Indian was Jim Thome, even though he had just left the Tribe to become a Philadelphia Phillie, for big bucks, of course. We had last seen the large left-handed slugger at Cinergy Field a few years earlier. He sent Karen an autographed baseball. The Browns even sent along a care package. However, the most interesting item Karen received was from a retired Browns wide receiver that wore #86, Brian Brennan. Brian had played with the Browns during the Kosar era when they lost the AFC Championship Game three times to the hated Broncos. Karen always loved her fellow Irishman. He was like a little leprechaun who always seemed to make the clutch catch on third down to keep the chains moving. Brian was now an investment management executive with McDonald & Company in Cleveland. He had sent Karen an autographed black and white game photo reading, "To Karen, Stay Cool, God Bless and Go Browns, Brian Brennan #86." Brian also took the time to pen a handwritten note to Karen on McDonald Investments stationery, dated June 25, 2002, which read as follows:

Dear Karen,

I was happy to hear I had a big fan in you. I was happy to hear that someone actually remembered me (just kidding, Ha Ha!). I know that you are in the process of going through some treatment. I wanted to write to wish you well during these tough times. When I played people thought I was too small and too slow. But every year I proved them wrong. I believed in myself. I live by 2 Quotes. 1) Life's Battles Don't Always go to the stronger or faster man (or woman), but to the man who knows he can. 2) Never, Never, Never, Never Give Up! I wish you well & I will keep you in my prayers.

God Bless,

Brian

We had both the photo and letter framed and displayed prominently in our lower level near the big screen television, with all of the other sports memorabilia we own as a testament to the virtue of perseverance. NEVER GIVE UP!

The day before I was released, Tommy updated the website again.

Tuesday, June 25, 2002 at 08:20 AM

First things first...Karen continues to respond very well to her treatments. Katie, the official oncology nurse for Team Volpe (all readers of this message are on the team, Congratulations, you made the cut), tells us that Karen is well "ahead of the curve." Yet we are all cautioned that Karen's recovery will not be a straight-line event. Hopefully, it will be less volatile than the stock market, but we should all expect some random up-and-down movements in both her physical progress and her spirit. The activity updates are appreciated and very interesting for Karen; please keep her posted on the people and activities she loves.

Allow an analogy…The game of chess can be very exciting at the beginning, before it settles into a second phase of more controlled and strategic actions of small moves here and there. With her chemo treatments behind her, Karen is soundly in the second phase. While the last traces of chemo are working the way out of her system, she has begun to receive a DNA protein, which regulates the production of white blood cells (WBC) in the bone marrow and reduces the possibility of infection. (Yes, of course, the last sentence was plagiarized.) So, within the next week to ten days we will begin to see Karen's WBC start to rise again.

A brief maintenance item here. Mark has asked the Coyne brothers to keep this page updated. Regrettably, for you, the avid reader, we accepted. Please let us know of anything you think we should post.

At this point, we would be remiss not to acknowledge the time, effort and selfless giving, not to mention the mowing, trimming, watering and mulching, that has been demonstrated by so many of Mark & Karen's friends. Especially their friends from the neighborhood and St. Louis de Montfort. Thank you all very much!

Now, since we know Karen is looking for info on activities…. This past Sunday, the Volpe kids went swimming with their cousins at Uncle Tommy's pool and then had a cookout, bonfire and sleepover at Uncle Kenny's. On Monday, Sam became a "Chadds Ford Shark" with her cousins, Katie and Timmy, and competed in her first swim meet. Brother Will rang-up Mom and gave her a strong play-by-play. Sam led most of the race, but succumbed to a longer girl in the final stretch, a strong second place finish in her first event, the backstroke. She later competed in three more events. Will has joined the junior golf program at a local golf course with cousin Sean and is on the course as Sam and I type this message to you. Mitch, well, Mitch is Mitch. He's one of the coolest guys you could ever spend time with. He's happy, funny, active, loves his books and a new Kinex set he received for his birthday. Later this week, we are going back to Lake Mohawk for a little boating, golfing and fishing with Aunt Colleen's family.

May God continue to bless Mark, Karen, Will, Sam and Mitch!

CHAPTER 19

Garden Gate Way

When I got to Karen, I thought she'd be happy to see me. I was all dressed up and looking good, but at this point, I was just beginning to figure out what had generally transpired while I was gone. At this time, I still didn't know that Dr. Samuels had diagnosed me as being bipolar. This was never explained to me until later. All I knew was that I was supposed to take my medications as directed and then everything would be fine. This was a condition that according to Dr. Samuels, "You'll have to learn to live with for the rest of your life."

Karen's view of the world had changed drastically. She had hypothesized that I would eventually lose my job at the Midwest ISO, and we would be forced to move back to Akron where we would have direct access to family support on a daily basis. She told me that one night, while I was at Community North, she had gotten up late, about 3:00 in the morning, and stared at her scarred and tired body in the mirror. She said to herself, "It's all on you, girl. You've got to get yourself together, get out of here, sell the house and get a job."

To me, this part of the story is totally remarkable and ironic. I believe God had a purpose in forcing me to be institutionalized for a week. I could now empathize with my wife, knowing what it was like to be confined against your will for an extended period of time and be at the mercy of those charged with your care. We were one, right from the moment our mothers lit the unity candle on the altar right before the bridesmaids made their way up the aisle on our wedding day.

Karen was very upset with the situation regarding who had access to her room. I wasn't there, and I take full blame for the ensuing turmoil. Family dynamics and the stress of the situation had left the door open for a lot of hard feelings, and Karen hated the upheaval. She despises conflict and always wants peace and harmony. Everyone has a different side of the story, and everyone wanted to do what was best for Karen; the problem was there wasn't any universal agreement as to how to accomplish this end. In my mind, based on the call I received from Katie Hincher, the protocols regarding the visitation were not being followed and it was my obligation to make sure these rules were followed to the letter.

I had to honor the "in sickness and in health" part of my vows and do everything possible to maximize the odds for a successful recovery. I fully believe that one day, I will have to answer to God for my actions during June 2002. I knew I would stand before him and the Lord would ask me if I had done my best.

Had I done everything possible to ensure my wife recovered from leukemia and came back home so that together we could continue to raise our children as husband and wife, consistent with our vows to accept children lovingly from God?

I was bound and determined to adhere to my part of the contract regardless of who or what got in my way. I know offended people, but to me the end justified the means. I knew that, in time, the wounds would heal. We all wanted the same thing.

I'll never forget what Karen's brother Kenny had said during a ride downtown on his brief visit, prior to all the shit hitting the fan.

"Mark, my friend, you don't have to be nice when it comes to Karen's care. You have to be a dictator!" he said.

Maybe I took his advice too much to heart.

More importantly, a significant milestone had finally occurred, as explained by Tommy in the Caringbridge update below.

Friday, June 28, 2002 at 12:19 PM

Elvis has left the building...

Karen has been released from the hospital and continues to recover at home. Mark and his parents picked Karen up and finished clearing her out of her room just about an hour ago.

Karen does in fact to seem to be ahead of the curve in regard to her recovery. So much so, that it caused the doctors/nurses to double-check their work so to speak. Karen's nurse has told her from Day 1 that if one of her blood tests reaches 500 (I forget which one), then she will be able to go home. The "problem" was that she got to that level much faster than any one expected. She is 16 days or so into her battle, but the doctors say that they would expect to see this type of progress around Day 31 or so.

Karen will continue to return to the hospital for treatments, but that is one of the many things that I am not clear on. Stay posted to this site though...

So, my Sister should be home as I write this. She is looking forward to being with her family, a hot shower and sleeping in her own bed. We're still not sure when Will, Sam and Mitch will get to come home, but I'm sure they will be visiting in the next couple of days.

Thanks to everyone for their interest, prayers, and efforts during the first part of this journey. We will keep you posted as Karen gets adjusted. Hopefully, she can write the next journal entry...

Love,

Tommy

Despite the unlikely odds, the woman was coming home several weeks earlier than Dr. Cripe and Katie Hincher had outlined. She didn't leave in her wedding dress like I had pictured. But to all of us, this was an amazing feat and could definitely be classified as a minor miracle.

"DO YOU BELIEVE IN MIRACLES? YES!"

Karen made her first entry into the journal after resting at home for a few days since I was still not on my "A" game yet. I was relaxing, trying to care for my wife, although I must admit, I don't think at this point I was doing a very good job attending to her needs. Thank God we had a great network of friends from our street, Garden Gate Way, as well as family and friends including fellow parishioners from St. Louis de Montfort. This journal entry was significant because she was still recovering mentally from the events of the month of June, and to me, this outlet of being able to express herself to everyone following her case on the website indicated her mind, as well as her body, were on the road to recovery. A major part of the battle in beating cancer depends on one's mental outlook.

HOW KAREN CONQUERED CANCER

Sunday, June 30, 2002 at 09:13 PM

Hi! It's Elvis. And I'm not dead.

I'm so very thrilled and blessed to be home, back with my family, that I am admitting to so many emotions that I am very much overwhelmed. I had been so very, very sick that a lot of what has transpired are details that I'm still finding out about. The power of prayer and the constant love of family and friends have seen my family through this tragedy. Not in my lifetime, will I ever be able to let each and every one of you know how your notes, cards, prayers, calls and thoughts have sustained me. My life has been forever altered. It felt very much like……..Three weeks ago I was walking down the street…………and then the sky fell…………

You all know that I do not have a medical or technical background. I have learned a lot about my condition out of necessity. I am basically in quarantine in my home until my next bone marrow biopsy on July 15. By the following day, we will know if I am in remission. If not, I go back for additional chemotherapy. If I am not in remission, this is a situation that I am able to consider because I absolutely hated the isolation unit at IUMC. It was scary and lonely, and I felt awful. Special thanks to those of you that wanted to visit and could not as I have to tell you, it just would have been too hard. Cancer, for me, has not been a very social event. I felt the need to dig deep and tough it out as best I could.

Our lives will never be the same. Mark and I just look at each other and cry without saying a word.

Saint Louis de Montfort, our neighborhood, our friends
in Cincinnati, our friends from college and high school,
friends, family, the friends of friends and family…….

Without the power of prayer, I promise to you as I tire and
need to call it quits for the day, I would not be here today.
I love you, Mark loves you, and my children……we thank
you from the bottom of our hearts.

Over the next few days, we had Karen resting comfortably in her own bed. Margaret Evans had flown in from Portland and she was a major help. One of the things I learned early on during this ordeal was how to manage the numerous friends and family who were so generous with their time. There were so many people who were willing to help, but one of the problems with this was that you didn't want to have too many resources downtown at IUMC with Karen or at our house at the same time. I referred to this as the "picket fence" approach to managing these very generous resources. It was better to space them out, than to have them tripping over each other, so on some occasions we'd have to tell someone we were covered for now and that two weeks later would be better. Pat actually tracked and coordinated the schedule for out-of-town family members who were able to come over and help. I did the best I could to deal with the local help in an attempt to maximize the precious use of everyone's time.

I was taking my medications and still having trouble assimilating. As hard as I tried, it seemed that I was slowed mentally and the medication dragged me into a state of lethargy that made me feel less than sharp. I had no trouble sleeping because the meds literally knocked me out for hours at a time. A few days later, I was coherent enough to write this journal entry.

HOW KAREN CONQUERED CANCER

Wednesday, July 03, 2002 at 10:06 PM

Everyone has heard the age old adage, "No News is Good News," and this is definitely the case with Karen as her progress continues to sparkle.

Karen's good friend and Will's godmother, Margaret Evans, was here the past few days to help out. We really appreciated her visit, and she is now on her way back to a new job in Portland, Oregon.

Four of the past five days Karen has traveled down to IUMC for her blood work. The latest numbers look very good. WBC is 6,300 where the normal range is 4,500 to 11,500. This number is expected to fluctuate at this point. More importantly her Blast is zero, where it was at 92-95 when she was at her worst prior to the chemo. Hemoglobin is up to 10; this allowed the doctors to remove the central IV earlier today. Her platelet count is at 103, which is the highest number I recall ever seeing for this measurement since this odyssey began. Normal range for platelets is 150,000 to 450,000, so we like this trend and so do her doctors. All of the projected future trips down to IUMC for her daily blood work have been cancelled. Restrictions on diet have been eliminated, but we are still limiting visitors to the house because she fatigues quickly.

The next big step will be the bone marrow extract and biopsy slated for July 15th. We all hope and pray that the results prove she is in remission.

Have a wonderful 4th of July and God Bless This Great Country of Ours

Nothing of any consequence happened over the next several days. Karen was on a neutropenic diet, and we had to be careful to watch what she ate. No fruits or vegetables were allowed—everything had to be cooked thoroughly. Bacteria and viruses were the primary concern due to Karen's compromised immune system. Karen took a subcutaneous shot of Neupogen, which was designed to have her bone marrow jumpstart the production of red and white blood cells and platelets. We were indeed blessed. A parade of friends and neighbors were ready, willing and able to help.

Margaret Evans brought the kids really cool presents, and her visit with Karen was helpful for both of them. Karen was resting comfortably at home and sleeping a lot. I had returned to work on a daily basis, but I was having trouble getting back into the swing. I tried to work through my dulled cognitive ability, but at this point, I don't think I was of much help to anyone. Luckily, Dr. Todd Arnold up the street and Amy Jackson's sister, Jen, a practicing nurse at Methodist Hospital, would stop in to check on Karen's vitals. Melinda Bruggemann from next door was very adept at giving Karen her Neupogen shots. The one time I tried, I bruised the hell out of Karen's arm so she fired me from this task.

Also, our children had returned to Indiana. We were a family unit again, trying to cope with the challenges ahead. Attaining remission was the goal, and things looked good. Karen's recovery, despite the odds, was nothing short of remarkable. I must admit that my own recollection of this general time period is still very sketchy and slightly warped.

A week after the 4th of July, I made another journal update:

HOW KAREN CONQUERED CANCER

Thursday, July 11, 2002 at 11:49 PM

Karen continues to rest in her own bed at home. Her spirits are good and her diet is improving, even though the chemo masks the real taste of the food. Earlier in the week, long time friends, Tom Lambright and Dr. Brian Wynne came in from Seattle and Philadelphia respectively.

In the middle of the week, Karen had discomfort with her left Achilles' tendon, of all things, and a trip to the ER was required as a safety precaution just in case the pain may have been a clot. The diagnosis was tendonitis due to a lack of activity, and ice, ibuprofen and more rest was prescribed. The good thing that came out of the trip to the ER was that the blood work revealed continued stable numbers—WBC remains at 6,300, hemoglobin is 9.7 and platelets are over 400.

The next hurdle is Monday's bone marrow extract and the biopsy results that will follow. Remission is the name of the game and is Karen's primary focus. If this is the case, then the following weeks consist of two weeks rest at home and five days in a regular hospital room, not isolation for more chemo.

Think and pray for remission.

Karen wants everyone to know how grateful she is for everything: the cards, guestbook entries, meals, help with the yard…. and wishes she could thank everyone for everything that's been done for her and her family.

On behalf of the entire Volpe and Coyne families all we can say is thank you from the bottom of our hearts.

Amen!!

CHAPTER 20

Charleston's

The day we had awaited for finally arrived; a scant 45 days after her ordeal had begun. Karen and I made the trek down to IUMC. This time, both of us were familiar with what the bone marrow biopsy procedure entailed. We finally met the invisible oncologist, Dr. Larry Cripe, whom we had heard so many great things about. Up until this point, we knew nothing about this mysterious man behind the curtain whom we had entrusted to save Karen's life. Dr. Cripe was totally charming and had a great personality, exactly the opposite of one of the reports we had found on the Internet. He explained the process, given the yet-to-be-confirmed possible remission. Dr. Cripe told us that based on Karen's blood counts he thought she was in remission, but only the biopsy results could tell us for sure.

I crouched down next to Karen on the opposite side of the bed while Dr. Cripe performed the procedure. This time everything was different. After applying the local anesthesia, the instruments were inserted without any probing and searching, as was the case the first time with Dr. Li.

As the syringe trigger was pulled back, it filled up immediately with bright red bone marrow. I could tell by the look on Katie Hincher's face and the wideness of Dr. Cripe's eyes that this was a good sign—it appeared that Karen was in remission. We still had to wait for the visual inspection of the blood smears on the slides and the lab analysis of the specimen, but we were all certainly encouraged.

I logged the following report out on Caringbridge.

Monday, July 15, 2002 at 06:34 PM

This morning Karen went to the IUMC Outpatient Oncology Pavilion in downtown Indianapolis where we met with Dr. Larry Cripe for the first time, and Katie Hincher, RN.

Karen's blood work showed WBC at 10,700, hemoglobin at 9.3 and her platelets are up to 382. All three numbers are viewed as positive. The bone marrow extract was performed, and the specimen slides were sent off to the lab for analysis. Dr. Cripe stated he would be surprised if the lab work showed anything, but that Karen was in remission. We will know conclusively early tomorrow morning, as Katie will call Karen with the results of the biopsy that went off without a hitch, other than a sore behind.

The prognosis is as follows: if today's test results are good after two weeks of prep work, Karen will check into a regular hospital bed in the oncology wing at IUMC, and not in the isolation, for 8 days of chemo at the same intensity as last month. She then gets a 2-month break from the chemo. After two months she will be re-admitted for a 5-day chemo treatment, but at a lesser intensity than the first 2 sessions. We hope that this plan can be executed with few complications, but we are aware that it is truly not in our hands.

We found Dr. Cripe to be very direct and downright charming; he answered our questions head on and is obviously accomplished. He was even interested in hearing about both of our careers, our children, and about this wonderful community in Carmel we call home. We're big fans of Dr. Cripe based solely on our half hour with him! He performed the bone marrow extract himself.

Karen's appetite has picked up and her attitude is great knowing that what lies ahead consists of more chemo outside the confines of isolation.

The prayers, cards, rosaries, and masses have all worked.

It's going to be impossible for us to thank each and every one of you, but we'll try.

She's not totally out of the woods yet, but there's at least a tunnel now and maybe some light at the end, if you squint really hard.

Faith, Hope and Love—the greatest gift is love.

We anxiously await tomorrow's test results and hope that we are not "jumping the gun." We'll update tomorrow with the actual scoop.

Love to all.

All signs indicated that Karen was in remission; her blood work numbers looked right. Dr. Cripe appeared very confident, and the bone marrow extract went much smoother than the initial biopsy performed by Dr. Li, in June when she was originally admitted. There was no problem finding the marrow. I told her I thought she was in remission on the way home. My opinion was based purely on the non-verbal cues I was getting from Dr.

Cripe and Katie. They both seemed positive. After all, they do this everyday, but in spite of my confidence, I was on pins and needles all morning.

Karen called me at my desk with the news that she was in remission right after Katie called with the great news. I cried a minute or so, said a prayer of thanks, and then started making phone calls and telling anyone I could find in the office the goal of remission had been attained.

She had gone from death's door to being cancer-free in six weeks. Karen made the entry below and announced to everyone that prayers do, indeed, get answered.

Tuesday, July 16, 2002 at 01:16 PM

……….Yahoo……Yipee…..Praise God………

………….REMISSION ACCOMPLISHED…………

Thank you, thank you, thank you! What a trip this has been. Yesterday I had my bone marrow biopsy. It was truly a pain in the behind. I am standing while writing this as a testimony to that fact. Dr. Cripe was wonderful and said, "Based on how you have responded to treatment, I would be surprised if you are not in remission when the test results return." The doctors at IU have been continually confused at how quickly I am recovering. They must not be reading this web site, and they must be unaware of all of the prayers and support that I am blessed with.

On August 5, I go back to IU for an 8-day stay for another chemo treatment. It will be the same as the last, without all of the complications of the last round, of course. Then I go back 2 months later for 5 days; this time the chemo treatment will be less intense.

This experience has been devastating and uplifting. Overwhelming and prayerful. Heartbreaking and motivating. We needed your help, and you were there. We are so thankful. How would we have survived without your prayers and support? God Bless each and every one of you. And I FELT each prayer as it was said.

I have so much to say and so many for which to thank God. Bless each and every one of you.

Love,

Karen, Mark, Will, Sam and Mitch

Karen, Tom, Pat and I went out to dinner at Charleston's in Westfield. It was the first time the four of us had ever dined at the same table. Pat and Tom had put their differences aside and were communicating on a regular basis for the first time in a long time. Karen felt this was one of the good things that came out of her ordeal. She always had a knack for finding the silver lining in any situation. Several times during dinner Karen said this was, indeed, a significant event.

When we made the left turn onto Garden Gate Way after dinner, at least 100 neighbors and parishioners were waiting for us, each holding a red balloon. Kimmie Wetzel and Amy Jackson assembled the troops, and they all released the balloons screaming "REMISSION ACCOMPLISHED!" It was hard to not get a lump in your throat. All of these people had prayed so hard, and worked so hard, and brought over so many meals, and mowed the yard, and done our laundry. It was truly a reason to celebrate. The achievement of remission in the wake of such odds and circumstances made this one of the most important days of our lives. A sign that read "Carpe Diem Karen" was draped across our front porch and signed by many of our neighbors.

There was hope, but there were still two more rounds of chemo and a two-year maintenance program to get through.

I fully understood everything that was going on, but the meds had left me a shadow of my former self mentally. I just couldn't react. I was slow and felt drab all the time. Karen observed and often remarked that I actually dragged my feet as I walked. I've looked back at the emails and documents I authored at work during this time period. They all read fine, but there's just not many of them. Everyone at the office knew it was going to take some time for me to come back, but only a handful of people knew about the bipolar diagnosis and the intensive medication program that had been prescribed. I knew if this became common knowledge, my career could hit a brick wall and I might need to leave. Jim Torgerson, Jim Holsclaw, Lori Spence, Donna Dare, Joe Gardner, Jeff Sprague and Steve Kozey were all very supportive, but at the same time I was concerned about losing forward momentum.

I spoke with Donna Dare often after I returned to my daily routine at my desk. Her office was across the corridor from mine. Donna is a senior paralegal and we had worked together on many FERC filings and other projects. Years earlier, before I really knew her, she had lost her young son, Tyler, to an inoperable brain tumor. She had unbelievable faith, strength and courage. Karen made sure Donna kept an eye on me, given all the meds I was taking, to make sure I didn't do anything stupid at the office. Donna always had wonderful words of encouragement; she always listened to me and helped me get through some rough days. I'll never forget the time she told me, "Heaven is more glorious than we can imagine."

We were working on a merger agreement at the time. Midwest ISO was acquiring the Little Rock, Arkansas-based Southwest Power Pool. I wanted to make sure that I did everything possible to make sure FERC approved the new tariff. This would help ensure that I retain similar job responsibilities in the new organization. I just couldn't concentrate or focus, my mind wandered or stalled in mid air. Jim Holsclaw covered for me throughout this time period.

On July 23rd, Karen and I visited Dr. Samuels at his office. When we walked into his office, Karen started to talk while I sat back and listened. She had been doing some research on the Internet and she told Dr. Samuels that we had misgivings regarding his diagnosis of me having bipolar disorder.

"I have been married to this man for 15 years, and he does not have the mental disorder you believe he has. I know him better than anyone," she said.

Karen went on to explain that she had been battling leukemia and was fighting for her life, and that when I had my episode, it was during a very stressful time. I had not been getting enough sleep. All during this time, Dr. Samuels started shuffling through his papers and looked rather perplexed, as though he was hearing this "whole" part of the story for the first time. In short, Karen was saying this episode of mania was an isolated incident and that her husband did not have bipolar disorder.

Karen explained that she understood I had a manic episode, but she said, "The research I have done says people suffering from bipolar disease have serious mood swings from near depression to extreme highs. My husband does not exhibit any of these swings and is seldom, if ever, depressed. The only time he's depressed is after the Browns lose and that usually lasts about an hour."

He looked at both of us and said, "I have never missed a diagnosis in my career. Are you doubting my diagnosis?"

And then he kind of looked down at his papers and seemed to be snickering at us.

After a long and uncomfortable pause, Dr. Samuels said rather smugly, "Most, if not all of my patients, are bipolar, and furthermore, this can be a very destructive disease. I've had one of my patients go off her medications, and she just took off to Georgia and bought thousands of dollars worth of carpet."

"When can I go off my medications? They are really making my mind dull," I asked.

"You're a smart guy, Mark! You can quit taking your medication any time you want. You're not on that high a dosage," he said.

"I'll make you a deal," he said. "You can stop taking the Zyprexa, but I want you to continue to take the Depakote and have your Depakote levels checked periodically at St. Vincent's."

"Fine!" I said, as we stood up to leave.

"Please set up another appointment for early October before you leave," Dr. Samuels said.

Karen was really angry at this point. She was sure I wasn't bipolar. She was sick and tired of seeing a doped-up, over-medicated husband dragging his feet. I had even been checking the Internet myself regarding the drugs I was taking. According to the information I received, the two drugs I was taking are more commonly prescribed for people suffering from schizophrenia and/or depression. Karen and I both knew I was not schizophrenic. These drugs were hardcore, and I should never have been put on them.

Karen was bound and determined to get her old husband back. She started making some phone calls to find a new doctor for me the following week before her second round of chemotherapy. She worked through our insurance company and found a psychiatrist named Dr. Dale Theobald. When she called the number, the lady who answered the phone said, "Indiana Cancer Care."

"I'm sorry," Karen said. "I was trying to contact a Dr. Dale Theobald."

The voice on the other end of the line said, "You have the right number. Dr. Theobald works here. Shall I connect you?"

"Yes, but wait, what did you say when you answered the phone?" Karen asked.

"We're the Indiana Cancer Care Center, specializing in counseling both patients and family members who are dealing with cancer," the lady said.

Karen started to cry as the receptionist connected Karen with Dr. Theobald. After Karen explained our situation, Dr. Theobald said he would be happy to meet with the two of us. We didn't keep the October 1st appointment with Dr. Samuels. Months later I would get my records from Dr. Samuels. Besides his bipolar diagnosis, he also notes his suspicions that I was using drugs.

Not true.

I drank on occasion, sometimes in excess, but I have never used any amphetamines or other illegal narcotics. His notes also stated I was a very intense person who talked very rapidly.

This was clearly a case of psychiatric malpractice, but unfortunately the State of Indiana has passed legislation making it nearly impossible to win a medical malpractice suit.

CHAPTER 21

Cape Hatteras, N.C.

Our family pulled together and buckled down for Round Two. We attempted to find some sort of routine, but knowing that the mommy was going back in for two more rounds of chemo, especially the corrosive duanorubicin, loomed at the forefront of everyone's mind. I was still on the Depakote and trying hard to get back on track. Karen was home preparing for the next two rounds. What made this part of the journey even harder for Karen was knowing the devastating effects of the corrosive chemo, and knowing that she had to take on these treatments twice more over the next couple of months. Chemo may have saved her life, but it also had literally scalded her mucous membranes from the inside out.

"If they had just shoved ground glass up both holes with a broomstick, it would have felt better than this," she lamented.

Her lips had turned black, and slowly over time the dead skin peeled away and ugly lesions lined the inside of her mouth. She knew what she had to do, but the prospect of enduring the treatments again and again caused her much mental anguish.

She made regular trips down to the IUMC to get transfusions of whole blood and platelets. While there she befriended a patient she had met while in isolation. His name was Ken Shiflett, and he had not been as fortunate as Karen, having never achieved remission. He came in for transfusions too. They talked and became friends. Karen worried about Ken and prayed for him constantly. He was about the same age as Karen, married, with one child. She couldn't understand why she was able to attain remission and Ken had not been able to get there. His counts just continued to escalate.

Once in remission, Karen received Neupogen shots daily as prescribed by Dr. Cripe. Eventually, her bone marrow started to produce healthy white and red blood cells, as well as platelets. Things were going as planned.

In the meantime, I was preparing my witness for my Christ Renews His Parish weekend, which was coming up in early August. I was the Christian Community witness, and the men on my team afforded me as much time as I needed to tell my story. I prepared eight pages of notes from which to speak and was definitely getting excited about my witness, while at the same time I was a little nervous.

Karen made the following entry on her Caringbridge website.

Monday, July 29, 2002 at 09:01 AM

Home……sweet……..home

It's so great to be home with my family. Mark has been able to start back to work. The kids haven't missed a beat. They have, each one, been helpful and supportive. I'm increasingly aware that my days till I go back are counting down. I feel the need to do as much as I can in this next week. Uniforms are ordered and school supplies have been bought. Today I need to plan Sam's birthday, which is Aug. 19th.

As I have been about town these last days, I have received questions regarding this web site. It appears that my opportunity to be dark and mysterious has passed me by. My life is an open book now. Here are some answers to frequently asked questions:

1) No, Camp Coyne is not a real camp and no you can't send your kids there. Coyne is my maiden name and my brother Kevin and his wife Colleen spoiled my kids rotten. (Sure wish I could have been there!)

2) Coors Light does taste good again. Thank God some things never change.

3) I am not completely bald just yet. I look like one of Jim Henson's Muppets. Do you remember Fragile Rock cartoons? I resemble a bad comb over.

4) I have a wonderful older sister, Kathy; and three younger brothers, Kevin, Kenny and Tommy. I love them each dearly. I am a very lucky woman.

5) Yes, my parents are divorced. They are wonderful parents. I have a very cool stepfather too.

6) Applebee's chicken oriental salad rocks.

All is well here. Dr's orders are to put some weight on. No problem!! I'm trying to get some strength back in my legs before I'm back in bed for a while. God is good. Please keep those prayers a comin'.

We then prepared for the Smith family reunion and were fortunate that Karen's Aunt Teresa and her husband, Rex Repass, had taken on the large task of hosting the reunion near their new home in Blue Ash, Ohio; a suburb of Cincinnati and only two hours from Carmel. For the past several years, Kenny had hosted the annual bash in Kent, Ohio, which would have meant a five-hour plus car ride versus the short trip over to the Queen City.

For our family talent, Samantha, Will, Mitch and I did a lip sync version of Bruce's song called "Glory Days." Karen was there, but she was still physically beat up and fatigued. She seemed to have fun and enjoyed being with the family. Everyone told her how much they were praying for her, and how they knew that if anyone could pull off beating cancer that it was Karen. The highlight of our performance was when Mitchell stepped up with my dad's old tenor saxophone and blew some loud squeaky notes through the mouthpiece with true grit and determination to make the big gold instrument produce something that sounded melodic.

It was hilarious!

Before leaving for the reunion, Karen had updated her website, and as usual, Karen expressed more concern for others back in isolation than she did for herself.

Friday, August 02, 2002 at 12:19 AM

> Tomorrow, we leave for Cincinnati for our weekend of our family reunion. It's my mom's side of the family and sure to be a riot. It always is. On Monday, I return to Indiana University Hospital, not isolation this time. It seems a shame to go back for any reason because I feel great!! I had always been told that my stay would be for 8 days, but it now appears that they are going to use a new kind of chemo on me that will get the whole job done but in less time. They are not certain if my system will tolerate it. If this new aggressive drug makes me too sick, I may have to do the 8 days. We'll have to see how it goes.

All is well here. Dad and Kathy are helping out this coming week, and Mom will be here the next week. Thank God. I am anxious to get in and get out and get on with life. I have a hell of a lot to live for and I am thankful for all of it. Please keep me in your prayers. Also, please pray for all those poor souls that I left behind in the isolation wing. I swear they haunt me. Some have been there three times as long as I was. It is a very difficult and unpleasant way to live.

Thank you; see you in a couple weeks!!

Karen

On Monday, August 5, 2002, Karen was readmitted to the Adult Cancer Care Unit at the IUMC, but instead of administering the very corrosive forms of chemotherapy we both had dreaded, Dr. Cripe decided to use a drug called ATRA, or retinoid acid. Recent research indicated ATRA was yielding great results in keeping patients with Karen's type of AML in remission. ATRA is a drug pioneered by Dr. Martin Tallman and others from a derivative of accutaine, a drug used primarily to control harsh cases of acne for teenagers. Dr. Cripe had been consulting with Dr. Tallman on a regular basis throughout Karen's case, and Dr. Tallman felt that Karen could tolerate ATRA given that she had dealt with the idarubicin and duanorubicin so well, in spite of the harsh side effects during round one when she originally achieved remission. The idarubicin and ATRA concoction became referred to as "designer chemo," which was a term Karen had heard Dr. Li say in the hallway one morning before rounds. I was all for it, and we were both pleased to hear that she would only be in the hospital for four days or so while the ATRA and idarubicin were administered. The nasty bright orange duanorubicin would not be used.

After returning home on Friday, Karen logged the following entry in spite of total exhaustion as the harsh effects of the chemo started to take hold.

Friday, August 09, 2002 at 03:34 PM

The Doctors decided to try out a new chemo on me because "I am young and strong". (The type of Leukemia that I have is most often found in 65+ year old men.) It is very hard on the heart, but they feel it is a "sure fire way to keep you in remission." For that very reason, I said, bring it on. The bonus is that since it's not watered down, they can do it in 3 treatments, three days in a row. I was warned that if I get nauseated, they might reevaluate. It's very weird to watch a bag that says HAZARDOUS—POISON on it flow into my veins. I feel fine, but weak and lethargic. I have started my hormone shots to get my bone marrow working again. To tell you the truth, my sister, Kathy, administered the shot. If only you could have seen me trying to get the stuff out of the bottle and Kathy sticking me. Too funny.

The summer has come and gone. Don't have a clue where it went. Our thanks and prayers to all of you who have spent this precious summertime with us in mind. I have so much to live for and I can't wait to get ON WITH LIFE. I go back in for the last scheduled chemo on the Tuesday after Labor Day weekend. So far everything is going as planned. Of course, if I were in charge, I would have planned it differently!

Karen

Karen returned home from her second round of chemo and rested. I was back at work, and the kids were going back to school in a few days. Karen's mother and her sister were able to spend time with Karen while she recovered. Karen was again on a neutropenic diet and was not allowed to eat any fruits or vegetables. Everything she ate had to be cooked, and no fresh flowers were allowed in the house.

Usually the mosquitoes bothered Karen just like they did everyone else, but during this summer Karen noticed the insects would land, think about it and then leave. It was as if they could smell the chemo.

"Bite me and you're dead!" Karen said.

All signs pointed to Karen's continued improvement. She was progressing and her overall health was improving. The words of a child tell it all.

Karen:

I swear to you my five-year-old son is an "old" soul. He says the most amazing things when I have the time to talk to him all-alone, usually at bedtime. Earlier this week, he said, "Mom, I noticed that Sam and Mitch look happier. I guess God heard me praying for them." How cool is that?

You have an amazing family...I can't tell you how glad I am that we have had the chance to get to know you, and how thrilled we are to see you smiling and "holding court" on Garden Gate Way!

All our best,
Tom, Shelly, Nick and Drew Thieme

Carmel, IN—Tuesday, August 13, 2002 at 02:43 PM

I must admit my recollection of this period of time is a blur for me personally. One significant event happened around the middle of August. Pat told us that one hot summer night at her condo in Ohio she was having trouble sleeping. Around 2:00 a.m. she went into the extra bedroom where Karen and I slept when we visited. She prayed at the window.

Moments later Pat heard a mysterious voice say, "She's going to live."

He does talk to us if our hearts are open to listening. It's not just wishful thinking. I asked Fr. Hellmann, on one of his many visits to our home, if it was generally the case in the Bible that when people encountered the Holy Spirit or angels that it occurred while they were sleeping or meditating. He said, "Yes, this is generally the case." I was trying to sleep when I was touched by the power of the Holy Spirit at the Ministry Center back in February.

The rest of the week went by quickly, and Karen wrote the following a little over a week after returning home.

Thursday, August 15, 2002 at 11:37 PM

Hello to all. I so enjoy hearing from you. I'm holed up in the house for a while now. My doctor's appointment today and blood work showed that the chemo has definitely done its job. While your white blood cells are at around 11,000; today my count is .42. The injections I am taking will start my count on its way back up over the next days, but as a result, I am basically in quarantine. The masked lady once again.

Sam had a nice birthday party yesterday, and the kids go

to school in the morning for just a few hours to take supplies and meet their teacher and to find out who is in their classes. Don't you remember those days? Mom and Mark will be taking them; I'll be here waiting to hear the stories when they come home.

I have become very proficient at sleeping; while standing, during a conversation, in the car.... I am the "napper of the year." Tired all the time but glad that you all have kept in touch by dropping by or calling. I am going to be one lonely soul when the kids are back in the swing of school and I am here. Oh well, this surely can't last forever. Love to all. It's past my bedtime...

On Saturday, August 24th, Karen's birthday, I broke away from home a few times during the day to help my CRHP team put on the weekend for the new Team #17 at St. Louis de Montfort. At about two in the afternoon, I began to speak on the subject of Christian Community. Here's a synopsis, based on my notes and my recollection of what I said to the group of men assembled. I spoke for a long time.

I started by talking about how my mother always admired St. Joseph because he took on his role solely on faith. He was awakened by the angel Gabriel who told him not to be afraid, to stay with Mary even though she was with child and they had never had relations. My parents had selected Joseph as my baptismal name.

Then I spoke of my early childhood memories of being the oldest of four children. I mentioned my now estranged sister, Lynn, who I'd talk about later, the middle child, David John or "D.J.", born 10/4/62, and the youngest, my brother, Paul, born on 11/30/64. Paul and I are commonly referred to by my mom as "The Bookends." Both of us have degrees in accounting. We look the same, sound the same and both of us are constantly talking.

The first significant day that I remember of my own existence began when I was four and a half years old. I was watching cartoons on an old GE 12" black and white TV when suddenly the cartoons were gone. My mom began watching intently, and then the neighbors started showing up to join us. Everyone was very quiet and serious as they watched Walter Cronkite on Channel 8, CBS in Cleveland. The day was 11/22/63 and JFK had just been assassinated in Dallas. This day marked the beginning of my own personal memory. I remember the following day and the day after that when Oswald was shot.

I witnessed lots of history on that small GE TV; it was my outlet to the world. I watched the early space missions, Peter Jennings daily on the Vietnam War, the assassinations of RFK and MLK, and the riots at the 1968 Democratic Convention in downtown Chicago.

In 1966, my parents decided to move to Stow, where they built a new house within walking distance of Holy Family Catholic School. So in second grade, I encountered the Sisters of St. Augustine, the nuns who taught at the school for the first time. Other fond memories from this era were my Grandma Volpe's big Italian dinners. Being Italian is a religion in and of itself. After all, the Pope is totally surrounded by Italians. We went on great family vacations; my fondest memory was the famous story regarding the blue marlin my dad and I caught off the coast of Cape Hatteras, N.C., back in August 1969. This was our big victory and was officially coined "The Catch of the Day," as none of the other marinas in the area could lay claim to such a fish at seven feet long and 70 pounds. I spoke about my Great Grandma Anne Vitarelli, who owned a bar in Dubois, Pennsylvania, and how she raised nine children by herself during the Great Depression.

My dad did a lot of out-of-town travel, so I spent a lot of time with my mother. I followed all the Apollo space missions and remember Neil Armstrong's walk on them moon, on our new 27-inch color TV. The nation had risen to meet JFK's challenge and NASA put a man on the moon first, before the Russians. I recalled vividly the shootings very nearby at Kent State University on 5/4/70; to me it was the day the '60s died.

We went to church every Sunday as a family. I grew up in a household that was very conservative politically. I enjoyed being the class clown, played CYO sports. I was a great catcher in little league—great defense, but I didn't hit a lick. In 1970, I built a Soap Box Derby racer and I launched model rockets. I did the minimum in grade school getting mediocre grades because I knew grade school didn't really count, and I also always just assumed I'd be going to Walsh Jesuit and then on to college.

I went to Walsh in September 1973, with 27 of my classmates from Holy Family. All the guys who were great rivals in grade school were now on the same team as many of the top athletes in the area decided on Walsh. I always received good grades keeping a 3.4 GPA. I played in all the bands, taking up the saxophone for jazz band. I played baseball until I got spiked in the face during an intra-squad game. It was a bizarre accident, spiked by my friend named Jeff Klein who also happened to be dating my sister at the time.

I found the Jesuits to be superior educators; they taught one a solid command of the English language. It was a premier college preparatory program where 98% of my graduating class went on to colleges like Duke, Case Western, Harvard, Stanford and Notre Dame. Walsh helped lay a great foundation. I learned how to study and think, and it was a truly great example of a Christian Community. I attribute lots of my success to those days at Walsh, and I'm thankful to God and my parents for giving me the opportunity to go there. These formative years had prepared me for life and the challenges I currently faced, both professionally and personally.

Then, at the point when I had been talking for about 20 minutes, I lost my train of thought. I stepped away from the podium to gather myself and take a drink of water.

The medication I was on had slowed my thought process. I apologized for rambling, and then I said, "I really don't know why I'm up here spending so much time talking about myself and my glory days from high school when I know the real reason I'm called to be here is to talk about my wife and her battle to beat cancer."

And then I continued on, although I must admit in retrospect, my mind was starting to waiver. I tried hard to concentrate and focus.

> I made no bones about the fact that I was very fortunate and was afforded such wonderful educational opportunities. My life has had its troubles, but I never served in the military or had to fight in a war to defend this great country and our freedom.

> My fraternity brothers were another example of how Christian Community had played an important role in my life. We watched each other's backs and helped each other get

through some tough classes. Even though I partied way too hard, I studied hard and still got very good grades.

I landed a job at Marathon Oil Company out of college for $19,000 annually. I was hired into the Information System area working as a Systems Analyst. I dated a lot; it was kind of like I was still continuing with my college lifestyle even though I had a job. I worked on an MBA from Ashland University, at night graduating with a 3.4 in their Executive Management Program.

I went through the painful review of the first real challenging moment in our marriage and talked candidly about the abruption of the placenta, while Karen was expecting Mitchell, and our steadfast refusal to abort a live fetus—how she laid on her left side constantly for four months in order to maximize the blood flow.

Then I spoke briefly, without going into all the details, about my estranged sister, Lynn, and how she was forced to make a decision to either stay with her husband or leave him if she insisted on being a "Volpe" and continued going to family functions. I talked about my wife's role as a peacemaker, and how together we tried to bridge the differences and salvage the situation.

Next, I invited one of my CRHP brothers to read the "Parable of the Prodigal Son" as found in the Bible under Luke 15:11-31. I closed this portion of my talk by saying that I believed there was still time for healing, and to never give up hope for there is always an opportunity for forgiveness.

Next, I transitioned briefly through my career moves and relayed how my family ended up in Indianapolis via our short stop in Cincinnati while I worked on the formation of the Midwest ISO during my brief tenure at Cinergy.

I paused for moment and said, "I have spoken in front of groups many times, but there is no doubt in my mind that what I am about to talk about will be the most important message I will ever deliver. I have spent more time preparing for this part of my discussion in order to assure that my message is clear."

Finally, I had arrived at the major point of my witness, and as I looked out at these men who had been sitting there patiently for at least 40 minutes, I could tell by the looks of anticipation on their faces that I had their full and undivided attention.

I reviewed the chronology of events that led to St. Vincent's, finally coming to the devastating conclusion that my wife had leukemia and our decision to take Karen to the Indiana University Medical Center to be treated by Dr. Larry Cripe. This decision making process was spearheaded by Karen's brothers. I could see some tears from a man at a table at the rear of the room as I spoke about having to ship my kids off to Ohio until the situation was under control, and I stated, "No father should ever have to tell their children their mother might die."

Finally, I relayed my conviction that it was about at this point in time when I witnessed the sheer power of the Christian Community kick into high gear in that all of our needs were met by family, neighbors and our fellow parishioners at St. Louis de Montfort. The lawn care, the meals, the prayers, the rosaries, and even a blood drive which was held in Karen's honor were all examples of the positive things that people wanted to do to help. This was the Christian Community in action!

I talked in graphic detail about the bone marrow extract and the devastating effects of the chemotherapy. Then I said, "It's been very hard to just sit there and only be able to watch as the chemo literally burned my wife from the inside out—the chemo had torched all of her mucous membranes."

As I looked down at the floor, I had trouble fighting back tears and I bit my lip while I thought to myself about how my wife's beautiful body had been burnt so horribly by the chemo.

I spoke briefly about my own problems with exhaustion or battlefield fatigue, and how I had to be hospitalized myself. I felt horribly guilty about not taking good care of myself rendering me unable to be at my wife's side during the most critical juncture of our married life. I updated these men on how Karen's situation continued to improve while she was in the isolation unit, and her miraculous recovery that allowed her go home two weeks earlier than planned, but more importantly, a bone marrow biopsy found her to be in remission on July 15, 2002.

To close, I told these men I was sure she would be cured and walk the earth as an inspirational cancer survivor five years from now. I spoke of her hair loss and the blisters in her mouth, and then I apologized for the fact that I needed to get back home to her because she was still in the middle of the fight, having just undergone her second round of chemotherapy earlier in the week.

I talked about my goals in life, to retire early and to write a book. I think I have a story to tell: Karen Conquers Cancer. It was my hope that someday I'd throw a blowout of a party, in the way of a wedding reception for Samantha, our only daughter. I'd welcome the chance to teach a business related class at the high school level, maybe even adopt a child and coach special teams for a high school football team.

To close, I said, "Someday, I know I'll travel to Rome with Karen. She had been to Rome before we met, and she insists that once you tour Rome and see the Basilica, St. Peter's Square and the Coliseum, there will be no doubt in your mind that Jesus

Christ has walked on this Earth, as the Father had sent his only Son, God made man, here to redeem our sins."

At the end, I played a recording of the title cut from Springsteen's *The River* album, one of Karen's favorites. I reminded everyone that we are welcomed into the church and introduced to the community for the first time through baptism, and in the Catholic Church, we use blessed waters in the administration of the sacraments. When we walk into church, we bless ourselves. Holy water is used at the last rites and at funerals. I asked the men to sit back and listen to the lyrics.

Then I said, "That's my story and I'm sticking to it. God love ya!" as the music began.

The room was dead silent. Even though it had been an hour and half, I could see a few of these grown men still had tears in their eyes. Many were deeply touched by what they had just heard. I quickly dashed out the door so I could get back to my ailing wife.

CHAPTER 22

Cedar Point

Karen went to the Cancer Pavilion on Monday, August 26th to see Dr. Cripe. Normally, Karen would first give them a sample of her blood for analysis and then she'd go back into the waiting room for her appointment. While we waited she was concerned about a pretty college-aged girl who was waiting all by herself. She wore a bandana and you could tell she had lost all of her hair. Karen was growing more perplexed and concerned for this girl, continuing to look over at her. I just glanced up at her when Karen pointed her out and then I went back to reviewing the baseball box scores.

"Never mind, that girl is going to be fine. There's an angel standing right behind her," Karen said to me.

"What does the angel look like?" I asked.

"She's radiant; she's absolutely beautiful," replied Karen.

I went back to reading the sports page of the *Indianapolis Star*. There was no doubt in my mind. Karen had really seen an angel watching over this young cancer patient. I could only hope Karen also had an angel watching over her.

She met Dr. Cripe's clinical nurse, Victoria Hunt, for the first time on this visit. "Victoria's no Katie; she's not very friendly," Karen said.

Later that day, I flew over to St. Louis for a two-day technical conference to compare and contrast the difference between the two transmission tariffs in use by the Midwest ISO and the

Southwest Power Pool, and the new tariff we were planning to file with FERC as part of the merger. Jim Holsclaw went with me to St. Louis, and we watched the Browns get drilled by the Packers in an exhibition game on *Monday Night Football*. While I drank a few beers and ate hors d'oerves, Karen was home and wrote the following update on the website:

Monday, August 26, 2002 at 07:55 PM

Well, the cycle continues. Today I got my "get out of jail card." My blood work at the hospital allows for me to leave the house because my white blood cells are meeting minimal requirements. My red blood cells are taking a long time to recover, so I tire very easily. This is the first day since my last entry as I wait for the nausea and side effects to begin to subside. My last round of chemo was so much more intense that it has taken my system twice as long to recover. That, and the fact that the chemo from the first round is still in my system so my side effects seem to intensify with each round. I hurt from top to BOTTOM; I leave the bottom emphasis to your vivid imagination. Chemo burns abound. Since I am still recovering, today I was told that my next chemo is being moved from September 3rd to the 9th.

We are spending Labor Day weekend in the Erie Islands, Kelley's, Put-N-Bay and Cedar Point. My dad takes our whole family to Cedar Point each year, and there are no words for how excited we all are. Especially me. Going in public is always interesting when you look like I do. One little boy asked, "Are you trapped in there?" (I was wearing a mask). A lady at a checkout counter was sure I had AIDS and didn't want me to use her pen. Bald and pale is beautiful!!

Mitch starts soccer tomorrow. He's a natural. Will's hockey will not be far behind, and Sam is still our gymnast. They are all doing well in school so far, the shock of being back is gone. Mark is back to traveling this week and giving his speeches. He has been and continues to be the World's Most Supportive Husband. I have my own private cheerleader. But then my next-door neighbor Amy has been known to do some cheers, but those are generally beer-induced. Let it be known that the Volpe's are fine, until the bell rings for round three. BUT............Round Three is the final round, please God, I'll be feeling better again then for the Holidays and the rest of the Browns' schedule. (That was purely for Mark's benefit).

Love to all from the appreciative Volpe Family

About 2:30 a.m., I woke up and could not sleep. I had no confidence that I could lead the discussion the next day in front of 150 various stakeholders who would be attending the technical conference on the SPP-MISO Tariff Convergence. Usually, I relish this role and actually look forward to being in front of a crowd. I tossed and turned. I thought I was going to have a panic attack in my very warm room at the Marriott. I was sweating profusely, so I called Karen and talked to her for 45 minutes or an hour. She calmed me down and let me know everything was going to be all right.

Karen was so reassuring and she said, "You can do this."

It wasn't like me to get nervous, but I really believe the harsh medications I was taking were starting to take a toll and really screwing with my mind. As I went to hang up, she told me I had done the right thing by calling, and that she was glad I had called.

Before the meeting kicked off the next day, I told Nick Brown, the man who would be my boss and the Chief Operating Officer of the merged company, that I was a little uncomfortable. He said that he understood, and that if I needed a life jacket, he'd be there to bail me out. As it turned out, I did just fine and after about the first 10 minutes I was at ease. It was a difficult crowd, and I had a tough time drawing them out on the issues. Finally, about mid-morning, the real issues began to surface and I felt some relief that I had succeeded.

Karen was getting stronger. You could tell she definitely had what it took to beat cancer—she was never worried only about herself. My struggles concerned her as well, but luckily we had latched on to Dr. Theobald. After hearing our story, he decided that I could be weaned off Depakote. However, he made it clear that if I had another episode, similar to what happened in the month of June that I'd be on medication for the rest of my life. I agreed to follow his program and over time we slowly reduced my dosage. I knew Dr. Samuels was dead wrong when he told me I could go ahead and quit taking my meds. I knew this was unwise, and that there was no way I should quit taking the medication cold turkey.

You could see Karen's strength and conviction in her September journal entries as she became more philosophical about life and the challenges we all face at one time or another. She went back in for her third round of chemo on September 8th, and while she was in the midst of the battle, Karen's resolve and internal fortitude shown through as she prepared for this next round.

HOW KAREN CONQUERED CANCER

Thursday, September 05, 2002 at 09:18 PM

A quote from my sister-in-law Paula Volpe: "People are like tea bags, you have to put them in hot water to see how strong they are." Amen!!

Is it tea yet?

Each day is a test, for all of us I think. As I have tried to keep in touch with so many of you, I quickly find that we all have our challenges. The Volpes are not alone in their daily struggles. For some of us it's health, for others, finances, relationships…

One thing of which I am certain, you have to use each day as a gift and make it count. I am so blessed to have this handful of days that I am feeling well before I go back in on Monday. I am anxious to have all of this behind me and to be able to concentrate on being a wife and mother again. My kids are so sensitive and are trying hard to be brave. They are old enough to be wise and to overhear conversations and to be scared. Will came home from school the other day upset because a friend at school had told him about a relative that they thought was cured of cancer and then he died. He wanted to know if that would happen to me.

God didn't make me sick, but God is choosing to heal me. I have children to raise. I have parties to attend. As Mark watches me get stronger, he gets stronger. When I am struggling with the effects of chemo, Mark struggles. Mark needs me too. This cancer stuff has got to end, and soon. I'm getting so impatient.

Thank you, God; thank you, family; thank you, friends…

My new favorite prayer is for a cure to cancer so that no other family will ever have to experience a summer like ours.

Bless you all,

Karen

Karen's final round of chemotherapy went well. She seemed to have gotten use to the treatments and knew what to expect. On Monday September 16th, I escorted Karen downtown to see Dr. Cripe at the clinic to receive a transfusion of whole blood. While she was getting the transfusion, I met Holly; another patient Karen had become friends with who also had leukemia. She was cute as a button with her colorful bandana. I'd guess her to be in her mid-30s. As I recall, she was married and had one child. The two of them hung out and chatted about their illness. Holly seemed to be making good progress, and her case showed promise. On the way home, I asked Karen if she wanted to go somewhere for lunch.

"South of the Border sounds good," she said. "I think the guy who donated my A negative blood was definitely Mexican, so a taco salad would definitely hit the spot."

Her sense of humor had certainly not been diminished by the ongoing battle with this disease.

Tuesday, September 17, 2002 at 04:34 PM

I've had so many blood transfusions that I'm craving tacos.

Chemo—behind me

Spending the night in the hospital—behind me

Knowing there is an end in sight—priceless

Looks like we are going to survive this fiasco, but it is as if we are a bit tattered from the trip. I should be feeling really crappy here in a few days as my blood counts drop for the final time. I will work my way back out of that, and I'll be put on a "Maintenance Program." It consists of a lot of drugs. At some point then, I'll get to have the port in my chest removed. I never have truly lost ALL of my hair. Mark calls me his little eaglet. I have just a smattering of hairs going every which way.

Prayer is a wonderful and powerful tool. I go back to the hospital several times a week to have my blood checked. I have many friends that have not responded to the chemo and have never reached remission. My friend Ken has just gone into his second 30-day isolation with chemo, and they are looking for bone marrow donors. Please keep him in your prayers as well.

I feel overwhelmed with this whole thing. I feel like I have 3 too many balls in the air. I'll probably write one more time before we close this journal up. I wish I could hear from everyone who opens it up and peeks in. You are all important to me. I'm no writer, but it is good to have this journey in black and white like this.

"Only the good die young"—now that explains everything!!

I truly do love and thank you all,

Karen

I seemed to be getting by, but I struggled and tried to be proactive in managing my own issues. I was working out at Lifetime Fitness in an attempt to keep from gaining weight; which was one of the side effects of the medicine. I tried to watch my diet, work out, and cut down on alcohol. The only good thing about the drugs was that they helped me get a solid night's sleep. The problem was it took a lot of coffee to get me going in the morning. I always felt I would be able to eventually return to normal having stumbled and fallen while rounding second. Karen had picked me up, and I had managed to crawl back on my hands and knees to second, just barely able to grab a corner of the base. I knew from my experience with the Holy Spirit that I was "safe" as the second basemen slapped the tag on me.

Karen finally got to me one night when she said, "Snap out of it, Volpe, you got me through it. I'm going to be okay, but you've got to understand you're not bipolar, you're fine. You did it. You saved me! Now please give me back the old Volpe monster I married."

When she said this to me, I instantly decided to be more assertive and start to be the leader. It was like a slap in the face. I needed to wake up, take charge and start playing quarterback again.

A couple of days later, the Browns made an improbable comeback to victory at Tennessee winning the game by scoring two touchdowns with just over five minutes remaining to tie the game while time remained in the final quarter and then win in overtime. A key play was a remarkable onside kick recovery where Phil Dawson hit a wedge with his left foot down the sideline opposite of the flooded side of the field and was recovered by a streaking Dennis Northcutt. Will and I went nuts as it reminded us of the comeback we saw in person down in Nashville,

B.C. a year earlier—B.C. meaning "Before Cancer," as Karen puts it. Even though Tim Couch was down by two scores with only five minutes left, they never gave up.

It was time for me to take to heart what my wife was telling me. I needed to battle back the same way she did.

On the last day of September, as Karen began her two-year maintenance program, she made what she truly believed would be the final entry in the journal on the Caringbridge website.

Monday, September 30, 2002 at 05:54 PM

Well……I wish that I could say that this experience has gifted me with endless words of wisdom and knowing. The "negatives" associated with cancer are quite obvious. Aside from the pain, fear and nausea, you have other concerns. I am now certain that the experience of cancer, or any illness, has impacted everyone around me in a type of rippling effect. Not only was our summer a complete washout, but my family devoted their summer to my getting well. Mom and Dad have been amazing and loving and supportive. My brothers and sisters have made endless trips back and forth and up and down the highway. Aunts and Uncles and cousins…………I thank God for my family and will never be able to repay them, nor will I try. My neighborhood support system has been the envy of many. We love where we live. I moved out here to the middle of nowhere kicking and screaming. Now it is home. On the day of my remission, my father took Mark and Mom and me out to dinner; upon our return, 100 neighbors were lining the street with red balloons. We got out of the car, and they screamed REMISSION and released them. I was moved with relief and love and amazement. Then we opened the champagne!!

I've heard from college friends and high school friends, my

church held a blood drive in support of me. Our three children have been loved and supported in our Catholic School Community. When we survive this as a family, I will have them to thank. Countless times I have been told that I was being prayed for and thank God that I was. There is truly no other excuse for my being here. I have so far beaten the odds. Why can't I do that in Vegas?

I have responded to treatment in a textbook fashion. While other cancer patients around me struggle, their families struggle and I am confused. Why did I get this, why did they? Cancer does not discriminate, and that is what scares me most. I drive my sister crazy; she has always told me that I should be more careful, lock my doors, live with caution. Never has that been my plan, and yet now I wonder how I will feel. Everything scares me now. I worry all the time about those I love. Illness, etc…But I know that worry is a waste of time, particularly at 3:00 a.m. when I should be sleeping.

Thank you, God, for Mark, Will, Sam and Mitch. Help me to count my blessings every day. Help me to know that there is always someone worse off that needs my prayers. Help me to use this life that you have returned to me with usefulness and purpose. Help me to leave this world a better place each day.

In three weeks I will go into a maintenance program, which will include lots of pills, including an oral chemo pill. I have every reason to believe that in 5 years I will be among the growing group of CANCER SURVIVORS. I thank you for tuning in and for caring about the Volpe family. We are alive and well and living in Indiana. Please stop on by!

God Bless and LIFE ROCKS!

CHAPTER 23

Oklahoma!

Jon Butler, one of my fraternity brothers, coined the phrase, "You've got to maintain!" At the time, he meant figure out a way to control oneself especially during that hedonistic period I fondly recall as those, good old college daze when sobriety and sound judgment were totally lacking. Jon was a low-key, quiet, very laid back and unassuming type of guy. He was a good student, majoring in electrical engineering. I roomed with him a couple of quarters or so and have never forgotten his words of advice. When I'd get out of control, he would always say, "Volpe, you've got to maintain!"

Now it was time for Karen to maintain her remission. For the next 20 months she would have her blood checked regularly; she would take a battery of pills and we would pray she remained in remission. Dr. Cripe told us about the odds in very straightforward terms. Eighty percent of the people with Karen's type of leukemia would lose their remission sometime within two years from the original onset of the disease. After that, the odds of the cancer returning were much smaller, as in a single digit percentage.

Our goal was simple. Karen had to remain in remission two years from the date of onset, or June 2004. We asked Dr. Cripe the obvious question.

"What would he do if she lost her remission?"

He replied quite confidently that if this were to occur, he would administer arsenic trioxide in order to achieve a second remission, but he felt that the odds were good that this would not be the case, given Karen's profile. Regardless, he was also sure the arsenic trioxide would work and get her into a second remission if this were the case. Things would get much more complex if this were to occur because Karen would need a bone marrow transplant, and this possibility introduced a whole new set of dynamics.

Karen was put on an oral chemo maintenance program, taking daily doses of methotrexate and Purinethal. She took an array of other pills as well, but these two were the mainstay drugs used to help keep the leukemia at bay. She was bald, but her hair was starting to slowly grow back in. Later, she went through a stage of hair growth; Karen jokingly referred to these as pubes, and then after a few months she referred to her tightly woven hair as Jerry Seinfeld hair. Will called her locks of hair "chemo curls."

We tried to resume having fun, and on the weekend of October 5th, we went back to northeastern Ohio to visit family and see the Browns battle the Ravens on ESPN's *Sunday Night Football* broadcast. Karen and I left the kids at Pat's, and we went up and tailgated with D.J. and his wife, Paula. Karen cut loose a little and actually had a fun time drinking a little and acting silly with Paula.

There was a sick moment in sports history, or at least Browns' history, that occurred right in front of "The Dawg Pound" this cool evening. The ball was snapped over Tim Couch's head, and as Couch scrambled to the errant football, Ray Lewis and a slew of Ravens crashed into Couch. Tim laid there motionless on the field, knocked unconscious, suffering a concussion. Those classless fans in the pound cheered because the backup, Kelly Holcomb, prepared to come on the field to take over as quarterback. There were more than just the fans in the pound cheering while Couch lay there prone on the field, not moving.

I was horrified!

It reminded me of the time back in the mid-'70s when Joe "Turkey" Jones had picked up Terry Bradshaw and thrown him on his head. The fans were going crazy with glee. Their antics were truly in poor taste, but it was the '70s and it was the hated Steelers quarterback twitching in pain on the ground.

It was bad enough to cheer when an opposing player was hurt, but this was our own quarterback who had taken an ass whooping his entire professional career and had played his heart out, with hardly a lick of pass protection or a running game the past three years. I was embarrassed at how the Cleveland fans presented themselves on national TV. It was the first time I had left a game early, and as we made our way out, Holcomb threw an interception in the end zone on the last play of the game that could have won it. He had rallied the Browns from a big deficit to pull within a touchdown of winning, but still losing 26-21.

We decided our kids would not miss school, so we drove down to Akron, picked up them up, and headed back to Indianapolis arriving in Carmel at five in the morning. It ended up being a wasted effort because when the alarm rang at 6:30, nobody moved including me. The kids were late getting to school, and I didn't get to work until 10:00 in what was probably one of my dumber moves. However in my mind, it was a significant event as we tried to get the family back to having some fun and traveling.

A week later, my CRHP team served as the seed team at St. Mary's parish in Alexandria, Indiana, 40 minutes northeast of Carmel. The men at St. Mary's wanted to start the CRHP program. To get it started, members from another parish were solicited to help the men at St. Mary's by putting on the weekend on their behalf. From there, the men at St. Mary's would take over establishing their own CRHP process. I welcomed the opportunity to give a shorter version of my witness on Christian Community that I had presented a few months earlier. After I was done talking about my wife's struggle to beat leukemia, a man from St. Mary's came up to me, and he complimented my wife and I, given our story of faith and courage.

Then he said, "Do you know our Holly?"

With that, the hair on my back stood up, and I became a little choked up as I immediately recalled meeting the young and pretty Holly at IUMC a few months earlier during one of Karen's transfusion visits.

"Yes, I have met her. She's remarkable and I know she's going to make it, too," I said.

At that I knew I had to get back to my wife, who was still suffering the aftermath from her third round of chemotherapy. Right before I left, one of my CRHP brothers lent me his copy of Springsteen's latest release, *The Rising*, which was written especially for the families victimized by the events of 9/11. In time, this album would also provide comfort to me—it was his most powerful album ever, or should I say CD, since *Born To Run*.

As I flew down the highway, I felt guilty having left Karen home alone for four hours with the kids. While I drove south, I also couldn't stop thinking about Holly. She too had a husband and family going through the same ordeal as ours. The lyrics to my new Springsteen favorite "Lonesome Day," were ringing in my head as I thought about my witness and Holly.

"Let kingdom come; I'm gonna find a way through this Lonesome Day."

It was one of those small world stories: St. Louis de Montfort had Karen to pray for, and St. Mary's had their special girl named Holly for whom the entire parish was rallying around. At the same time, it was hard for me to not also think about Karen's friend Ken Shiflett who had never made it into remission. I had never met Ken, and on one of our recent visits to IUMC, Katie Hincher told us Ken had passed away. Karen went to the calling hours and talked with Ken's wife.

Karen and the kids had been trying to convince me to get another dog. We had a dog after we moved to Indy. It was a black lab we found out on I-74 on our way back to Mason to visit our friends near Cincinnati. We named her Mason, but she kept running away. One time Karen had a choice between picking up the kids or chasing the stupid dog. The kids won out, and the wild animal was gone for good. A new puppy, my family reasoned, would be wonderful company for Karen while she recovered. She dragged me down to the Animal Protective League of Indianapolis one afternoon, and before I knew it, I had the credit card out to get a cage and shots for our newest addition to the household, a cute little female mutt named "Jessie." She was adorable, but this animal would only last six months before we would be forced to take her back to the pound.

We were unable to housebreak the charming little doggie. I spent my 44th birthday steam-cleaning the carpets throughout our home. The dog had a case of diarrhea all over the house. I ended up on my hands and knees cleaning up the carpets for hours when I should have been eating a steak and opening presents with my family.

On Thanksgiving weekend, we headed back to northeastern Ohio for what was indeed a special and emotional Thanksgiving. There was so much to truly give thanks for because we all had weathered a horrific storm. Karen just wanted to move on and was tired of everybody telling her how great she looked, when she felt she looked terrible. Her hair was slowly starting to grow back in, and over time she was looking less frail. While she was back in Ohio, she relayed a story that had happened to her in Indianapolis one day as she drove a friend, Jackie Graham, who was dealing with her own cancer, down to IUMC for her transfusions and blood work.

As the two of them were waiting at a stoplight, some redneck in a pickup truck spit on my wife's minivan. Karen surmised that the man who spat on her minivan probably thought the two of them were lesbians, and Karen was the "tough dyke" with the short hair. She was sick of people looking at her strangely at the bank and at the grocery store once she tried to resume having a life.

We had a nice Christmas, and Karen sent a Christmas card to everyone who had sent her a card, present or flowers while she dealt with the wretched leukemia. We wrote a quick note on the back of our family photo that was taken in front of our Christmas tree to more than 300 well wishers, including family and friends. Karen kept every return address, and her mom wrote out page after page with names of the people who had touched our lives and prayed for Karen's recovery. As I look at the picture today, it's hard to believe how far we have come, how far we have climbed. In the photo, the children are fine and happy. Karen looks drawn, but her beautiful blue eyes shine with hope.

In the meantime, Karen had spent some time on the phone to see whether the trip to New York City she had purchased at POWWOW back in 2001 was still salvageable. All of the expiration dates had come and gone for the airfare and hotel accommodations while Karen was sick. We had outbid everyone who was interested in this trip back in 2001, and Karen had planned on taking the trip in 2002, but cancer got in the way, and this little adventure was put on the back burner. I had mentally chalked this expenditure up as a lost cause and one of the prices we had to pay for her getting so sick. The forfeited money didn't matter to me because Karen had made it through the ordeal and was on the road to becoming a cancer survivor. However, it mattered to Karen and instead of taking her sister or sister-in-laws; Karen decided it would be much better if the whole family went to the Big Apple.

Karen played the "cancer card" very well. When she called Continental Airlines and told them of her predicament, they said, "We'll be happy to honor the certificates even though they are past the expiration date."

Next, she called the Edison Hotel on Times Square.

They were unbelievably nice and said, "Mrs. Volpe, we would be happy to have you stay at our hotel, subject to availability, on any date you can make it to New York City."

As a follow-up, the hotel even sent a nice gift package with a note saying they looked forward to seeing us soon. I booked three more airline tickets, and from there the entire Volpe family was set to head out to New York City on January 2, 2003.

Karen and I didn't buy much at all, and our Christmas presents to one another were pretty simple. We had gone through a lot of unbudgeted cash due to insurance co-pays and miscellaneous deductibles, but we decided the family trip to NYC was priceless. This would be a special family present. Karen needed to get back on the road and have something to look forward to. In spite of going through some cash, our situation didn't keep me from giving her a simple gold bracelet engraved with three words: "The Adventure Continues."

When she saw the words, she knew they now had a much more significant and deeper meaning than when we originally coined the phrase in Calgary.

Our family made it to the airport and boarded our flight over to New York's La Guardia without a hitch. When we hit the ground, we quickly found a cab and made our way to Times Square. The children were amazed at all the traffic and the skyscrapers; there was so much to see and so much to do. We checked into our room at the Edison Hotel, unusually large for a hotel built in the 1920s. The friendly bellhop gave us all sorts of tips on where to go and what to do. As soon as we had organized and unpacked, we went quickly down to Times Square. I took the kids for a quick bite of pizza, while Karen waited in line for bargain-priced tickets to a Broadway show. When I returned to relieve her in line, Mitchell was about ready to crash. Karen didn't mind waiting in line while I took him back to the Edison for a nap.

While Mitchell and I were at the hotel, Karen scored five tickets to see Patty Duke as Aunt Emma in the Rodgers and Hammerstein's classic *Oklahoma!*

Out on the street near Times Square, Karen, Will and Samantha also met David Blaine, the outrageous magician we had all seen on HBO. He looked at Karen and said, "You are a very troubled person, aren't you? And you have not been well."

He pulled out a deck of cards and asked Karen to pick one, look at it, and place it back in the deck. Seconds later, she looked in her purse when requested to do so, and her card was in her purse. He did the same trick again, and this time the card appeared inside a nearby storefront window.

As Karen, Sam, and Will departed, the magician grabbed Will's shoulder, looked him square in the eye and said, "Take good care of your mom. She needs you!"

They were all amazed and burst into the hotel room to tell Mitchell and me all about their bizarre encounter with the magnificent magician.

The five of us had dinner at this old-fashioned '50s-style diner, where our waitress had just come to New York City to find stardom. Samantha was fascinated, and then we dashed off to the show. *Oklahoma!* was excellent, a good family show including numerous old familiar songs. After the show, we were shocked to find we were all allowed to stop in at a bar right by our hotel in a hotel complex called the Waterfall. We're not in Kansas anymore, Toto!

Karen and I had a drink, and then we went back to the hotel because we had to get up early to see Matt Lauer and Katie Couric. We woke up at 6:00 a.m. and managed to pry the kids out of bed. We dressed quickly and then took the long walk up to Rockefeller Center for *The Today Show* on NBC. It was very cold, so cold that Karen took one child at a time into an adjacent coffee shop. We waited an hour and half with our Ohio State flag in front of us to be on one of the camera shots when they pan the audience and everyone screams. I was bummed because Katie Couric had the day off. Finally, we were on and a good long shot of our Samantha was seen across the entire country at about 9:00 a.m. EDT. Then we ran across the street into the warmth of the NBC's gift shop.

There was the long cold walk back to the hotel for a quick nap, and then we were off again, even though the kids liked the idea of a warm hotel room and two TV sets. We took a cab over to Martha Stewart's for a private tour of her enterprise. We were there for more than three hours and saw Martha's business from top to bottom. We saw the entire mail-order catalog product development complex. I had no real appreciation of all the time and research for product development that went into such an undertaking. They were already working, a year in advance, on products for the 2003 Christmas catalog. The entire magazine production process was very interesting, and we also witnessed first-hand the kitchen where her fabulous recipes are developed. We spoke with a number of women who worked on *Martha Stewart's Living* magazine about the horrific events of September 11, 2001.

Unfortunately, we weren't able to see a taping of Martha's television show, because of Martha's legal troubles. I just couldn't believe that Martha Stewart was about to go to jail, while a man like O.J. Simpson walked the streets and played golf every day, like any other retired pro-football player. All five of us were beat, so we had a pretty simple dinner and then hit the sack.

On Saturday, we dragged our kids all over Manhattan. First we took a subway to the Staten Island Ferry, and then we took the ferry ride across to the island, got off and then right back on again. We had a great view of the famous bridges and the Statue of Liberty as we cruised out on Hudson Bay. Then we walked around Chinatown for a while. We never took a break as we headed back to midtown Manhattan for a jaunt through Macy's, which was still decorated for Christmas. Next, we went to a place where we could get a good view of the Empire State Building, figuring we would freeze if we went up to the observation deck.

We went to St. Catherine's Cathedral, Toys-R-Us and Saks, all on Fifth Avenue. For dinner, we grabbed a cab up to Little Italy and had some pasta at Sorrento's. While we were at dinner, we watched the first half of the mythical National Championship Game of college football between our Ohio State Buckeyes and the Canes from Miami of Florida.

Then we stopped by at the site where the Twin Towers had toppled to say a prayer. It was a very touching moment, and although it was night and we couldn't really see the huge cavern left there, it was still hard to imagine the horror that had transpired on September 11, 2001.

In my mind, I compared what happened there with our own miniature version of 9/11 in Karen's fight to beat cancer. However, there was one big difference with Karen.

She had hope.

After visiting the site of the tragedy, the cabby took us back to the ESPN Zone near our hotel on Times Square, where we watched the end of what was one of the most exciting college football games I have ever seen. The huge underdog Buckeyes managed to pull out the win after a questionable pass interference call. I was happy, but in my mind, I was bummed because the Browns were taking on the Steelers the next day in Pittsburgh in the NFL playoffs, and I knew there was no way two underdog teams from Ohio could win big games on the same weekend.

The next morning we slept in. Karen took Samantha shopping while the boys and I stayed at the hotel to watch the Browns. The Browns got off to a fast start and had the Steelers on the ropes the entire game. Cleveland's quarterback Kelly Holcomb passed for over 400 yards as the Browns built a 12-point lead. But as usual, head coach, Butch Davis, relaxed the defense the last eight minutes of the game and allowed Pittsburgh to move the ball slowly, but surely and without a pass rush the Steelers prevailed. Total frustration set in again; it was like the jinx of The Drive and The Fumble had happened again. When we settled in at home, the kids headed back to school, and we resumed the winter grind.

It was a trip to remember. Karen loved every minute it, as did the kids.

A few weeks later, we hosted a large cocktail party for the neighbors, who were going to the first annual Mardi de Montfort Gala Dinner/Auction. We rented a stretch limousine so none of our neighbors had to be concerned with drinking and driving. Our neighbors were very generous in attending, as we were the only ones with children attending the school at SLDM. However, the Thieme and the Crisci families had younger children just around the corner from starting kindergarten. Karen spent a good part of the day at the school decorating the gym and transitioning the gym into a New Orleans-themed outdoor garden. Karen and Father Dave Hellmann had been the visionaries who had approached the pastor, Fr. Tim Kroeger, with the idea to begin the school's major fundraiser, but due to her illness, she had been unable to plan how the inaugural event would unfold. Cindy Kelley had taken over as the main event planner and Karen was impressed with the décor and the numerous items that had been procured from area businesses. The gracious parishioners and friends ensured the event would be a success.

After Fr. Tim gave the blessing, and Cindy Kelly thanked the numerous people who had served on the many committees to make the inaugural event happen, she then started to talk about my wife. I don't remember a word she said, but at the end everyone attending was standing, applauding Karen. She sat there in her seat looking straight down as Cindy and her husband walked down to present Karen with a dozen beautiful red roses. Many of the women at our table and I were so touched by the ovation that we couldn't hold back the tears. Karen just shook her head and looked down.

She finally looked up at me with tears in her eyes and said, "I just want it to be over. When will it be over?"

CHAPTER 24

Paradise Beach

The biweekly trips to the Cancer Pavilion continued, as did Karen's oral chemo maintenance program. One of the side effects we had to keep an eye on due to the methotrexate was Karen's liver function. Victoria Hunt was charged with continued monitoring of Karen's liver enzymes every time she came in. Her white blood count had returned to a normal range of around 6,200. There were no signs of any Blasts, and the level of her platelets had settled in around 175,000, which was low, but still within the normal range. She no longer needed transfusions, and she was gaining weight.

She was beating the odds so far and still dealing with the fact that she had cancer. When she was in the hospital, researchers who were trying to find out how Karen had contracted the disease interviewed her a few times. Unfortunately, there has never been enough data to statistically link the disease with a cause. Some studies suggest a correlation with exposure to the chemical benzene. Karen never was exposed to a plant setting where constant exposure to this chemical would fit. She researched the disease on the Internet.

Was it caused by indoor house paint? We had just painted the lower level when Karen became so suddenly ill. Could there be something in the chemical dyes that are in the fabrics she handles for Karen's Kurtains?

I had my own far-fetched theory that this whole saga was related to a virus she picked up in Europe while backpacking in the early '80s that had remained dormant in her body for 20 years before the change in her DNA makeup manifested itself with the leukemia. She searched for an answer, determined only on becoming a full-fledged survivor; that is, someone who has been living cancer-free for five years. Regardless of how she had contracted the disease, at this point we made baby steps toward returning back to a normal life, both physically and mentally.

Karen had begun a class in Pilates at Lifetime Fitness after finding the classes helpful in restoring her flexibility and stamina. Her skin was still ailing from the effects of the chemo and was extremely dried out from all the treatments. While she attended her class, I continued to hit the treadmill, do my sit-ups and lift weights. At the end of January, I had finally been totally weaned off the Depakote, and I was determined to get into some semblance of shape.

Karen had decided to participate in the Indianapolis 500 Festival's Mini-Marathon the first week of May, and she had invited her brothers and sister and their spouses to join in. Tommy and his wife, Diana, played indoor soccer and were also in-training. Kenny and Anne also signed on to walk "The Mini" as everyone in Indy called it. Her dad also signed up to make the long 13-mile hike through the streets of downtown, out around the track at the famous Speedway and back. I was somewhat confident in being able to at least walk a 15-minute mile 13 times in order to complete the half-marathon. Naturally, I was worried that in spite of setting such a lofty goal, Karen might not be able to finish the race given the brutal side effects of the chemo that had devastated her body.

In the meantime, I decided we needed to go on a long weekend to get away to somewhere warm for Valentine's Day.

February, to me, was always such a lousy month: football was over, baseball hadn't really started, and March Madness was just around the corner. We had been given a package of free hotel accommodations in St. Thomas with the purchase of our timeshare condo in Vegas. I found a nice deal for the airfare on ATA to St. Thomas, so we decided to spend Thursday through Sunday, including Valentine's Day, in the sunny Caribbean on one of the Virgin Islands. Pat came out to watch our children while we bathed in the sun.

When we arrived at the little airport in St. Thomas, a nice lady greeted us with free strawberry daiquiris. The whole scene was a little too much for Karen to handle. She cried in disbelief as she sipped the drink and even went back for seconds while we waited on our transportation to the Holiday Inn. Then she disappeared to the ladies room. When she came back I noticed that she had taken off her heavy sweatshirt and was wearing a more appropriate top for the 86-degree climate. Then she said, "I also took off my bra; let's get outta here."

While we were on the tropical island, we went out to eat and drank a few rum-oriented drinks at one of the local bars. Early on, we found a real fun waitress at the Hard Rock Café who had given us the scoop on the island. We scouted around and did some shopping. We just hung out at the pool a little while each day. Our room overlooked an ugly body shop and baseball field. If we looked out to the left, we did have a view of the water where yachts, cruise ships and seaplanes parked. One day, we went off to Meggen's Bay, but as it turned out, it was one of those days when an all-day cloud hovered above our part of the island, but it didn't matter to us as we continued to drink rum and listen to the local talent sing mostly Jimmy Buffett songs, including my favorite "Margaritaville."

We ran into a retired couple we had seen on the shuttle bus a few times. Their names were Ron and Sherrie and they told us the best beach on the island was a place called Paradise Beach, but that it took a long 40-minute taxi drive to get there. We took a long ride through some poverty-stricken areas of the island. When we got there, we saw what was, without a doubt, the prettiest place I had ever seen on the planet. Paradise Beach was appropriately named.

Karen, never a stranger to anyone, struck up a conversation with a family on the beach. As it turned out, they were from Akron, Ohio, of all places! The trip to St. Thomas was an important milestone for both of us. It indicated we had turned a corner and were starting to have fun again, to be a married couple. The romance had resumed.

We weren't patients anymore.

Our flight home was delayed due to an ice storm, and we ended up flying back early Monday morning, arriving just in time to get Karen to her appointment with Dr. Cripe at 10:00 a.m. Karen's blood work checked out fine, but she did complain of a constant nagging headache. Dr. Cripe attributed her headache to the oral chemo drugs she had been taking for the last five months. Karen was also being treated for keratosis, which required some blisters or minor dry patches on her skin to be burned off. These were skin cells that in time could prove to be cancerous. The chemo had brought out the potentially dangerous skin cells in advance and a wonderful oncology-dermatologist named Dr. Wolverton helped Karen deal with these areas of her skin.

At work, the SPP-MISO merger never materialized, so I turned my efforts toward developing a tariff that would include the necessary provisions for implementing a competitive energy market in the Midwest region. I worked closely with Rick Drom, who was the former General Counsel at the Pennsylvania-Jersey-Maryland (PJM) Interconnection, the organization we were trying to emulate that had been running a tight power pool for 20 years.

Anna McKenna, an associate of Rick's with whom I worked on a daily basis in developing the tariff, had an undergraduate degree in economics from McGill University in Montreal. She was born in Sicily and had moved to Canada at a young age. Besides her law degree, she was also fluent in five languages. I relished the opportunity to work with and learn from the best in the business. I also found out, by accident while in Washington D.C., that Jim Torgerson had hired a new vice president named Ron McNamara, who would be my new boss, as the Midwest ISO went through the arduous process of designing and developing the largest competitive energy market in the world. Ron is very well accomplished, having implemented energy markets in Australia and New Zealand. He had a PhD in Economics from the University of California at Davis and had worked for Duke Energy, American Electric Power, and Enron prior to the debacle that led Enron down the path to financial ruin. Ron held a passion for developing energy markets. He's an energetic guy and was a welcome addition to the Midwest ISO.

On a more personal front, I went to see Dr. Theobald in late February. He was happy with my progress. I had been off the harsh medications for more than six weeks, and, according to Karen, the old Mark was slowly returning. The challenge of the energy market, and more importantly, the fact that my wife remained in good health, had me feeling pretty good about life. I was proud of how my family had handled Karen's ordeal. Now,

I was more concerned with moving on. I really tried to believe it was over and that it was time to forge ahead.

However, not a morning that went by, as I sprang out bed to turn off the alarm, I fell into the terrible habit of thinking to myself, "God, is this the day my wife loses her remission?"

I always believed it was over and behind us, but I couldn't change the fact that Dr. Cripe had told us 80 percent of the patients with Karen's type of leukemia would lose their remission within the first two years. We were rapidly approaching the one-year anniversary and as the days passed it meant we were halfway to this milestone.

Finally in early May, Karen, Kenny, Anne, Tommy, Diana, Tom and I went downtown on a cool Saturday morning to walk the 13.1-mile course. Will had planned on being in the race, but his baseball commitment prevented him from attending. Karen had been battling bronchitis for most of April, and by race day she was ready to press on. Karen and I walked with Kenny, Anne and Tom, Karen's father. We were making pretty good time walking at a 15-minute-per-mile pace. Tommy and his wife, Diana, were the only ones who actually ran the race. A few days before the race, Will found out Pat Carlini from WTHR Channel 13 would be covering the race, and he wrote her the following letter in the hope his mom would be on television.

Dear Mrs. Carlini,

I wanted to send this to you because I have seen you on TV and you seem nice. My name is Will Volpe and I am 12 years old. This Saturday is a big day for me. I will be walking with my mom in the mini marathon. Our family has had a hard year. Last June, my mom was complaining of an ache in her stomach. After lots of pain, she went to the hospital. She was there for 3 days. They said that she would be ok. We all thought that she would be ok. Life went on as if mom was on a vacation. My dad was Mr. Mom until the news hit my family. I remember when dad called us to the family room. I was sitting in the very left seat of the couch. That night was the worst night of my life. Dad told us that my mom had CANCER, one of the worst six lettered words. He didn't know what kind of cancer but we found out that it was Leukemia. She spent the summer at IU hospital. Now she is in remission and our lives are getting back to normal. She calls pictures of herself, BC before cancer or AC for after cancer. Her hair is growing back and it is very, very curly. She is a miracle because she was 99% leukemic. Now almost a year later, we will be in the mini marathon together with my Dad too! If you see the race on TV, we'll be the ones in last place; my mom is the one with the crazy hair.

Thank you Mrs. Carlini

Will Volpe
thank you for your time

Karen's dad had to stop, at least seven times, to take a break. Karen started to feel some pain at the 11-mile mark, but she managed to push on and after three hours and 40 minutes we all made it to the finish line. Samantha and Mitchell came over the fence and crossed the finish line with their mom, who had accomplished an improbable feat when you consider all the destruction her body had encountered the prior year. Exhausted, we returned to Carmel for some top sirloin steaks, a few beers and plenty of sleep.

Indiana Life Insurance Company sponsored a contest called Celebrating Life in which anyone could submit a letter to the company explaining how someone he or she knew in the race was celebrating life, having beaten the odds in one way or another. The winners would receive an award, and Indianapolis Life would donate $500 in the name of the winner to a charity of his or her choice. I decided Karen's story merited an entry. Little did I know that her dad and sister, Kathy, had also submitted entries on her behalf as well. My entry was far from concise, and I sent it in via e-mail to Indianapolis Life on May 16th, a week after the mini and right after Karen's most recent appointment with Dr. Cripe, who was mildly shocked when told that Karen had walked the entire 13.1 miles.

Celebrating Life

No one person celebrates life each day the way my wife Karen Volpe celebrates life. Being somewhat new to greater Indianapolis, she heard about the Mini-Marathon in April 2002. It was too late get in shape to participate in 2002, so Karen set the 2003 race as her personal goal and invited family and friends to join her.

In June 2002, Karen was diagnosed with leukemia and she proceeded to receive three rounds of chemotherapy at the Indiana University Medical Center. Fortunately, in July, she was found to be in remission; however the effects of the treatment had taken a devastating physical effect. Despite the trauma, she continued to train for the mini by taking Yoga classes, hitting the treadmill and going on regular walks. About a month before the race, she contracted bronchitis, which made her final training even more difficult. On Friday night before the mini, still bound and determined, Karen hosted a carbo loading spaghetti dinner that was attended by family members from here in Indianapolis as well as a throng of Karen's family who traveled over from northeast Ohio to be in the race.

Over the course of the thirteen miles, Karen kept a brisk pace for one walking the mini, averaging around fifteen minutes per mile. Karen walked with her husband, Mark; her father, Thomas; her brother, Kenny; and his wife, Anne. At about the eleven-mile mark, she was beginning to feel some wear and tear, but the finish line was only two miles away—Karen pushed on. As we neared the finish line, two of Karen's three children, Samantha and Mitchell, ran out to give her a hug and they grabbed her hand as she pushed across the finish line. Karen's oldest son Will had planned on walking with his mom, but his commitment to his baseball team precluded him from being there. Will had sent Pat Carlini at WTHR TV13 a letter explaining how he admired his mom in her courageous fight with cancer. Karen crossed the finish line wearing Will's race tracking device #25072, so he was there with her in spirit.

Karen has plans to participate in other races around the country and will be on hand for next year's race too. The Monday following the race Karen had her regular checkup and blood work with her oncologist, Dr. Larry Cripe. He admits that there is still the possibility that the cancer could recur given that Karen was 99% leukemic when she was admitted to IUMC last summer. At the Volpe home, we "Celebrate Life" every day knowing that there are no guarantees with this type of cancer. Karen continues to be vigilant in taking the medications Dr. Cripe has prescribed for her two-year maintenance program.

If Karen's story and celebration of life were deemed worthy of one of this year's $500 award, she would donate the proceeds to IUF/Leukemia, Lymphoma and Multiple Myeloma Research headed by Dr. Cripe here in Indianapolis. All of the donations made to this nationally recognized cancer center would go for further research aimed at the development of treatments for patients with these diseases.

Sincerely submitted by Karen's husband Mark J. Volpe on May 16, 2003.

The contest entry written by her father is included below. His letter to Indianapolis Life is quite remarkable.

It would be fruitful for one to try to determine the height of a man by viewing his shadow at night, as it would be to reveal with any degree of specificity the courageous, characteristics, strength and determination of my daughter, Karen Volpe. Karen stared fear in the face, refused to blink, and beat it.

Coming off ovarian cyst surgery one day, pneumonia the second day, double pneumonia the third, Karen while still bleeding badly from surgery, was diagnosed with the real problem. Karen was 99.6 percent leukemia-ridden upon arrival at the IUPUI Medical Center on the fourth day of her sudden illness.

World class IU doctors, nurses and staff upon admission, June, 2002, told me Karen's chances of survival were somewhere between zero and non-existent. They had not yet learned with whom they were dealing. Karen is a fighter, and she practically invented the power of positive thinking!

We are from Ohio, unfamiliar with exciting Indianapolis traditions such as the Mini-marathon. The day Karen learned of its existence, she told me of her intent to walk. She did not walk alone! Husband Mark, her brother Ken, sister-in-law Anne, another brother Tom III, sister-in-law Diana, and dad walked with her. (One other brother and her only sister had planned on walking but were unable because of family considerations in Ohio.) With considerable help from neighbors in Carmel, Karen's mother babysat the grandchildren. The Mini-marathon walk was completed by all and qualified as a wonderful family affair, but here is the important part: had none of us walked with Karen, she would not have walked alone. Karen walks with God, and He understands she must remain to raise William, Samantha and Mitchell.

We are not sure whether it is God the Father, God the Son, or God the Holy Spirit that intervened on Karen's behalf. Regardless, He knows to check with fellow Trinity members before changing the plan as Karen plans on going nowhere until and unless her three children are grown, educated and on their own, after which she intends to be with Mark. Count on it! I am.

Respectfully submitted,
Thomas J. Coyne, Ph.D.

(The $500 donation shall be directed to Dr. Cripe for the leukemia research he does.)

And Kathy wrote straight from the heart.

Celebrating Life Award

I am nominating my sister, Karen Volpe, for the Celebrating Life award. Karen lives her life with such an incredible passion. Karen is passionate about everything that she undertakes. She is a phenomenal mother and wife. She is the glue of our family and gives of herself in every role she plays: daughter, sister, godmother, daughter-in-law, sister-in-law, etc. Karen is the altar lady at her church and personally decorates the altar for every holiday and season. This past January, while taking chemo, she took down 18 Christmas trees from the altar at her church. The entire time she has been battling leukemia, she has been more concerned about how her illness was affecting everyone else in her life than she was about her own situation.

Karen has always celebrated life and has continued to do so while battling leukemia. Karen is a "doer" and has not let this disease keep her down. Throughout my life, Karen has been the wind beneath my wings, and I am so proud to be her sister.

I am grateful to Dr. Cripe and the entire oncology unit at IUPUI for saving Karen's life. I had the honor of spending time with her while she was in reverse isolation and everyone with whom we came in contact was superb. I believe that if had Karen not been on 5 North, she would not be here today.

May God Bless Dr. Cripe and his team of professionals.

Sincerely,

Kathy Bergh

(I am hoping that a $500.00 donation will be directed toward Dr. Cripe and the research he does.)

CHAPTER 25

Virginia Beach

For the rest of 2003, we settled into a sense of normalcy. On July 15th, I sent Karen a dozen red roses to commemorate one-year of remission. We were over halfway to having made it to June 2004, where the statistics indicated she had a very good chance of remaining in remission for the long haul. I signed the card "Carpe Diem," which mimicked the awesome sign Shelly Thieme and the other ladies of the neighborhood had put up on the front of the house when she had achieved remission one year earlier.

We made it down to Virginia Beach for two weeks. This was important to the kids because going to the beach every August was like Christmas Day for them. It was a gleefully anticipated major event each summer. During the summer of 2002, there was no Christmas for the Volpe children as their mother's illness had forced us to go without the annual trip in the sun and sand.

In early August 2003, we had returned and it was a celebration. The children sensed all was right with the world because the five of us were together again, back at the shore. We went out to our favorite restaurant, Rockafeller's, down on Rudee's Inlet, a couple of times. My parents were there for part of the time, allowing us to have solo use of their condo for more than a week. My wife and father walked the boardwalk down to the pier and out to the end. This is a pretty good hike, about a mile or so from the condo and back. They vowed to return together after my dad turned 70 with Karen, totally cancer free, and my dad having dealt with his own scare involving his heart. They had both faced most difficult circumstances and came through—now they vowed to meet the test of time.

I was surrounded by the serenity of the seashore and I started to write this book. Didn't Hemingway do his writing from near the shore in the Florida Keys? When we left, I had typed 70 pages. My writing was intended to be a tribute to my wife and it was my hope others could learn from the things we did correctly, as well as our mistakes. Maybe this inspirational story could provide some benefits to others facing an extraordinary medical challenge. It was also a good way for me to vent. I had no grand illusions that my book would ever make it to the *New York Times* bestseller list. However, it was fulfilling and yet a perplexing project, given the nature of the story.

How would I know when I was done?

Karen continued to see Dr. Cripe once a month, generally on Mondays, and kept up with her oral maintenance program. Her nagging headaches continued, but Dr. Cripe felt they were related to the oral chemo drugs. One day Karen received a phone call from an Indianapolis Life Insurance Company representative. Somehow, out of the more than 1,000 regional entries, our family's three separate entries had each come back as winners. The company representative told Karen this was so remarkable that they decided to increase the donation to Dr. Cripe's ongoing research from $500 to $2,500. Karen was asked to go downtown for a photo shoot to receive her award. Think about it. What are the odds that our entries would end up in separate batches, reviewed by three different sets of judges who independently concluded the same thing?

In the fall, we continued along with our typical family activities. Samantha had considered quitting gymnastics, but Jane Deveau, who owned the school, wanted her to reconsider. So, Karen and Samantha collectively decided to rededicate their efforts towards Samantha's gymnastics career.

We also found out why Tom had stopped to use the facilities so often while we walked The Mini. He had prostate cancer. The ailment was treatable because it was caught early. Tom was like his daughter. He was determined to beat his disease. They now shared another common bond, cancer.

In mid-October, I took all three kids to Cleveland to show them how to tailgate, and we saw the Browns beat the Oakland Raiders. It looked as if Halloween had come early—Raider Nation fans showed up wearing their Darth Vader outfits. Samantha said to one guy cruising by, in full makeup with silver lightning bolts coming out of his head, "You've got to be kidding me, right!"

A few weeks later on one rainy Saturday morning all five of us went to Bloomington to see the Ohio State Buckeyes beat the Indiana University Hoosiers. About 80 percent of those attending the road game were clad in scarlet and gray. Buckeye fans were everywhere. When the entire stadium did the O-H-I-O cheer, with each side of the field and each end zone shouting its respective letter in order, the handful of home crowd Hoosiers had to be slightly embarrassed. We tailgated after the game as traffic let out, and we were very impressed with the Indiana University campus. It wasn't flat like the cornfields of central Indiana near where we lived. There were rolling hills and lots of trees.

Indiana University has a good business school, and after all, we had become big fans of IU. It was the IU Medical Center up in Indianapolis, led by Dr. Cripe and Katie Hincher, who had saved Karen's life. It was hard not to be a fan, even if Samantha wasn't impressed with the athletics of the Hoosier cheerleaders. My children heard the "f" word a few too many times from the Hoosier student body near where we stood for most of the game in the end zone, but Karen and I weren't about to let this ruin a wonderful day.

A few weeks later in early November, we returned to Bloomington to watch Samantha in her first big gymnastics meet. She did very well and her all-around score, the total for all four events—floor, beam, vault and bars—exceeded 35, high enough to qualify for the state meet in Mishawaka near South Bend later that year. We were so proud of Samantha. She had gone from quitting gymnastics altogether to qualifying for the state meet. Even though she was a little older than the majority of the girls competing at level 4, she set her sights on doing well at the state meet and then moving on to level 5.

Another fun holiday season came and went. We hosted a big party for the neighbors where a Chinese gift exchange was the rage. Karen made the mistake of scheduling the party during the second half of a Browns game that they lost in overtime to Denver, of all teams.

Samantha continued competing in several gymnastics meets, while Will was forced to move up a level in hockey to Pee Wee after only one season at Bantam due to a change in the age cutoff date. Will gave away some size and is not the fastest player ever to wear skates, but he thinks well and is seldom out of position as a defensemen. Mitchell continued to do well in indoor soccer, a sport he had come to love. He's very coordinated and has great skills, plus a pretty good leg, scoring many goals. Our youngest was pretty tough and resilient given all that he had to deal with at such a tender age. He never backed down and he dominated play in a very humble way. Mitchell was always the first player to congratulate another player on a goal, and he always reacted rather casually when he scored a goal himself, which was often.

For Christmas, I could think of only one present that seemed fitting for my bride. She was shocked to open up a single very heavy box and find a black mink jacket.

She looked at me and said, "I never saw myself as a person who would wear a fur."

I told her I wanted her to be warm, and she deserved something special, having just beaten cancer. When I bought the jacket using a coupon from Lazarus (getting a super deal at the before-Thanksgiving sale), I told the ladies in the fur department I was buying it for my wife who had just undergone 15 rounds with leukemia and had come out on top. The sales lady told me she had met many women over the years in a similar situation that had come in to buy a fur or put one on layaway.

She said, "Only one never returned to pick up her coat!"

In January, Deveau's Gymnastics hosted the Circle of Stars meet in downtown Indianapolis at the Convention Center. As parents, we were required to do our share of volunteer work or pay a large fee to help subsidize the costs of putting on the competition. It was a cold day, and the Colts were playing the Patriots in the AFC Championship Game so the city was all abuzz and excited about the possibility of Peyton Manning taking the Colts to the Super Bowl. Luckily, the game was in suburban Boston, otherwise, the area near the Convention Center immediately adjacent to the RCA Dome where the Colts play would have been very crowded and parking would have been expensive. The Convention Center had provided a number of big screens in the concourse for fans to keep up on the game. Unfortunately, Peyton threw too many interceptions, and in spite of a last minute gasp at a comeback, it was the Patriots that went on to eventually win the Super Bowl. Samantha didn't fare too well either that day, but we were still very proud of our daughter.

Karen had decided to join the "Team-In-Training" efforts with the local chapter of the Leukemia and Lymphoma Society, which was sponsoring runners in the Mini-Marathon and other races around the country. She had set a goal to raise $5,000 for the Leukemia and Lymphoma Society, and she decided to send a letter to a select group of family and friends. Here's the touching letter she sent out to everyone.

Dear Friends and Supporters,

It seems almost criminal to ask for any more support from you. Your support has been so amazing and appreciated. I wouldn't even be able to make myself do it if I were not so aware. So personally aware of the need for continued Cancer Research. To the complete shock of my family and friends, I was diagnosed in June of 2002 with Leukemia, AML—M3. I have a very rare form of the disease. At 42 and as a woman it was basically unheard of. Less than two years before my diagnosis 80% of the patients died, the survival rate was grim. Due to Cancer Research I was offered a new drug called ATRA. This, in addition to the standard fare of chemo, chemo and more chemo has allowed me to write this letter today. Research is our ONLY hope. For every affected patient there are Mothers and Fathers and children that pay a very dear price. Cancer and its devastating affects can follow you around for a lifetime.

In June of 2002, my husband and I were busy planning our exciting summer, our 3 kids were in their last days of school, it was a gorgeous day and all was right with the world. I had complaining of a stomachache and flu like symptoms. I was WAY to busy to stop our busy schedule for a stomachache. Additionally, it would be helpful to know that Leukemia is a frequently misdiagnosed disease. It has symptoms very similar to other ailments. By the time it was discovered what I had, I was very, very ill. A trip to the emergency room later our roller coaster ride had begun. I had double pneumonia and a collapsed lung and was 96% Leukemic. I was in isolation for 30 days as the initial step of my treatment. When I was finally able to go home, I was anxious to attempt to get my affairs in order because I knew more Hospital stays and Chemo lay ahead. I opened my checkbook and found the LAST check I had written in June had been to the Leukemia and Lymphoma Society. Blood related cancer will be the diagnosis for 106,000 people in the U.S. this year and will claim the lives of 58,000 this year. Research is changing the numbers! I am a prime example.

Team-In-Training is the tool that I choose to use to give back to those that have saved my life. They count on our research money. I want to keep the money flowing, 80% of the money I am able to raise will go directly to research. The other 20% will go to support patients and their families. Our family needed, and took, all the help we could get. That was another hard lesson to learn. Previous to my cancer diagnosis I was strong and active. I am trying to regain that strength and my mentors in Team-In-Training are going to help me. I will be run/walking the Indianapolis Life Mini Marathon in May of this year. I walked the Mini last year and it was a very rewarding experience. Family came to town and joined me in a marvelous show of support. It was amazing. This year I want to do it for those who can't and for the families of those who can't. On this day, at this moment, due to research, I have my life back. I don't know what the future holds and neither do you. I am in remission. In May, not only will I complete the Mini, but I will complete my chemo treatments. At that point it will be wait and see. Time will tell all.

I am asking you to contribute toward my personal goal of $5,000. This is your opportunity to change the future of the patient diagnosed with Blood Born Cancer. Please donate whatever amount that you are able, $20, $50, $100 are just suggested amounts, larger amounts will be smiled upon as well. The contribution is tax deductible. Please make checks payable to the Leukemia and Lymphoma Society and return them in the enclosed envelopes by April 1, 2004. Thank you so much and may God watch over you.

Karen Volpe

She raised more than $6,000. A handful of donors wrote personal checks for $500. The impact the letter had speaks for itself.

As 2004 dawned, our main focus was making it safely into the month of June because the odds of Karen's ultimate recovery hinged on the calendar turning to June, without a loss of remission. As every day came and went, we felt the tide turning our way. It was only a matter of time before the statistics were on our side.

Of course, I was well aware of the saying, "There are liars, there are damn liars and then there's statistics." However, I kept this quirky little saying to myself as I had every confidence that Karen's cancer would soon be totally behind us.

CHAPTER 26

Vail

As the months rolled into February rapidly approaching June, we decided that skiing somewhere out west for Spring Break might be an excellent way to transition from the chemo maintenance program and back into the mainstream of being a soccer mom. I spent some time on the Internet looking for potential places where one of our numerous banked weeks from our Vegas condo could be used somewhere in the mountains. One day, from out of nowhere, as I continued my database searches, rooms suddenly became available in Vail and Avon, Colorado. I jumped on a room at the Christie Lodge in Avon, just 10 minutes from Vail. Plus, we were arriving on the first day of the off-peak season—lift tickets had dropped from $79 a day to $27 a day. What luck! Free accommodations and cheap lift tickets, good at five area resorts. Then I managed to find bargain airline tickets, which worked nicely into our budget. It was a time to celebrate and live for today. One of the things I remember Pat's husband, John Bird, telling me one day in reference to his first wife, who had died a few years earlier, was that there was no sense waiting to travel until later in life, he said, "Do it now while you have your health!" This advice always stuck with me.

Karen's constant headaches were getting to her. She had just gone through her own CRHP weekend in March. A friend of hers, whom she had met through women's CRHP at St. Louis de Montfort, who was in pharmaceutical sales, told her she thought the methotrexate dosage was very high and potentially damaging. Two weeks later, Karen met a doctor from church who told her that her life was over, due to the saturation of methotrexate throughout her body. She contemplated cutting back on the methotrexate

The month of June was just around the corner. It was important to her that she would be able to have a good time in Vail, in early April, and not be a drag on the entire family. When she told me that she was contemplating cutting back on her meds, I told her I would support any decision she made, and that it was entirely up to her. After much thought and consideration, she decided to cut back on her methotrexate in the hope that her constant pain would eventually subside. This decision was made without consulting with Dr. Cripe. Karen decided she would eventually tell him of her decision, but she was not going to actively seek his permission.

Her remission had gone smoothly. Slowly weaning herself off the meds to the point of quitting the treatments 30 days or so prior to two years did not pose any major risk, I thought. Otherwise, I would have tried to talk her out of it. It's easy to play Monday morning quarterback and second-guess if things went awry, but I was not the person that was so miserable with the grinding headaches. To me, she had made it. June was practically here; and if she was going to lose her remission, it would have happened by now.

The trip to Denver went pretty well. Will was a trouper and helped haul our clothes and ski equipment. As for Mitchell, he had received an advance on his birthday present, a new Salomon snowboard that was on sale, of course, at the end of the season.

We grabbed our Mitsubishi four-by-four rental at the airport and headed west on I-70 toward Vail. As we drove west, the snow got deeper and the Rockies shimmered against the first sparkle of moonlight. When we got to the Christie Lodge, at about 11:00 that evening, everyone pitched in to move the luggage and equipment into our cozy, but clean accommodations. The room had brand new furniture and carpet. Karen was elated. All of the old furniture was still in giant dumpsters in back of the lodge's parking lot.

The next morning we got up, and by 10:00 we were at the base of Vail to get Sam and Will's rental skis. The people at the ski shop were very helpful, and they made sure we had everything we needed. Next, we were off to the gondola for the ride up to the top. The kids were fascinated by Vail's grandeur. The bottom of the hill was typical spring skiing conditions, warm and mushy. As we zoomed to the top, we could see the clouds come up to greet us, and then it became obvious that the better snow was in the higher elevations. It was the craziest weather. One minute it would be bright and sunny and then within minutes, a squall would set in and pelt us with sleet and horizontal snow as the wind kicked up.

For the first day, we spent a lot of time at lift number 15. This was really a beginner hill, but to Mitchell, this was a nice place to learn how to control his new snowboard. He was frustrated at first, because it took some getting used to. Karen volunteered to stay with him until he got the hang of it while Sam, Mitch and I took off for some real hills. We had walkie-talkies so it was easy to page the other party to find out where everyone was heading. The first thing Karen taught Mitchell was how to stop. This was a very good idea, but after Karen showed Mitchell how to lie down on his butt cheeks when things got tough there wasn't anything else either of us could show Mitchell. We knew how to ski, but had no clue how to teach Mitchell anything about his new board. One of the instructors gave Mitchell a quick lesson, and his level of frustration slowly diminished. Mitchell has amazing foot coordination.

Samantha had some problems initially, but eventually she also got the hang of it. She's very athletic. At the end of the day, we all skied together, and after five or six hours, we were spent and decided to call it quits. We headed back to the lodge and had a few Coors Lights. Karen did well despite her lingering headaches. Given all that she had been through, she still was able to ski well carving beautiful turns as she spun her way down the hill.

We worked the hills of Vail for six straight days at least seven hours a day, with only a 45-minute lunch break. Now we were a family that skied together. Vacations in the future could be planned around the slopes, not just the beach. This was a little ironic given the circumstances where we first met and how I popped the question years earlier.

At the lodge, we had the family hot tub outside our room and down a level. This was a wonderful way to whisk away the pain of a day on skis. Will set the pace! His transfer of hockey skills to skis, combined with the vigor of youth, allowed him to lead the pack. Mitchell was improving rapidly on the snowboard, although there were times when we literally had to drag him along. Karen had the technique down for putting Mitchell out in front of her and scooting him along many of the trails.

The weather cooperated for the most part. There were lots of days with plenty of sun, and then there were days when the cold fronts would roll in and the sky would be gray followed by hours of snow. It even snowed a few times at night making the next day's conditions more acceptable. Many veterans of the spring skiing scene said the conditions were the worst they had seen in years on the lower parts of the mountain. One day we were forced to ski all the way to the bottom because they had closed the lifts due to thunder. It never rained up on top, but having to ski through the mud and mashed potatoes versus taking the gondola down at the end of the day was a challenge.

We found that the best snow, and the longest run our whole family could negotiate, was on the west side of the resort called Lost Boy. It was a pretty long ride, and Mitchell grew to hate it, but the slightly challenging hill pushed Samantha to the point where she was fearless and had no trouble negotiating some pretty steep terrain, especially at the bottom.

There were a number of authentic Mexican restaurants in the area, and we dined at several of them. A few nights we saved money by using the little kitchenette in the room, where we cooked some pretty simple meals like spaghetti.

The last couple of days, Will decided he had mastered skiing and the snowboard would be another winter sport he would easily adapt to, so we fitted him with a nice rental, and he took to the hills. It was a much more difficult transition than he had assumed. We held up and waited for Will while he dealt with the same learning curve that Mitchell had endured earlier in the week. One of the highlights of the week was meeting up for lunch with Nora Wilson's father, Dr. Haas, whom Karen and I had skied with in Austria some 16 years earlier. He seemed to be getting along just fine despite losing his wife almost two years prior.

We had to catch a 10:00 a.m. flight from Denver to Indianapolis at the end of our wonderful week in Vail. We woke early to avoid a winter storm front that was moving in. About 45 miles out, we drove right into the storm. Luckily, we were able to keep moving at around 40 miles per hour, and we made it to the airport with plenty of time to spare. With lots of hands for all our gear, luggage, and souvenirs, everything fell into place. Samantha was happy in her new white sweatshirt with VAIL in pink letters and the rest of us remarked on how memorable this vacation was.

The next day we celebrated Easter.

Later in April, Samantha was a junior bridesmaid in Karen's cousin Katie Captain's wedding in Huntington, West Virginia. Our daughter looked absolutely stunning! She was the first person up the aisle.

After the wedding, as Karen and I waited to cross the street across from the student union on Marshall University's campus where the reception was held, Karen said, "It was really nice not to hear my name when they prayed for those members of the family who had passed away and weren't able to be here today."

Aunt Ellen and Uncle Mike were the proud parents of the bride, and somehow, once again, I ended up leading a chorus of men singing "Thunder Road" to Katie at the reception.

A few weeks later, Karen and I went to see Dr. Cripe. Karen told Dr. Cripe of her decision to stop taking the methotrexate due to the chronic headaches and the advice she had received from several people.

"That's fine, but I wish you had felt comfortable enough to tell me," he said.

Karen was somewhat apologetic about not informing him earlier of her decision, and Dr. Cripe felt that she had gone long enough with the maintenance program.

The bottom line finally had arrived, and we heard the words we had yearned to hear for so long.

Dr. Cripe said, "I believe you are done. You have beaten the leukemia, and you will never be on chemotherapy again."

"Really!" Karen said, "Well if that's the case, then give me a hug!"

She also hugged the remarkably compassionate Katie Hincher, who had been so instrumental in getting Karen into remission. It was hard for both of us to not break down and cry right there on the spot. We waited until we got to the elevator.

"Did he really say what I thought he said? Is it really over?" Karen said.

I said, "Yes! He said it's over. You have beaten leukemia, and you can move on with the rest of your life."

"Thank God," uttered Karen.

"Right, and we should do that right now," I replied.

We held hands and said an Our Father as the elevator sped down to the first floor.

While we drove home, I thought to myself, "This is great, the last chapter of my book, *How Karen Conquered Cancer* will be called "Vail." And how fitting, "V" for Vail, "V" for Volpe, and most importantly, "V" for Victory."

Karen had been collecting decorative versions of the letter "V" and she had at least 20 of them scattered strategically throughout her lovely home.

CHAPTER 27

ER

During the middle of May, Karen's headaches moved to neck pain, then evolved into a slight ringing in the ears and her overall fatigue gradually increased. In the middle of the month, she called Dr. Cripe's clinical nurse, Victoria Hunt, and told her about the pain. Unlike in the past, when it generally took her a few days to return Karen's calls, Victoria returned Karen's call the same day. Victoria told her that she had set up an appointment with a neurologist for June 24, 2004, almost six weeks away. Karen then consulted with our family doctor, Dr. Neil Wanee, in order to try to figure out what was causing her pain. Dr. Cripe preferred that we work through these issues with our family doctor. Dr. Wanee sent Karen to Community North Hospital for an MRI and an MRA. The tests were negative. A hearing test revealed that Karen had a minor loss of hearing with low-range tones. This was not the type of hearing loss that would require a hearing aid, but it was certainly disconcerting. Karen was being proactive in trying to manage her way through this latest turn of events.

We had always felt that Karen's pain was caused primarily because she had stopped taking the oral chemo medications, methotrexate and Purinethal. Maybe her body was going through some type of withdrawal. As the month of May wore on, the pain worsened, although Karen was able to be the master of ceremonies again at the SLDM Teacher Appreciation/Reverse

Raffle. She had just learned that another family at St. Louis de Montfort was also battling cancer. She had received permission from Laurie Stark to announce the Starks' family predicament and Karen did so right after grace. Tom Stark was stricken with a large cancerous growth that needed radiation before surgery could even be attempted. The barbershop quartet entertaining at the party sang a very solemn version of the "Our Father" right after Karen made the announcement. It was hard for me not to think about Karen's ordeal and just be thankful that it was over. I felt very bad for the Starks and prayed our God would be as kind and merciful to the Stark family as He was to us.

Karen was getting some mild relief from ibuprofen for her headaches, but the ringing in her ears was "almost maddening." Still, she was content to wait another four weeks for the appointment with the neurologist that Victoria had set up for the latter part of June. Karen would not keep this appointment.

She was experiencing a lot of discomfort, school had just let out and Pat drove out to help out with the kids. At about 4:00 a.m. on June 2nd, Karen popped up out of bed, like a piece of toast, startling me to the point that I was immediately fully awake. She sat on the side of the bed looking out the windows toward the Wetzels' house across the street. Earlier in the summer, Marty Wetzel had installed exterior landscape lighting that illuminated their home and the small trees down near the street.

Karen sat there silently looking toward the windows away from me, and then she said very quietly and without any panic in her voice, "I can't see anything at all out of my left eye."

"It's better now, but why did the Wetzels put up green Christmas lights in the middle of summer? All their lights look green," she said ever so softly.

"This is the last straw; we're going to the ER downtown first thing in the morning," I said.

I took a shower, and by 5:00 a.m. we had called Victoria Hunt's pager. The call was returned in five minutes. The voice at the other end wasn't Victoria. She was on vacation, and Katie Hincher was taking her calls.

What a blessing!

We had a competent voice that understood our case and would take practical steps to help us through these issues. Karen explained the situation to Katie and she told us to come straight to the ER.

As we left, Karen's mom said, "Make sure you get a blood test," and I replied back, "Trust me, we will."

Karen and I always had a long-standing date on Thursday nights at 10:00 p.m. to watch NBC's long-running, Emmy-winning drama *ER*. As we drove downtown on Meridian Street, past all the stately homes, to the Indiana University Medical Center's Emergency Room, her pain was glaringly obvious, so I drove briskly.

Karen kept saying, "I can't believe we're going back there. I don't want to do this."

I tried to remain calm and assured her that there had to be a simple explanation for what was going on, and that we would get it figured out.

There weren't any signs of the rush hour traffic yet so we made good time, even though every stoplight seemed like an eternity. Springsteen was playing softly in the background. "Please turn it off!" she said, writhing in pain, unable to find any comfort. We said an Our Father and a Hail Mary while holding hands as I maneuvered the black Pontiac Bonneville southward to IUMC.

While we drove, I thought to myself, "I only want to know one number from her blood chemical analysis and that's the Blast." I prayed that the Blast factor be a low number between zero and five.

The ER reminded me of a typical scene from the Thursday night show we had watched together so many nights. The nurses were so sweet and very attentive saying, "You just need a tune-up. We'll have you out of here in a couple of hours as good as new."

They drew some blood, and the attending doctor stated they were going to try to attack Karen's symptoms in baby steps. He surmised that the headache was potentially a migraine variant, and he gave her a shot of medication to try to get her some relief.

Her right arm bruised up in a deep shade of purple almost immediately.

They left us alone in the little room for awhile, and then the doctor came back in and said the back pain could be the early stages of arthritis, probably brought on prematurely due to Karen's two-year battle with leukemia and all the meds she had been taking.

A little while later, the attending doctor came back and told us that Karen's white blood count was elevated at more than 19,000. Just a month earlier, she was at 6,600.

"Don't get panicked," he said. "We really won't know anything until we get a look at your cells under the microscope and get a look at the differential."

"Differential, what does that mean?" Karen asked.

"The shape of the cells," he replied.

Karen and I held each other and said another Hail Mary.

"Hold on! Keep the faith, this doesn't necessarily mean what we think it might mean," I said.

Then I told her I needed to use the men's room. Instead, I ran to the chapel and begged the Lord for his continued compassion and mercy so that my wife would not have to go through this again.

About 30 seconds after I returned and sat down on the bed next to Karen, she said to me, "Volpe, we have to figure out a way to get this place more money; what they do here is amazing."

Then the door popped open and in walked Katie Hincher with another young doctor right behind her.

We knew she had lost her remission.

Katie did not mince her words: "Karen, I hate to have to tell you this, but your Blast is 86, and we've got to take another bone marrow biopsy."

The doctor behind Katie carried the case with all the instruments used to perform the biopsy.

Brave Karen just rolled over onto her side and said, "I can't believe this! Tell me this isn't happening!"

We were so close. We were so sure that we had beaten the odds, even though we had always understood that there were no guarantees. Dr. Cripe had always been very forthright in citing that 80 percent of patients, with this subtype M3 of AML lose their remission within the first two years. We were still in shock, as the doctor gently started numbing Karen's hip to perform the biopsy. This procedure was required even though we were pretty sure it was the same form of leukemia. It still had to be confirmed because in some cases where relapse occurs many years after the initial remission, the form of leukemia can be different than it was with the original onset of the disease.

The doctor performing the biopsy was very considerate and asked Karen repeatedly if she was comfortable. He was very gentle and quickly had the small piece of bone and a sufficient amount of marrow for each of the blood smears that would be sent off for analysis. She was so brave, and 10 minutes later, she seemed to have at least on the surface accepted the fact that she had relapsed.

Katie told us a room would be available on Five North, back in the isolation unit, in a half hour or so. Once I was sure Karen was settled, I told her that I needed to go home, tell her mother the news and gather her things for her hospital stay.

Karen told me that the children would remain near home; no sending them back to Camp Coyne.

Katie said that Karen would be treated with arsenic trioxide for eight to 10 days before going home again. Then Katie explained that a bone marrow transplant could be performed down the road, and that we would need to get Karen's siblings typed for a potential donor match.

When I got back to my car in the parking deck, I called my boss, Ron McNamara, and told him, "Ron, this is Mark. I'm at the IU Medical Center. My wife has lost her remission, and I'm sitting here in my car in this ugly parking deck trying not to cry."

"How does a thing like this happen?" Ron asked.

I told him, "It's beyond my understanding. We don't understand how people gain their remission, and at the same time, we don't know how they lose it."

"What can I do to help?" he asked.

"Just assure me that I have a job. I need to keep my job at all costs." He promised me that he would explain my situation to Jim Torgerson.

Deep down, I knew my job wasn't in jeopardy. I was just a little paranoid because there were a lot of changes going on at the company, as we approached the launch of the energy market.

On the drive home, the next dilemma that I wrestled with in my mind was how to tell Pat that her daughter's cancer had returned. I was also concerned for my children. Samantha and Mitch were already on summer break, and Will still had a few days left at Clay Jr. High. As I drove, I thought carefully about picking the right words, and I was confident that being direct was the best way to do it. When I arrived home, Pat was in the backyard with the kids and the Bruggemann children were on the swing set. Pat came up to me. She was talking on her cell phone to Colleen. She looked at me and said into the phone, "They're home! Where's Karen?"

"Please hang up and call her back," I said.

I put my arm around her and walked her away from my kids.

"Pat, Karen's not with me, they're admitting her. She's lost her remission, the cancer's back," I said with my voice cracking slightly.

Pat was so strong and courageous. I was always impressed with her strength, but I don't think she was really all that surprised as I remembered her telling me to make sure they do a blood test when we walked out the door five hours earlier. Next, I had to tell Samantha and Mitchell for the second time in two years bad news about their wonderful mom.

I brought them into the house and sat the two of them on the steps in the front hall, and said, "The reason Mommy has been having all of those terrible headaches is because she's lost her remission and the cancer is back." Samantha had tears streaming down her face, and Mitchell just sat there with a blank stare of stunned disbelief.

"This isn't fair! Some families never have to go through cancer once and now we have to do it twice," Samantha said.

Pat comforted the two of them and told them we had to be very brave and she assured them that their mommy was going to be okay. I went to the front hall closet and pulled out Karen's new Ohio State flag, a gift from her sorority sisters. Old Glory needed to come down off the flagpole because Memorial Day weekend was over. It was time to rally around Karen again, time to put up the scarlet flag with the big gray letter "O" and the buckeye leaf in the lower right corner.

I realized the fight was on again, fighting the back tears, as I hoisted up the flag and said to myself, "It's time for the Buckeye girl to fight again."

> *Drive, drive, drive down the field, win scarlet and gray,*
> *Don't let them past that line, we're gonna win this game today.*
> *Smash through to victory we'll cheer you as you go.*
> *Our honor defend, we will fight to the end for O-HI-O.*

A year or so earlier, while decorating Will and Mitchell's bathroom, Karen had written the words from the fight song high on the wall above a picture of OSU's Eddie George in a 1995 win against Notre Dame.

Then I made some phone calls to my parents and others to tell them of Karen's setback. I went upstairs and tried to pull together all the essentials she'd need for the next few days. It was hard to go through her dresser and closet. I couldn't believe what I was doing; it was starting to sink in with me. It was all too surreal.

It was another month called June.

The fight was on again.

I remember running over to tell a few of the neighbors the news. I talked to Joel Jackson, and he assured me that the neighborhood stood ready to help us through this thing again. Then my thoughts turned to William. He was still at school and I needed to get back downtown, but I really felt that the news should come directly from his father.

When I arrived at Clay Jr. High, all the buses were lined up in their designated locations awaiting the students who still had a few minutes before dismissal. After asking a few questions, I found out that bus #48 serviced our neighborhood. So I wandered down to the bus, hung around in the grassy area out in front and waited a few minutes. A few minutes later, a slow steady stream of giddy junior high students started making their way out. I spotted Will walking along the sidewalk talking with a classmate. Will had his oversized book bag slung across his back. He didn't see me, and I needed to intercept him before he made his way onto the bus.

He looked up at me in a kind of amazement and said, "What are you doing here?"

"How 'bout if I give you a ride home?"

"But I really like going home on the bus with my friends."

"I know, but there is something I really needed to talk to you about," I said.

And he looked up at me very seriously and said, "Mom's screwed, isn't she?"

"Yes," I said, "but let's talk in the car."

So we made our way traveling back against the wave of students to the parking lot where the Bonneville was parked. When we got in, he was still stunned, trying to take it all in. He got a little teary-eyed, and I told him that it wasn't going to be like last time when everyone got shipped back to Ohio, and all of our summer activities ended. This time it was important that we stay together as a family unit and that baseball, gymnastics and soccer would all continue. I wanted this to still be a summer vacation in spite of the fact his mom had relapsed. We would work through this illness together.

As I drove him home, I told him that I expected him to remain my rock, and to continue to be the leader—his brother and sister would be leaning on him. These are the types of responsibilities incumbent upon the oldest. I dropped him off and he headed off to find his grandmother. She told me later that he cried. I think that he wanted to prove to me that he was man enough to take the news and not cry, but when he saw his grandmother, knowing that it was her daughter and that she had to go through it all again, he couldn't help but to let it loose.

I drove to the hospital with Karen's pajamas, slippers, robe and toiletries. Later on, after trying to get her room organized, Dr. Cripe and Katie Hincher came by to see Karen.

Dr. Larry Cripe sat in the big blue lounge chair next to the bed.

Karen looked over at him and said, "How are you doing, Dr. Cripe?" and he just looked back at her and said, "I knew you were going to ask me that."

For the first time, I could read the emotion on Dr. Cripe's face. He was very down, looking contrite and distressed. It was hard not to cast our minds back to that joyful moment a month earlier when she had said to him, "Really, it's over—give me a hug!"

The conversation turned to Karen's relapse.

"The plan is for her to be here in isolation for eight to 10 days, and she will receive infusions of arsenic trioxide, a new substance for Karen, and not the forms of chemotherapy she received two years ago," Dr. Cripe said.

He explained that this treatment would not be as harsh as the idarubicin and duanorubicin she had been on before. Then, the plan called for her to go home and get the remainder of the treatments on an outpatient basis over an eight to 10-week period before we would get into the bone marrow transplant stage of the process, assuming she achieved another remission.

The protocol with a patient that has relapsed is much different. Instead of wiping out all the white blood cells, including the good along with the bad, the arsenic trioxide throws a switch that tricks the immature Blast cells into maturing, which causes the white blood count to increase for a few weeks. Then, as the white cells reach their full maturation process, they begin to slowly die off.

"This time the number will go up way up to as high as 150,000 before it will start to trend back down and if the count increases too rapidly we might "blunt" the effects of the increase with the traditional chemotherapy," Dr. Cripe said.

Katie Hincher asked us to fill out some forms so that Karen's siblings could be tested for a possible match for a bone marrow transplant. I took the forms and promised to get them back first thing in the morning.

Karen was so apologetic and couldn't believe that we were back in the isolation unit. "You're like family to us, please don't feel that way," Katie said. "We're sorry you're back here again."

Karen told Dr. Cripe her head felt a little better. They had given her Ativan and it seemed to be helping, but the ringing in her ears was not any better. If anything, it was even more maddening. More MRIs and visits with the neurologists were scheduled for Thursday.

"So when do we start with the arsenic?" Karen asked.

"Well, we don't have the full results from the bone marrow biopsy back yet, but it wouldn't hurt you to start on the treatment yet tonight," Dr. Cripe said, adding that the arsenic trioxide wouldn't hurt her.

The arsenic trioxide or ATO, as we came to call it, was ordered up, and Dr. Cripe and Katie departed. Karen was carted down to the basement for the first of what would be many

MRIs. We called and got Karen something to eat: slow-cooked turkey and mashed potatoes.

She ate some, and rested for the remainder of the evening. Soon the phone calls started to roll in. Word of her relapse had spread quickly, and everyone wanted to call and wish her the best. After the phenegren, to help with the associated nausea was administered and the ATO was started up, I headed for home at about 11:30 p.m., knowing that I needed to rest. Karen was very cautious about making sure that I got sufficient sleep given the ordeal we went through in June 2002, when my inability to get enough sleep had such devastating results for me personally.

After spending most of the next day with her at the hospital, I sat down, thought for a long time and then made the following entry in Karen's journal on www.caringbridge.org.

I carefully pondered every word I wrote. Breaking this type of news to friends and family was not a duty I took lightly.

Thursday, June 3, 2004 8:38 PM

> A few weeks ago, Karen and I discussed deleting Karen from this wonderful website given the news that Dr. Cripe expected Karen to remain free of leukemia. Karen's chemo maintenance program of methotrexate and Purinethal was over and had worked as designed in keeping Karen in full remission. Unfortunately, over the past few weeks Karen began to have extreme headaches, ringing in the ears, nausea, trouble with her vision and lower back pain. We worked through our family physician to address these issues; however, yesterday morning we went back to the ER at the Indiana University Medical Center to try to figure out the source of Karen's assorted pains. All along we had attributed the symptoms to Karen going off the numerous medications she had been taking as part of her mainte-

nance program and that her body was going through an adjustment or type of withdrawal from almost two year's worth of assorted chemotherapy.

Initially, the ER physician thought it was a migraine variant, and the back pain was attributed to arthritis; however, the blood chemical results taken Wednesday morning revealed that Karen's white blood cell count was at 19,100, significantly elevated from the 6,600 recorded one month earlier. The rest of the CBC results were not good, the Blast factor was at 86, a sure indicator that she had relapsed. A bone marrow biopsy was performed and the early indications are that Karen has lost her remission. The AML subtype M3 had inexplicably returned. We always knew this was a possibility, in that 80% of patients with AML lose their remission, but a month we ago felt that we had gotten past the two-year hurdle and that the numbers were on our side.

Karen was admitted and has undergone the first dose of chemotherapy. This time Dr. Cripe has prescribed arsenic trioxide. This form of chemo seems to be not as harsh as the barrage of drugs she was hit with two years ago. She will have regular EKGs in order to monitor her heart.

Today, Karen slept most of the day and battled the side effects associated with extreme nausea. Her spirits are good—she has seen several neurologists and the ophthalmologist as we try to get a handle on the swelling of her brain that is exerting pressure on the optic nerve, which is obviously the root cause of the headaches. Her WBC is now at 24,100, however this is to be expected as this count will rise over the next few days before the chemotherapy takes hold.

Naturally, we are disappointed by the turn of events. Will, Samantha and Mitchell all took the news as well as can be expected. It is a shock, but Karen remains bound and determined to beat this disease. The long-term plan is to get her back in remission and then do a bone marrow transplant.

For now Karen will be in the hospital for 8-10 days and then she will do the remainder of her treatments on an out-patient basis.

She is an amazing woman—she beat this terrible disease once and she will do it again.

Keep the faith!!

CHAPTER 28

The Sea of Galilee

Karen's new room in the isolation unit that was to be her home for the next 10 days was isolation room #5827. This room was in the exact opposite corner of the isolation unit where she spent so much time in June and July of 2002 in the Adult Cancer Care Center. I liked the location of the room because it was slightly secluded and was at the end of the hall, versus the room from hell two years ago that was literally just through the heavy double doors immediately adjacent to the nurse's station, where I had smashed the computer monitor during my delusional rage. Most of Thursday and Friday were spent getting Karen acclimated to her new routine and coming to grips with the fact that she had relapsed.

She constantly said to me how sorry she was for putting everyone through this the first time and now for a second time.

My answer was always the same. "Karen, you would have something to be sorry for if this was the result of a willful act like smoking, drug abuse or alcoholism."

I have always felt that this was a major part of Karen's predetermined purpose that our Lord had in mind for her long before she was born. He had hand-picked her as a shining example of how to remain strong, courageous and to persevere in the wake of all obstacles, the ultimate test of faith. I kept telling her that God was here with us.

She was not alone.

Prior to her dinner arriving one evening, Fr. Tim Kroeger arrived and we all chatted. He brought her a little locket filled with water from the Sea of Galilee. Fr. Tim described it as one of the most beautiful places on Earth. He prayed over her that the Lord's healing powers be brought upon her and mentioned that everyone was praying for her.

Her room was a constant hubbub of activity; in addition to the nursing staff, there was a series of visits from specialists in neurology and ophthalmology who were in and out, running various tests to check Karen's neurological functions and her eyesight. Her nurse during the day was Kristen. She was very diligent, capable, upbeat, talkative and pretty.

In the afternoon, I remembered that there was a computer on the sixth floor near the ICU. I meandered up there and made the following entry.

Friday, June 4, 2004 2:01 PM

Karen did get some sleep and still battled nausea, however this seems to be subsiding, as she was able to eat some breakfast. Her WBC is still increasing. This is by design, until the chemo reverses the trend at some point and takes her back to zero and ultimately remission. I got the impression from talking with Dr. Cripe that this would take a few days or even a week. Last evening, she had an MRI and today her head doesn't hurt as much. There is still concern regarding her eyesight. The blood vessels at the rear of her beautiful blue eyes are of concern, as the leukemia has caused her brain to swell, pushing on the optic nerve and altering her peripheral vision. Her left eye is slightly swollen. This is a fight. Her brothers Tommy and Kevin are on their way—be safe.

I was spending a lot of time on my cell phone with Karen's brother, Kevin, giving him updates that he would pass along to the family. I also talked with our good friend from SLDM, Kim Santucci. Kim is wonderful, funny, reliable and, most importantly, Italian. I knew I could trust Kim to handle anything I asked. For now, I told her that this was going to be a long process, and that I'd need her mostly in July to help coordinate Karen's outpatient treatments. This would require chauffeur-type service on weekdays down to IUMC for her transfusions.

The only big thing we had going on was to make sure Mitchell made it to his tryout for the Carmel United Soccer Club. Mitchell is a very good player, having scored approximately 30 goals between his indoor and outdoor leagues over the past few months. Several coaches had told us that his soccer skills merited a higher level of play. I gave Kim the assignment of making sure Mitchell made it to his tryout for the travel squad on Saturday morning, June 12th.

Kevin and Tommy arrived from northeastern Ohio in the early evening on Friday and checked in at University Place, the same hotel Lance Armstrong used in 1996, immediately adjacent to the IUMC. Their appearance definitely lifted Karen's spirits. Tommy cracks me up. He makes Karen laugh too. When I came back into Karen's room, he had added several items to Karen's progress calendar in the form of important dates for Kevin. These rather humorous notes read something like the following:

June 14—Kevin Pick Up Prom Tux
June 20—Kevin Volunteers at Women's Prison
June 24—Kevin Scab Removal
June 27—Kevin GED Ceremony

On Saturday morning, Pat was running around the house gathering up various items for Karen. She was heading down to IUMC to help Karen get cleaned up and spend the better part of the day with her, while I spent some time with the kids. As she went down the basement steps, I heard a loud thud and then heard her gasping for air.

I found Pat face-down breathing very hard, with her glasses wedged between her face and the carpet. Her right arm was trapped under her rib cage in an awkward position. It didn't take me long to figure out that she had tripped on a toy and had literally flown through the air from at least six steps up through the large opening to the right at the bottom of the steps, landing just inches short of the pool table.

At first, I was careful not to move her head for fear of a head or spinal injury. She was short of breath, but eventually she told me her head and neck was okay. I tried to get her to sit up, but her ribs and back hurt too much. I told her I was going to call 911 and she said, "No, call my brother Bob; he'll know what to do."

I ran upstairs and called Bob, explained the situation, and he was over in 10 minutes. While we waited, I rubbed Pat's back; she complained that her right shoulder blade really hurt. Once Uncle Bob arrived, we tried to get her sitting upright, but only managed to get her onto her left side.

Bob looked at me and said, "Call 911!"

I went over to the bar phone and talked to the dispatcher who asked me what the problem was, and I said, "My mother-in-law has fallen and can't get up!"

Pat started laughing and said, "Don't make me laugh anymore; that's not fair."

The dispatcher told me not to give the injured person anything to eat or drink.

Pat yelled to me, "Tell them no sirens, I don't want to wake up the entire neighborhood, just because I'm such a klutz!"

So I passed Pat's request along, thanked the dispatcher and hung up. Pat was upset that she had injured herself right when Karen needed her the most. Uncle Bob, Aunt Patty and I tried to calm her down.

Pat asked for a Diet Coke and I said, "No way. They said no food or drink."

Thirty seconds later you could hear the sirens; that upset Pat even more. I went upstairs to flag down the EMT. My children slept through the whole thing. Once the emergency squad arrived, they checked her vitals and put her on a body board and then hoisted her up the steps.

One of the EMTs said, "We're going to take her over to St. Vincent's in Carmel, okay?"

And I said, "No, you're not! If you take her there, my wife will kill me."

They said, "How 'bout Community North?"

I said, "That will be fine."

Uncle Bob and Aunt Patty grabbed Pat's purse and her suitcase. I leaned over to my Aunt Patty as she got into the car while they loaded Pat into the emergency vehicle and I jokingly said, "They know me real well over at Community North; maybe Pat can get my old room with the nicely padded walls."

I called Tommy, who was already in the isolation room with his sister, to let him know the situation and told him not to tell Karen.

Eventually he called back and said, "We need to let Karen know the truth; keeping it from her will prove to be a bad thing."

Pat had cracked four ribs and broken her scapula, something one of the nurses at Community North had never seen before. Pat was hospitalized for two nights. I called Pat's husband, John, in Akron and kept him apprised of the situation. Once the kids got up, I gave them a little lecture on the danger of leaving items on the steps.

Mitchell said, "But Mommy does it all the time!"

I took a deep breath and then further reminded them this bad habit was at the heart of the problem, and now our MaMaw got hurt, and it's got to stop. The toy Pat had hydro-planed on was a Mylar hovercraft Mitchell had received a few days earlier at a birthday party that the Bruggemanns threw for Mitchell and their son, Bennett. I had told Mitchell to take it to the lower level. I was growing tired of seeing him launch it throughout the family room. Instead, he launched it only halfway down the steps. Pat would have seen it, but she missed the light switch as she was rushing around the house.

Murphy's Law strikes again!

I mowed the yard and did a bunch of stuff around the house. Then, later on around noon, Karen called and said that she wanted to see the kids. Right after Will's 3:00 p.m. game, he came home and grabbed a shower, and then the four of us headed downtown for the first time to see Mommy since the relapse.

Later that evening, I added the journal entry below to Karen's website.

Saturday, June 5, 2004 10:55 PM

At 5 p.m. this evening I could hardly believe my eyes! Will, Sam and Mitch were all lying in the same cramped hospital bed, each vying for their own little space next to and in front of Karen. All four were wearing the yellow protective masks to guard against passing along infection while watching Nickelodeon on TV. My four little banditos all snuggling together!! It was quite the scene.

Actually, Karen didn't pay much attention to the TV; she was very intrigued with the 17 pages of e-mails from the Guestbook. She just said, "WOW, this is unbelievable." Keep them coming—they really pump her up. I must admit I get a little misty reading them as well.

Karen continues to make great strides. I was a little surprised by her sudden request and elated to haul the kids downtown to IUMC after Will's baseball game.

The WBC increased to 39,000, but again this is not an alarming number, and in fact, the percentage increase actually declined compared to the prior two days. She was given some platelets, just because her blood is so thin. The headache and ringing in the ears are now tolerable, and she's eating well, except things don't taste like they should. This is an indication that the medication employed to reduce the swelling of her brain is doing the trick. Her constant nausea has subsided, and she's sleeping when she wants to instead of out of sheer exhaustion.

She really looks great, her eyes are clear, her color is great—all the vitals are fine. She had to trust me on the "looking great" account because I forgot to bring her a mirror and cream rinse. Sorry dear, but I had a busy morning. For some of the details see Ellen Captain's recent entry in the Guestbook. Also, I want to extend a special thanks to the Carmel Fire Department, Uncle Bob and Aunt Patty for all their help today. Her brother Tommy spent most of Friday evening and into the wee hours of Saturday morning making sure his sis was okay. This was awesome and allowed me to spend Friday night and most of today concentrating on quality time with the three little Volpes.

We brought down the TV/VCR and a bunch of movies for Karen to watch. Kevin has been in town as well. Yesterday both Tommy and Kevin had blood samples taken which will be screened for a potential bone marrow donor match.

Which sibling will be a match? This certainly would make for better drama than *The Bachelor*.

Kathy and Kenny will get theirs done soon, and according to Katie Hincher, the results will take about a week.

I also heard that Father Dave Hellmann visited with Karen. He's an awesome priest. Father Tim Kroeger and Father Dave have both been a source of strength. Healing waters from the Sea of Galilee were delivered to Karen's bedside in a beautiful little locket on Thursday by Father Tim, and from my perspective, these waters work.

Special thanks to the wonderful Santucci family for bringing dinner over to the Volpe house. Garlic is such a wonderful ingredient!!

Rest in peace, Ronald Reagan.

CHAPTER 29

Tour de France

Tommy always had some great ideas as we ventured along on this journey together. Sunday night on the sixth of June, he and Kevin had to make the 300-mile venture back to Ohio to resume their day jobs. Late Sunday afternoon, Karen's main nurse Kristen came into Karen's room with the blood work kits that were needed to draw samples from her brothers to determine whether their bone marrow was potentially compatible so it could be used as donor marrow for Karen.

Once Tommy's draw was complete, he pulled out a $20 bill, laid it on the table and said to Kristen, "The 20 spot is yours if you can guarantee me that you'll have to do both of Kevin's arms instead of just one."

Kristen laughed and said, "I doubt that we will require drawing from both arms."

About halfway through the draw Kevin's left arm went dry, and Kristen had to switch to Kevin's right to complete the draw. Karen, Tommy and I all found this very amusing—Kristen left the money on the table and felt bad that she had to spike each of Kevin's arms.

Tommy had paid for an additional night at University Place, and even though he wasn't going to use it because he was heading back to Ohio, he suggested that I spend a few hours sleeping over there, and that way I wouldn't have to battle rush hour traffic on Monday morning in order to make it to the important early morning meeting with Dr. Cripe and his team. Tommy and everyone else were concerned about my sleeping patterns, given the little problem I had two years prior. Tommy also suggested that I catch a nap at about 8:00 p.m. so I could see the season ending finale of HBO's hit series, *The Sopranos*, which had evolved into my favorite show on television. Even though it's about crooks from New Jersey who happen to be Italian, I love the writing and character development. Oddly enough, Karen and I had also been following another series on HBO called, *Six Feet Under*, which is all about a dysfunctional, but very entertaining family that ran a funeral home in Los Angeles. This mini-series had a little bit of everything including drug abuse, infidelity and homosexuality.

Karen was still having vision problems, and the ringing in her ears was still unbearable. The headaches were barely tolerable. She was dealing with the arsenic trioxide treatments pretty well and was having only minor trouble with nausea. I was constantly doing the best I could to get food into her. And after *The Sopranos* was over, I cruised back over to her room.

She said, "Is there any way you could get me some fresh pork fried rice from a Chinese place?"

"Consider it done," I said, remembering that there was a little eatery called A Taste of China nearby.

I was proud of myself for being able to find the pork fried rice at 10:00 at night, but then I had to sneak it by the nurses because Karen was back on the neutropenic diet, which meant that all her food was supposed specially prepared from the hospital's kitchen. She ate about four or five bites, and I considered this progress given the miniature amounts of hospital food she was eating whenever her tray arrived.

At one point during the evening she asked me, "Who do you think will be a match?"

I said, "Kenny," thinking that Kenny always had a flair for the dramatic.

Karen replied, "I know who it will be."

She paused, her tired eyes lit up and then she said, "Tommy will save me!"

I went back to University Place, stopped in at Chancellor's and had some wings before hitting the sack. Tommy even left me a fresh golf shirt for the morning. At 6:30 a.m. I was up, showered, and within minutes over to Karen's room. To get to Karen's room I used the same walkway Lance Armstrong used to get from the hotel to the hospital when he received his treatment for testicular cancer. Karen's father was manning the ship at home and had a handle on the kids; he planned on leaving on Thursday when the plan called for Kathy to head over for four days or so.

I'll let the journal entry below tell the story of what transpired on Monday.

Monday, June 7, 2004 11:00 PM

It was back to the "A Team" early this morning as Dr. Cripe's oncology team visited early in the morning with Karen and myself to review this weekend's progress and map out a plan for the next couple of days. We saw Dr. Li for the first time in two years. He was instrumental in Karen's battle to remission almost two years ago, and we understand that he will only be at IUMC for two more weeks. The prime focus is on making sure that the clotting agents in Karen's system are sufficient. More "kryo" was prescribed and Karen's platelets are now at 45; our goal is 50 so she's getting close. This number was down to 17 last Wednesday when Karen returned to IUMC, so this represents solid progress.

As a precautionary matter, another CAT scan was scheduled in order to insure that there are no further problems with swelling or minor bleeding in the brain. The WBC is up to 72,000, and while this is obviously a high number, Dr. Cripe and his team are convinced that we must "stay the course" with the arsenic trioxide. This form of treatment tricks the white blood cells into maturing too quickly, so an increase at this point is expected. Katie Hincher has indicated that this count can go well into six figures before the cells actually start to die off, so no changes to the original strategy will be undertaken. Dr. Cripe did stop by late in the day and discussed the "stay the course" approach with Karen. Medicine is an art, not a science.

Karen's ongoing headaches, ringing in the ears, and back/neck pain are all "tolerable" at this point. She rates them at "6." Last week when she was admitted, her answer to the rate the pain question was a "10."

The staff the IUMC has been most diligent and very vigilant in monitoring all aspects of Karen's health. An EKG was performed today with no signs of any abnormality, and the neurologists have been keeping close tabs on Karen stopping in to conduct the same tests several times a day.

We are so fortunate to be in the finest facility in the world for dealing with this type of leukemia.

Karen's dad will be here tomorrow. Will has a doubleheader, and Sam has her first day in Level 5 gymnastics. For those of you who didn't hear, she finished 10th in the whole Hoosier state last year among all eleven year olds competing in Level 4.

As for my wife, she's simply the most amazing, courageous, thoughtful and loving person I have ever met.

The luckiest day of my life was February 23, 1988, when on a sunny ski slope in the Canadian Rockies, she said, "yes" after I popped the question.

We need some more lucky days!

During the day Tuesday, the traffic in Karen's room picked up considerably, with numerous visits from neurology and ophthalmology, as more and more concern over her vision and headaches became apparent. Neither of us had a clue as to what the next turn on the roller coaster would be like. We just had to trust in the Lord and Dr. Larry Cripe.

Earlier in the week, Margaret Evans sent us two-dozen yellow wristbands that were inscribed with the word LIVESTRONG. The literature that accompanied the wristbands explained that the "Wear Yellow" program was a joint venture between the Lance Armstrong Foundation and Nike to raise $6 million for cancer research. The wristbands were selling for a buck each and could be found at sporting good stores, running shoe stores and bike shops. The LIVESTRONG inscription was Lance's mantra dating back to when he successfully battled testicular cancer at the same hospital. The yellow color was picked because the leader of the Tour de France wears a yellow shirt to distinguish him from the rest of the field.

Karen had read Lance's first book, *It's Not About the Bike*, and she thought it was a great inspirational story, but she also felt Lance had it much easier. Lance was famous, he didn't have children and his form of cancer was generally curable. The wristbands were instantly popular on Garden Gate Way, in Ohio, among our supporters at SLDM and at the Midwest ISO. The program was popular nationwide and many stores were unable to keep up with the demand for the hot item, which symbolized courage, faith and perseverance. Margaret Evans sent our entire family the black T-shirts with the Nike logo on the sleeve, and the words LIVESTRONG in yellow on the front.

These little bracelets had become the symbol of our rally cry and helped inspire Karen to press on in spite of her unbelievable predicament.

CHAPTER 30

The Rotunda

Just prior to leaving for Wednesday morning's consult with Dr. Cripe's crew, I made the journal entry below

Wednesday, June 9, 2004 6:25 AM

Karen had a difficult Tuesday and most of the concerns revolve around her eyesight in her left eye. The ophthalmologist confirmed that the swelling in the brain, pushing on the optic nerve, has exerted pressure on blood vessels within the eye. Karen can see fine in her right eye; however, there are distortions in her vision in the left. I am of the understanding that there is no permanent damage.

To treat this, they are prescribing a new medication for Karen called mannitol. This drug is more aggressive than the diox, and should help reduce the swelling. There has not been an increase in the swelling, it just hasn't gone down. No invasive procedures can be performed due to the leukemia.

All three children dropped in for a brief visit yesterday.

Dr. Cripe is a brilliant and caring man. We have put all of our faith and trust in him. He has difficult decisions to make—every case is different.

Remember him in your prayers.

On my way down Meridian, as I battled traffic in an attempt to be in Karen's room when Dr. Cripe's team made their morning rounds, the phone rang. I looked at the display on my cell, and it said KAREN, but when I answered it was Dr. Metha, one of Dr. Cripe's associates. He explained to me that various experts were up well into the late-night hours, and that they had explored all the options. The consensus was to perform "routine" brain surgery, to install a VC shunt, later in the day, in order to relieve the pressure in her cranium that was causing her discomfort. I immediately expressed concern about bleeding, and Dr. Metha further explained that prior to the surgery, they would load Karen up with plenty of platelets to aid her clotting abilities. He also said that the procedure generally did not involve a lot of bleeding. Dr. Thomas Witt, who had met with Karen the night before, would perform the surgery.

I called Kevin, Kim Santucci and my parents to let everyone know of this latest turn of events. The rest of the morning and into the mid-afternoon, I was amazed at the precision of Karen's team of nurses as they ordered up what seemed like at least a dozen units of platelets that were required prior to the surgery. A little later on, around 11:00 or so, Dr. Witt came by to explain more details regarding the procedure. The nurses continued the flow of platelets with the goal of getting Karen's counts up to at least 100,000 prior to performing the surgery.

An apparatus resembling a cage would be placed around her head, which would allow Dr. Witt to pinpoint where to insert the shunt into Karen's brain. The first order of business, to relieve the intra-cranial pressure prior to the surgery, Karen would be given a low dosage of an anesthesia that would allow her to remain conscious, but not totally aware of all that was going on. This was being done in order to place the apparatus about her head that would allow Dr. Witt to dial in on the exact coordinates where they would drill into Karen's skull for proper placement of the shunt. An MRI would be performed, with the helmet-like apparatus in place, and the doctors would actually draw where to drill on her head.

Once in place, the shunt would be used to help vent the excess spinal fluid that was building up in Karen's brain, causing the headaches and problems with her vision. The excess fluid would be sent down a tube, back behind her left ear into her stomach where the fluid would be absorbed as part of the normal digestive process. This all happened very fast, but everyone seemed very confident that this was the course that needed to be taken in order to get Karen some level of relief

Later in the afternoon, Tom came down to visit with his daughter and then headed back to Ohio. Karen's sister, Kathy, arrived about 4:00, just as Karen was going into surgery. After Tom left for Ohio, I went back to Karen's room to do whatever I could do to assist in the installation of the apparatus. At about 10 minutes to three, a team of three technicians and Dr. Witt arrived.

They were all business.

The team administered the mild anesthesia and started building what resembled a perfectly square erector set around Karen's head. They put little pads and then a round shaft gently into each ear to form a line of reference. Karen sat up in bed and would occasionally ask the technicians how they were doing. Slowly, over the course of about 20 minutes, the contraption resembling a square football helmet's facemask, called a stereotactic frame, took on its geometric shape. Once the rectangle was in place, it had to be secured and a local anesthesia was administered at points on Karen's forehead directly above her eyebrows—parallel points at the rear of the head were also hit with the numbing effects of the anesthesia. Then these blunt bolts were screwed into her head with a level of pressure that noticeably dimpled her forehead.

After a few minutes, a slow trickle of blood ran down Karen's forehead and into her eyes. She just sat there taking it all in. Karen seemed somewhat aware of what was transpiring. When Dr. Witt was satisfied, Karen was transferred from her bed to the transport gurney, the blood still streaming down her face. I helped push the Christmas tree device that housed all of her IVs as we made our way toward surgery.

Then it dawned on me the true imagery I had just witnessed. I was Simon helping her carry this cross. As we rolled down the hall, one of the transport assistants wiped the blood from her eyes.

I got goose bumps.

No one was mocking or jeering Karen, and no impression of her beautiful face was left on the patient care assistant's towel after she wiped the blood from Karen's eyes.

During the day, Julia Mattei, our new neighbor, made the entry below in the guestbook. Mitchell had spent three straight nights at their home, and I had stopped by a few times to check on him.

Karen,

Your network of friends and family is so amazing. I have been able to keep posted on your progress through so many loving people. I must say the best and most informative status report came from the most adorable, recently buzz cut, precious, young man. He came over to play bball with Michael, and sat down next to me to update me with all this medical terminology, white count #'s, on and on. I was so impressed with Mitch. He was so happy to have just seen you at the hospital. He was so casual and confident. Hey, he was happy to sit and talk to this old Mom!!! What a terrific boy you have. We laughed at the fact that it was a good thing you didn't smell the gift Michael gave Mitch for his birthday. You can ask him the details.

Well, you and Tom Stark are kicking me out of bed in the wee hours each morning. Just when I think I don't want to jog, and I want to sleep in, I think of you two, and know that is the peaceful quiet time to jog around the neighborhood and say prayers for the both of you. Are prayers heard more clearly if I say them while passing your house?? Please know I think of you 100x a day. Two years ago I knew and prayed for you as a Mom at our school, now you are my friend and neighbor. My family is here for you whenever you need it, and I have these 4 little ones yelling up to God to watch over you!! Get out of there quick. Remember, I owe you a beer at my house! Love, Julia

Julia Mattei
Carmel, IN—Thursday, June 10, 2004 8:00 PM

Once down in the basement, Karen was rolled into the MRI machine, and I saw Dr. Witt place a level on the apparatus in order to ensure that everything was congruent. Prior to starting the MRI, exact precision was essential. Then I went to the cafeteria to get some soup. I planned to sit in the surgery waiting area during the three-hour procedure.

As I finished my soup, my cell rang. It was Kathy and she was a little lost downtown near the restaurant, Malibu on Maryland, a nice jazz-themed place where Karen and I celebrated our 12th anniversary a few years earlier. I gave Kathy directions back northwest a few blocks to the hospital. I was glad that I wouldn't have to sit and play the waiting game all by myself.

I greeted Kathy at the information desk, and we made our way briskly to the basement, hoping to catch Karen coming out of the MRI before she went into surgery. We missed her by about 10 minutes, so we headed over to the surgical waiting area, where several other families were waiting.

The television was turned on, and everyone was watching the state funeral for Ronald Reagan, whose body had just arrived in Washington D.C. from California. The scene of the rider-less horse, with only the black boots in the stirrups and the flag-draped coffin, immediately made me flashback to when JFK had been assassinated in 1963. As a four-and-a-half-year-old, I remembered watching everything. The similarities were striking. Reagan's life with Nancy had been its own special Camelot, unlike the Kennedy ordeal having never been fulfilled. The commentators kept talking about how much in love they were with each other.

A nice waiting room coordinator came around to help ease anyone's anxieties. He explained that it was near quitting time for him, but that he could be contacted at home if anyone had any questions. Sitting directly next to Kathy and me, as we watched the procession slowly move toward the Rotunda, was a family from Evansville, Indiana.

The patient's husband was Harold, and he was there with a few of his children and his only granddaughter. I asked him whom he was there for and he said his wife, Mary, was having one of her kidneys removed because of cancer.

I wished him luck and told him I'd remember his wife in my prayers. He had to have been in his late 70s and he was very cordial.

The surgical waiting room coordinator came over to talk to the family from Evansville and said, "It's more complicated than just the kidney; there are other organs where the cancer has spread, and it's going to be another three hours, at least."

I said a quick Hail Mary for Mary and wondered what was going on with my own wife. A little while later, the coordinator said to Kathy and me that they had had just started and all of Karen's vitals were good, but that they really hadn't done much yet. By now it had to be near 6:00 p.m. I found a wall outlet to recharge my cell, resigned to a long night ahead.

Kathy grabbed a salad from the cafeteria and we chatted about her boys. Ryan, her oldest, was entering high school and would be attending Archbishop Hoban High School. Even though I was partial to my alma mater at Walsh, Hoban was a good fit for my first godson. Kathy also explained to me that they were taking their son, Adam, out of Holy Family for the eighth grade. The school had slipped quite a bit from what it was when I had attended some 30 years earlier, and he was getting picked on often. Too bad we weren't able to stay in the area.

Will would have stuck up for his cousin because he's full of courage. I've seen him get annihilated on bang-bang plays at the plate, and never drop the ball in spite of getting taken out by players that weighed a good 50 pounds more. He's tough as nails.

About 20 minutes later the doctor who had been operating on Mary came into the waiting room and introduced himself to the family from Evansville.

I knew this wasn't a good sign.

"We'll give you some privacy," I said to Harold as Kathy and I went into another part of the waiting area. I went upstairs and called Kevin and Kim Santucci to update them on Karen.

When I returned, I ran into Harold, who was walking very slowly with his head down. We made eye contact so I asked him about his wife.

He just sighed and said, "It's not good, the cancer is everywhere, and she's only got about six months maximum."

I told him that I was very sorry to hear their news and hopefully she would have comfort and dignity for the rest of her days.

Harold said, "We've been together for 56 years, married for 52." I thought to myself, that's a pretty damn good run; I'll gladly exchange 40 more years of marriage for a healthy Karen right now. Where do I sign? With that we shook hands and I wished him my best as they left for the recovery room. I felt very bad for his granddaughter; she was heartbroken with the news that there was no way to fix the cancer that had proliferated Mary's body.

Kathy and I settled in and continued to watch CBS News' coverage of Reagan's funeral. By now, his remains were lying in state at the Capitol. It had been a long day. I was tired and a little hungry. When you're under the gun, you have to coast as best you can.

Suddenly, Dr. Witt appeared and told us everything had gone smoothly. Karen would be in recovery for a few hours, and then we would be able to see her in the neurological ICU. Kathy and I were delighted with the positive news, and I suggested we head over to Chancellor's Sports Bar to celebrate. Kathy drank tons of lemonade. After about an hour, long enough for me to catch *ESPN's Baseball Tonight*, we headed back to the hospital to see Karen.

CHAPTER 31

Neurological ICU

When we arrived at the ICU and found our way to Karen's room, Kathy and I were amazed to see a perfectly radiant Karen with a neat white bandage wrapped tightly around her head. She recognized us right away and said to Kathy, "Is it really you?" We were somewhat bewildered because we expected a much less coherent Karen to still be dealing with the anesthesia. She seemed perfectly fine. Kathy and I were in shock. Initially the effects of the anesthesia didn't seem to bother Karen, and then she started saying things like, "Get me out of here, I don't like my nurse; she doesn't know what she's doing."

Maybe, Karen thought she was still at St. Vincent's.

Kathy was willing to spend the night with Karen, but once we were convinced that Karen was stable and had calmed down, I convinced Kathy to follow me back to Carmel so we could both get some much-needed sleep. When we left, Karen's nurse, Angie, gave me the number to call to check on Karen's progress. I also had to pick a secret password. I chose "Coldfish." And then we left without Karen seeing us. She was in good hands and Kathy had already driven five hours from Ohio.

When I got home I quickly scribed the following journal entry.

Thursday, June 10, 2004 1:33 AM

Early Wednesday morning it was decided that the only way to relieve the pressure on Karen's brain and simultaneously preserve the vision in her left eye, was to insert a permanent shunt into one of the two large ventricles comprising the brain cavity. The shunt would drain off excess spinal fluid from the brain, which was the root cause of the swelling. Most of the morning was spent giving Karen additional units of "kryo" in order to maintain her clotting capability, although we were told the procedure normally does not include lots of bleeding. Dr. Thomas Witt performed the three hour-long neurosurgical procedure after an MRI was performed to pinpoint the precise location for the shunt. A large helmet-like apparatus was affixed to Karen's head for the MRI to ensure accuracy.

The surgery went very smoothly, and Dr. Witt said there was a lot of excess fluid and pressure on the intra-cranium that should now be alleviated. All of Karen's vital signs are good. She's a little feisty as she deals with the post-operative effects of the anesthesia. With some therapy, we expect Karen to regain full vision in the left eye.

Kathy and I were there in the waiting room and spent some time with Karen in the ICU.

Mother and brain are doing fine!

So for Wednesday it was just some routine brain surgery, and tomorrow we'll turn our focus back to the leukemia.

We're likely to resume those treatments (arsenic trioxide) as soon as practical given the extensive surgery.

Kenny and Anne Coyne will be here mid-afternoon. John Bird also arrived today to help with Pat's ribs and scapula.

Yes, this is really happening.

Time for some sleep!

The next morning I woke up early and called to check on Karen. She had a good night, her vitals were good, and there were no signs of infection. Karen spent two uneventful days in the neurological ICU. While she rested comfortably, I enjoyed some quality time with our children. I told them that it looked like going to the Virginia Beach was doubtful for 2004, but the kids took this in stride and they fully understood that Karen came first. Karen was released back to the Adult Cancer Care Unit late in the day Friday, and her dad was there to coordinate the move.

Luckily, Karen was able to get back to her original room, #5827. We had to vacate the room when she went in for surgery in the event that someone else would need the room. I liked it for its privacy, but it was very cold, and there was no way to adjust the temperature. It was on the north side of the building, so it never got any sun; it was very dark and depressing. All of the isolation units were on the same air filtration system and this included the air conditioning system.

Tom, as well as Karen, were both happy that we were back in the Adult Cancer Care Unit. Karen had a male nurse for Saturday night named Thad, and it took Thad a long time to get Karen back on her medications. We had taken a two-day hiatus from the arsenic trioxide for the brain surgery. Her intra-cranial pain and the ringing in the ears had subsided. The wound site where Karen had a letter "C" etched into her head, above her left eye just into the hairline reminded me of the Chicago Cubs logo. This was the primary source of her pain, as one would expect. The left half of her head was shaved, but she still had hair on the right side. The incision in her stomach to run off the excess spinal fluid also caused her some pain. At this point, she was pretty beaten up, but it appeared that the procedure had worked without a hitch.

Now it was time to get back to attacking the real problem, leukemia.

Between Kenny, who had just arrived in Indy, and myself we managed to do enough prodding that Thad was able to get Karen back on the ATO, but it took us about two hours. It was very frustrating. We had to do a lot of "suggesting" for Thad to finally get with the program.

Once I arrived home on Friday evening, I put together the following update on the website.

Friday, June 11, 2004 9:56 PM

Karen continues to make progress in her fight to beat leukemia and is resting comfortably. She had a degree of restlessness over Thursday night dealing with the wound site on top of her head from Wednesday's brain surgery. She left the ICU and is back in the Adult Cancer Care unit on the fifth floor. A minor fever was detected mid-afternoon on Friday, but by early evening the fever had disappeared. She continues to take antibiotics and platelets are being administered in order to maintain the clotting process.

Her WBC is up to 129,000; however Dr. Cripe is not at all alarmed by the escalation in the count. The big news is that Karen's Blast factor, a measure of the bad white blood cells as a percentage, has decreased to 80. When she arrived at IUMC last week the Blast was 86 and rose quickly to 95 the next day. The arsenic trioxide treatments resumed Thursday and the downward trend in the Blast is certainly positive.

Karen's Aunt Ellen drove over from Huntington, West Virginia and the impeccable John Bird visited with Karen, as did Karen's Mom, Patricia.

The kids all had a great day with baseball practice for Will; gymnastics for Samantha and Mitchell's Carmel United soccer tryouts were postponed until tomorrow due to flooding.

Uncle Kenny took a minivan full of cousins down to Jillian's to hit the arcades and do a little bowling.

Got to go; the kids are back!

When Saturday morning came along, Indianapolis was experiencing a classic summer thunderstorm with heavy rains. It had rained most of Friday evening as well, so when I talked with Kim on Saturday morning, we both agreed that there was no way the soccer tryouts would take place, given the lightning. Besides it was about a 35-minute drive to Shellbourne where the tryouts were taking place.

Saturday, after I left Uncle Kenny and the big group of cousins at the Indianapolis Zoo, I went back north a few blocks at around 3:00 to check on my bride. Everything seemed to be going very well; I helped get her some dinner although Karen still wasn't eating much and was at this point still really dealing with the postoperative effects of the surgery. At about 7:00, a young resident named Annie, whose rotation included keeping tabs on Karen, came in and explained to us more about the M3 type of leukemia. She educated us on some of the terminology regarding cell development, but most importantly she brought us significant news, that even made Annie cry a little. It was nice to see a young doctor deliver such promising news and then act like a normal human being by displaying some low-key emotion.

I announced the great news on the website early the next morning, needing a night to sleep on this one!

Sunday, June 13, 2004 8:27 AM

Yesterday we learned that Karen has NO BLAST CELLS! This is amazing and proves the arsenic trioxide is working its magic in spite of the two-day diversion when the brain surgery was performed and the cancer treatments were put on the back burner. When Karen's sister Kathy called and told me earlier in the day on Saturday, while I was at the zoo with the kids and cousins, that her Blast was 8 and now it's two. I was very puzzled and I told Kathy, "That can't be true it was 80 yesterday; you mean 80 not 8." I was wrong and am happy to admit it. Based on notes Kathy took while discussing the situation with Dr. Metha, a key member of Dr. Cripe's oncology team and other reference materials, here's what we understand.

When the body reproduces white blood cells, which is always occurring, the cells start off as Blast (myeloblast) or immature white blood cells. With acute myelogenous leukemia (AML), of the subtype M3 that Karen has, the cells remain "frozen" in this early stage of development. We all have Blasts that eventually mature into healthy white blood cells. A normal cell divides, matures and dies all within about 72 hours. In a leukemic cell, the ability to divide and die off isn't there; hence the increase in the WBC.

The arsenic trioxide flips a switch and makes the Blast cell grow into a healthy cell or promyelocyte, which is the next stage in cell formation after Blast. The mature cell then eventually dies off; this is why we expect Karen's white blood count (WBC) to come down even though as of yesterday it was at 140,000. It may still continue to increase over the next few days. With the arsenic trioxide, we are not "killing" off all the white blood cells, both good and bad, like they did two years ago with the much harsher idarubicin and duanorubicin forms of chemotherapy. The goal then was to get Karen's WBC to zero for her to be considered to be in remission; this time the approach is much different.

The paradigm is switched, this time remission is defined as a WBC in a normal range of 4,000 to 10,000 and when they see few if any breaks in the chromosomes, they will consider her to have reached remission. Dr. Cripe does not want to see the 15th chromosome attaching to the 17th chromosome. Another factor to consider is Karen's ability to deal with infection; last time this was measured as ANC and when it reached 500 she was safe. At this point in time, the ANC is not at a sufficient level and the WBC count is still high.

Once this all lines up, the bone marrow transplant will be scheduled, but this is way down the road because Karen will come home at some point, hopefully soon and will continue to receive the arsenic trioxide treatments on an out-patient basis for several weeks prior to surgery.

I understand there's a prayer service at St. Louis de Montfort, our home parish in Fishers, Indiana at 6:30 p.m. this evening. I will try to stop in before going downtown to be with Karen for the evening. Special thanks to Grace Hineman for organizing the service.

Karen's sister-in-law Colleen, my fellow outlaw, will be here with her daughter Katie holding down the fort for next week. Drive safely, ladies!

The power of prayer is amazing, and Karen's string of five good days in a row are evidence of God's healing powers all working within her, all invoked by prayer. The entire family knows that somewhere, someone is praying the rosary in Karen's name 24/7.

All I can say is thanks and please keep it up!

On Monday morning, I got a call from Kim Santucci, and she sounded kind of sheepish. She told me that the Carmel United website had just posted the names of all the boys who had made the soccer team that Mitchell was supposed to try out for over the weekend.

When I told Karen the news she said, "I'm going to be sick!"

Tryouts had taken place even though the website still said that the tryouts for Friday had been postponed. I could only surmise that the tryouts had been held on Saturday or Sunday and this was announced verbally only to those parents who drove out to the fields during the thunderstorm on Saturday morning. Long story short is that we were assured that Mitchell would get a tryout in August with all the boys who had made the team. There still was room on the squad, but the coach felt, and rightfully so, that an individual tryout for a sport like soccer didn't make any sense. I trusted that Kim would stay on this issue, as I had bigger fish to fry. However, Karen was not happy with me for dropping the ball. I knew that Kim would get the situation rectified.

Throughout this entire odyssey, if I needed something out of the norm done, Kim Santucci would get it done. Kim was awesome and at times I felt bad for her because in a way, I knew she was reliving the loss of her mother. She was bound and determined the outcome for her friend would be different.

On Sunday night after Mass at a prayer service for Karen and Tom Stark, I spoke briefly for about five minutes and thanked everyone for taking more time after church to attend the prayer service for my wife and Tom. Then I relayed to everyone what I had witnessed several days earlier when Karen's head was adorned with her "crown of thorns" prior to the MRI, how I realized that my role was so similar to Simon. I had to help her carry this cross and then I told everyone about the remarkable moment when one of the transport assistants wiped the blood from Karen's face.

Then I sped off to grab Karen a burger and a frosty from Wendy's. Occasionally, we had to sneak in some non-hospital food. I spent a very restless night with Karen, but trying to get quality sleep in the big blue chair was not practical. Every time I'd come downtown, I'd bring a hardcopy of the latest entries and well wishes from Karen's website and read them aloud to her. I know Aunt Ellen did the same when she was with Karen.

The remarkable item to report from Monday was that Karen was able to get out of bed and make a couple of laps up and down the hall. I found this very significant given the fact that she had just had brain surgery four days earlier. However, the journal entry I made late Tuesday evening summarizes the progress after just about two weeks since the relapse from remission was discovered and the brain surgery.

It was somewhere near this point in time when I remember chatting with Katie Hincher as we walked down the hall. I expressed to her our dissatisfaction with the attention to detail Victoria Hunt had given Karen. I told Katie I knew in my heart that Karen had to have the shunt inserted in her head because Victoria was negligent in her job. She did not pay attention to the details of Karen's case! Katie was so politically correct. She just listened and let me vent. Deep down I don't think she disagreed with me.

When I made the frequent journal entries onto the website, I tried to keep the content concentrated on four areas. First, I tried to convey Karen's medical prognosis with two other thoughts in mind: to respect her privacy and not alarm friends and family, while trying to remain objective. Secondly, I felt it was important to acknowledge those members of the family and our friends who were working so hard at great personal expense to help our family. Third, I tried to convey to the reader the children's activities and let everyone know that for the summer of 2004, things were much different than June 2002 when everything for them in Indiana came to a complete halt. And finally, I always wanted to say something spiritual regarding faith in the Almighty watching us from above, as He was the one really calling all the shots.

We think we are in control of our lives, and as much as we would like to think we are in control, it is Jesus Christ who is really in charge.

On Tuesday evening, I wrote about what appeared to be a step in the right direction in the battle to beat the cancer that had besieged our lives.

HOW KAREN CONQUERED CANCER

Tuesday, June 15, 2004 11:13 PM

Karen's remarkable recovery from brain surgery and progress in dealing with leukemia continues. She has made several walks up and down the halls, multiple times a day for the past few days. There's even an exercise bike in her room for her to peddle when she doesn't feel like suiting up in the gown, gloves and duckbill mask, which are required for walking the hall. Besides we also have to unplug her IV and tote these along as well, so this requires an escort.

On to the numbers, where we are very happy to convey news of her first WBC drop. On Sunday, she was at 180,000, then in the morning on Monday up again to 191,000 and in the evening on Monday up yet again to 212,000. Remember, this trend has always been expected; then finally today, on Day 11 of the arsenic trioxide treatment, because we skipped two days last week due to a little brain surgery, THE WBC WENT DOWN TO 191,000 AS OF TUESDAY MORNING!!!

Dr. Cripe is very pleased and even more importantly his visual inspection of recent blood smears under the microscope reveal 30% of the mature white blood cells were indeed dying off. This is significant because on average patients, in a similar situation to Karen, did not experience a decrease in the WBC until Day 17 of the arsenic trioxide treatments. A factor contributing to the increased WBC were steroids and dexa "something or other," which she was receiving 4 times daily, to help with the swelling of the brain. This has now been cut to twice a day.

The men of the house all visited Karen today as William and Mitchell escorted their mom up the hall and back four times. Tomorrow, Samantha, Cousin Katie and Karen's sister-in-law Colleen will travel south for a visit.

Special thanks to Aunt Ellen for all she did here the past few days. She spent the night with Karen twice and has headed back to Huntington, West Virginia hopefully not by way of Chicago. (Sorry Ellen, but I just had to get that in.) Ellen and her husband threw quite the party in April to celebrate their daughter Katie's wedding. Samantha was a junior bridesmaid.

Mitchell received straight A's on his report card. Will's GPA was 3.143 and Samantha's grades were all A's and B's. Good job, Volpe kids—report card dinner on me, but only when our mom returns home!!!!

Please remember the family of Tom Stark in your prayers as well. For those of you who don't live over this way, the Starks are fellow parishioners at SLDM and Tom has started his own battle with cancer. He will win. They are a wonderful family.

I hope there's no rioting in Motown tonight, although there's bound to be a few cars on fire.

Good night John Boy.

Katie Hincher came by Wednesday afternoon with the best news I had heard since Karen achieved remission on July 15, 2002.
We had a match!
I ran to the PC on the sixth floor and quickly typed the following on the Caringbridge website and hit enter after Karen

tracked down her brother, Tommy, on his cell phone. He heard the magnificent news first, directly from his sister.

Wednesday, June 16, 2004 4:59 PM

The bone marrow screening results have been completed.

Karen's youngest brother Tommy is a "perfect match" to donate his bone marrow for Karen's eventual bone marrow transplant surgery. Kevin and Kenny were also compatible, but only Tommy was perfect.

God does answer our prayers.

Colleen, Katie and Samantha all went shopping to buy Karen some things, and then went down to the hospital for a visit. I had warned cousin Katie that her Aunt Karen might not look the same as she remembered. I told her there was a little bit of blood in the white of her right eye, and that she would be wearing a pretty bandana because they had to cut off Aunt Karen's hair to do the brain surgery. Katie smiled and seemed to understand what to expect.

I had planned on going downtown mid-afternoon after their visit.

Suddenly the phone rang about 11:00 a.m. with Father Dave Hellmann on the line. He spoke very gently as if not to alarm me saying, "I just visited the hospital and you need to go to Karen. I think she just got some bad news from the ophthalmologist, and she just wanted to be alone."

I drove too fast, almost getting into an accident. I couldn't help think that Karen's vision was permanently impaired. I prayed as I drove, "Okay, Lord, if we have to swap her eyesight for her life, then it's a deal. And besides, the kids have always wanted us to get another dog."

When I got to the hospital, Karen asked me to just lie there in bed with her; she was very sullen. I was somewhat dismayed that Colleen, Katie and Samantha weren't there, but I didn't ask any questions. So I just lied there next to her and waited for her to say something. Her energy level was very low. Finally she explained what happened.

"This morning was a disaster"

"What happened?" I asked.

"Poor little Katie came up to me with her mask on, took one look at my eyes and fainted, with her head smacking the floor," replied Karen.

"Is she okay?" I asked.

Karen said she had a little bump on her head and was a little dizzy, but she's all right.

Later on that day we turned our attention to her vision. The ophthalmologist, Dr. Brownstone, was convinced that the leukemia had infiltrated the spinal fluid and the leukemic cells had made their way behind the eye and would continue to wreak havoc with Karen's eyesight.

Dr. Brownstone said, "I really have no basis for saying this, and I really don't know that much about leukemia and its affects on the patient's eyesight if the cells infiltrate the central nervous system."

Prior to brain surgery, Dr. Cripe had a heated conversation with the ophthalmologists who wanted to perform either a spinal tap or a lumbar puncture to determine whether the leukemia was also present in the central nervous system. Dr. Cripe was adamant that such a procedure not be performed on his patient, who could potentially bleed out if they punched a hole in her back. Besides, it's virtually impossible to gather a sample without contaminating the sample with a drop of blood, which contains white blood cells that were already known to be leukemic. Even if we were able to ascertain whether the malignant cells were there, the treatment protocol with the arsenic trioxide remained the same. Dr. Cripe was vehement that no such procedure be performed on his patient who would certainly have clotting complications.

When I visited Karen that afternoon she was down. She remained very concerned about her counts not decreasing as quickly as we had hoped. I focused on the positive news and told her the numbers would eventually come down. I had found out that her white count had actually climbed to 229,000 but I knew that if I told her this number she'd be very upset. I kept this to myself and didn't post this number on her white board for her to see.

It took me awhile to convince her that this news of a perfect match was a big, huge win. We would find out later in the summer that Kathy was also a match on all factors. However, she had a different blood type than Karen, making Tommy the ideal potential donor. We were fortunate to have these options. Many people in need of a match never find a compatible donor.

Karen was also concerned about my mental and physical welfare. She insisted I talk with Dr. Theobald about her relapse. She was concerned about me taking good care of myself and getting sufficient sleep.

I am such a good husband and I always do what I am told, but in some cases there can be unintended consequences, even when motivated by the best of intentions.

CHAPTER 32

Methodist Tower

I did exactly what my wife asked and contacted Dr. Theobald's assistant, Donna Butler, about getting in to see him. I knew deep inside that I was having trouble getting adequate sleep. I had spent too many evenings downstairs in front of the big screen watching and listening to the words from Bruce Springsteen's *The Rising* concert tour in Barcelona, Spain from a DVD my old friend, Brad Winkler, had left me back in May when he was in town for the Indy 500. The power, energy and words from The Boss motivated me and the lyrics to "Lonesome Day" had become my personal theme song. A hospital can be a very lonely place.

The words, *"Let kingdom come, I'm gonna find a way through this Lonesome Day,"* just constantly stuck in my head. The title cut is all about the promise of the Resurrection: *"Come on up for the rising tonight."*

Some people get their strength from the Bible, others from poetry and others from classical music or the opera. My inspiration comes from the raw energy of Bruce's music, his vision and his dream of happiness for all, especially the working man. Yes, I'm a conservative Republican, definitely a white-collar guy, but Bruce is one of just a few Democrats I can think of whom I truly admire.

On Thursday, June 17th, I was able to see Karen Isenmenger PHD, FNP, an associate of Dr. Theobald's. We met at Methodist Tower, which was on Capital Street downtown at 3:00 p.m. and most convenient for continuing on to IUMC after the appointment. Karen Isenmenger listened to my story from 2002, in which I described my problem as sleep deprivation, not bipolar disease, and that Dr. Jerome Samuels had put me on Depakote and Zyprexa for nothing. My wife realized that Dr. Samuels' diagnosis and treatment were wrong, and eventually got me in to see Dr. Theobald in November or December. By the end of January 2003, I had weaned myself off all the hard drugs used to treat schizophrenia. I had suffered from sleep deprivation and I'll take it to my grave.

I was not bipolar.

I explained to Dr. Isenmenger that I was there at my wife's request because she wanted Dr. Theobald to know that she had relapsed and she was concerned for my overall well-being. I told Karen Isenmenger I had been taking half a Unisom, actually a Benadryl equivalent, which I used at home some of the time, and often on business travel as a sleeping aid. She said she didn't like Unisom because it doesn't eliminate the rapid eye movements that allow us to get into a full restful sleep cycle. I also told her that the Restoril 30-milligram tabs Dr. Theobald had given me back in early 2003, after I was finally off the Depakote and Zyprexa, helped me to relax, but did not really help me get into a deep sleep. Unisom worked fine for me prior to Karen's relapse. I explained that I usually got five to six hours of sleep per night and was functioning fine.

She prescribed what she described as a light dosage of a medication used for depression called Trazadone, requiring me to take 75 milligrams right before bedtime. A light dosage helps most people get some real sleep, and she wanted me to take it for at least three straight nights to build up the serum in my system.

She had consulted with Dr. Theobald on this plan and he fully concurred.

The pharmacist at IUMC where I got the prescription filled explained the dosage to me and also encouraged me to read the pamphlet listing the numerous side effects, which I glanced at quickly. It listed at least 25 things that could occur in some patients. This pamphlet had everything under the sun listed: numbness, sweating, anxiety, restlessness, bleeding of the gums, constipation and prolonged erections.

Who needs Viagra, when there's a wonderful drug like Trazadone?

I took the Trazadone from June 17th through 19th as directed. It didn't help me sleep like I thought it would. I'd sleep for two hours; then be awake for two or three hours. I was very restless. Later as the sun would come up, exhaustion would kick in, and I'd get maybe two more hours of poor quality sleep that resembled a long nap. Then I would start my day.

Here's my best recollection of what happened the following days.

As of June 18th, I decided to consume no beer or alcohol at all because of the warning on the prescription. I had another very restless night. Colleen Coyne spent the night with Karen, who vomited often all night, getting little sleep because of the arsenic trioxide. They had cut Karen's dose of phenegren in half, which was helping with the nausea. We both had very bad nights that evening. I hardly slept at all, watched some more *SportsCenter* on ESPN, and *Bruce in Barcelona* during the early morning hours. I was downtown at 6:30 a.m. because I couldn't sleep and wanted to be there when Dr. Cripe's oncology team made their 7:00 a.m. appearance to review Karen's progress.

Then on June 19th, I had a very busy day. Will had an 11:30 a.m. game, Colleen took Sam to a gymnastics exhibition at Lawrence Central High School, and then she left for Ohio after cutting back west to the hospital to see Karen. I took Mitchell to Will's 3:30 p.m. game just north of our house in Noblesville at 161st Street. I spent Saturday night with Karen in her room. I had one Dewars and some wings at Chancellor's prior to trying to get some shut-eye. The warning on the side of the Trazadone said to take caution in drinking alcohol with this medication; it may cause drowsiness. The warning clearly did not prohibit use of booze; in fact, I thought the drowsiness effect was a good thing, given that I was in a noisy hospital room trying to sleep in a big and somewhat uncomfortable blue lounge chair. I dozed a little bit, and Karen had a decent night.

It was a typical night in room #5827. Noises, nurses taking blood samples at 4 a.m., and the infusion unit beeping every 45 minutes; just some light sleep was all that we were afforded. I thought I was behaving normally. Karen's hospitalization had now gone beyond the projected eight to 10 days after her relapse. She would be in the cold, depressing room much longer than we originally believed. The room was freezing cold, and this didn't help either of us get any solid rest. I spent many nights in the blue lounge chair adjacent to her bed, as did many members of the family and a few close friends.

I made an entry in the journal the next morning:

Friday, June 18, 2004 8:43 AM

Karen's WBC continues to hover around the high 190,000 mark for the past few days and the doctors wholeheartedly believe that the count has topped off and will soon start to drop. I believe that this will occur on Father's Day, as was the case two years ago. History has a habit of repeating itself.

For the past couple of days, in spite of the great news regarding "PERFECT T," she remains a little down mentally and last evening the nausea returned. She's frustrated and just wants to get back home. Dr. Metha told her that he thought she'd be home by the end of June at the latest, but they need to see her WBC move downward first.

We had cut back the anti-nausea medication, but from here on out, we'll return to the same dosage that kept her comfortable earlier in the week. She is getting some sleep and eating a little. And today they're doing a CAT scan just to double check on the placement of the shunt. She continues to take her little walks and ride the bike.

Colleen and Katie have been wonderful, and we are glad they were able to spend so much time here right after school let out. Nora Wilson and PERFECT T will be in over the weekend. Colleen and Katie will head back home tomorrow.

Until next time!

I took the Trazadone again. I slept a little, but started seeing lots of colors and a bizarre kaleidoscope of colorful effects or fireworks on the back of my eyelids.

Eventually, I fell off and slept for two hours, and then I was awake again for two, and then a light sleep for two hours before showering. I felt like I was just getting by; some people do this all the time, but given the stress and my history, I was beginning to get a little concerned.

Although I was holding it together, my journal entries were starting to get a bit long-winded and repetitive, definitely an indication that my mind was churning and that I was far from settled.

Saturday, June 19, 2004 1:50 PM

After a rough night on Thursday when Karen was very restless, somewhat agitated and nauseated, the CAT scan performed on Friday morning revealed why, as it detected some minor bleeding around the cylinder that is a component of the shunt inserted 8 days ago. Over the course of the day more kryo, platelets and steroids were administered in order to slow the bleeding. Karen spent a very quiet and restful day on Friday, as she didn't walk the halls or hit the bike at all. We wanted to minimize any pressure to the brain. Her symptoms subsided, and she ate lightly, except for lunch when she finished off a grilled cheese sandwich.

Her WBC had gone up on Friday to 209,000, partially due to the steroids. Dr. Cripe informed us that he has been in touch with a world-renowned colleague named Dr. Tallman who pioneered the use of ATRA to treat patients with AML. As he consults with Dr. Tallman and other colleagues, the advice remains the same: stay the course with the arsenic trioxide, but the high WBC remains a concern. Later in the day on Friday, he stated that he fully expects Karen to reach remission, but if the WBC remains high, there will come a point when we may have to consider switching to the traditional form of chemotherapy, idarubicin, that was used two years ago to achieve remission. He had no way to anticipate the problems with Karen's brain that had required surgery and obviously complicated the matter.

I stayed with Karen through the night on Friday, and she got some sleep and there were no problems with any side effects.

Saturday morning, Karen's vision in her right eye remains blotchy in the peripheral while the left eye is fine. Prior to the brain surgery last week, it was the right eye that was fine and the left caused her some problems. This is due to some blood, but we don't know and do not have a good way to test to find out if this is attributable to continued post-op swelling or the infiltration of the leukemia into the central nervous system. Regardless of the cause, the treatment is the same: continue with the arsenic trioxide. If we fix the cancer, the vision problems will be alleviated in time. Dr. Cripe has always looked at this as treating the two problems in parallel. Cure the cancer and the eyes will follow.

Another CAT scan was done on Saturday morning to double check the bleeding in the brain. I just talked to Tommy, and he didn't say anything about it, so I'm assuming that we've weathered another storm.

At about 9:00 a.m. this morning I received another early Father's Day present. My godson sent me a cooler, that will only be used for non-alcoholic beverages (ha ha!) and some Polo aftershave from my parents. The third gift was received from the Big Man above and Dr. Cripe of course, as Karen's WBC COUNT DROPPED BY ALMOST 30,000 to 180,000!!! This was as of her 4:00 a.m. blood draw.

We both cried; we're at second base with nobody out—a single sends her HOME!! I believe this will be before the end of June, but this is just my opinion based on the encouraging comments made by Dr. Metha two days ago.

A WBC, taken at 8:00 a.m., shows a very slight increase to 184,000. I explained to Karen before these results were known to not be surprised to see the drop continue to happen in a jagged pattern over the next few days. The drop won't be smooth or linear if one were to graph the trend over time. The key is that this overall trend will need to continue to move downward. Keep in mind the body is always adjusting its production of white blood cells; it stores them up as it senses a need to build some reserves to fight off infection.

We both cried with the news of the big drop. I was only expecting a 10,000 drop. We've got Karen to second base with nobody out—a single sends her HOME!!

She also had the rest of her hair shaved off; the left side was done for the brain surgery. Now Karen has a Demi Moore look from the movie GI Jane, only Karen looks much better than Demi.

Her long time friend Nora Wilson (formerly Haas) and Tommy (old Irish name meaning Perfectionist) are here.

Samantha just participated in the Gymnastics Fantastics exhibition about an hour ago, and Will's playing in a tournament with two games today and two more Sunday.

Sam and Mitch will visit Karen shortly

On June 20th, Nora arrived and spent the whole day Sunday with Karen. I relieved Nora after spending the day at home mowing and watering the yard. Then I saw Will's 5:00 p.m. game. I showered fast, went out to dinner downtown with all three kids for about two to three hours, after visiting with Karen for an hour and a half, and spent the night at home with the kids. We all had a huge dinner at TGI Friday's with Tom.

Nora and her family left, after watching the end of the U.S. Open on Sunday evening, and at this point, there was no out-of-town help from the 21st through the 23rd of June. So I spent only a few hours at the hospital in order to tend to the kids needs as best I could. Thank goodness Aunt Patty had been at the house the last few days. I still wasn't sleeping well, even in my own bed, especially with no Karen to cuddle. I took the Trazadone again; this would be the last time. I experienced the same colorful side effects as I had earlier.

Finally, it dawned on me, and I got up in the middle of the night, at 2:00 a.m. or so, and went back to review the pamphlet as suggested by the pharmacist. I looked at the warning label review, as it seemed like it was worth checking again.

The little pamphlet included wording something like the following: This medication may cause, among a longer list of other things, the following (which I believe I was experiencing): anxiety, restlessness, blurring of the vision, tiredness, nervousness, insomnia, dry mouth (I was drinking tons of water), hostility and anger.

Later, I found more information from a variety of websites regarding Trazadone. This explained why I was being basically an angry horse's ass to my kids. They knew I was under a lot of stress, but at one point, I said half-jokingly to Will, "Pick up your clothes or I'll break your cute little nose."

This is not how I typically treat my kids. My fuse was very short, but this is just one example of how the drugs were affecting my personality.

At this point, I stopped taking it and went back to Unisom with only moderate success, still getting about two hours of sleep, then three restless hours, followed by two hours of sleep—an ugly pattern. At about 2:30 in the early morning of the 22nd I called my dad to talk about my concerns with Karen.

All of us, including Dr. Cripe, were getting very concerned with the high white blood count, and I was worried that she might never make it to remission and never get the chance at the bone marrow transplant. I asked my dad if he thought that maybe God had just given us a two-year reprieve, an opportunity to do some traveling and have some special time together as a family. My theory was the Lord was kind enough to give us a long two-year goodbye—we just didn't realize it, assuming the battle had been won. We were granted a gift that the victims' families on 9/11 never had.

My dad had a very calming effect on me, and we talked for about 45 minutes. My mind was at ease, and I was finally able to get some sleep. His advice was very soothing, and he let me know that what I was thinking was not too far-fetched. He was relieved that I understood and had accepted the fact that my wife might die. I was being an unwilling realist. I told him the part of the Lord's Prayer that caused me the most consternation was the phrase, "Thy Will Be Done."

What was His Will, and when would it be done?

My dad sent me the Prayer of St. Ignatius; it really helped put things into perspective for me. The prayer in essence says turn your life over to God: "Dispose of it wholly according to your will."

When you stop and think about it, this is a very difficult thing to do: total trust. My dad had always told me to call any time day or night, and it was one of the best conversations I have ever had with my father. I'll cherish the memory of that conversation and his candor forever.

I then called Dr. Isenmenger the next day to let her know the Trazadone experiment wasn't working. She called back a few days later. I was somewhat angry that it had taken her three days to return my call. I was a hurting unit and needed real medical help. I had even started to think that maybe Dr. Samuels was right and maybe I was bipolar.

Could it be this condition was brought on by stressful situations?

I hate incompetence and our experiences with the medical profession during our marriage made me even more skeptical. I wasn't as concerned with my own medical care; my focus was on matters of much greater importance, my wife's cancer.

Dr. Ross is still on my shit list for not getting me an MRI that would have immediately revealed my ruptured Achilles.

I asked him back in 1993, the day after my injury to my ankle area, "Are you sure this isn't a ruptured Achilles?" and he made me feel like I was being a big wimp. Well, I had a rupture that required major surgery a year later. "It's only a torn calf muscle. You'll be fine in six weeks," was his brisk reply.

He was wrong!

Now I walk with a slight limp and can't run very well at all. I have pain in that ankle just about every day.

Then there's Dr. Marino, who basically told us to abort Mitchell. And more recently, Dr. Samuels had decided I was bipolar for life, and he put me on drugs that made me a semi-functional zombie, so my patience with these "know it all" MDs who see themselves as being above reproach was about out. They were both wrong!

Have I failed to mention Karen's care at St. Vincent Hospital in Carmel two years prior? Dr. Reisman wasn't wrong. It just took them too damn long to be right.

Okay, sorry for all the Italian emotion. I'll shut up now.

I constantly thank God, that when we needed a spectacular doctor with my wife's life at stake, we had found Dr. Cripe and Katie Hincher.

On the 23rd of June, I had a conference call with Steve Kozey at MISO and some of our customers. We had an hour of preparation to discuss a list of questions prior to the call. Mr. Kozey could tell I was slightly agitated and he managed to calm me down. I took a deep breath and walked down the hall to get a drink of water. I was able to do fine on the call, but I really had to concentrate. The power marketers on the call were full of compliments and appreciative that I would take the time to answer their question given my personal situation. This was one of my FERC filing projects that I had to delegate. Things had changed and I was even impressed with my ability to recall details while on the call. Steve Kozey was there, and he was very aware of what happened two years ago, so under this pressure I think I did well enough to convince him I hadn't lost it.

I played a round of golf with Will on the 24th as he drove the cart; I walked so I could sweat a bit out on the course. We had a great time and he hit the ball very well. His short game needs work, just like his old man.

I talked with Aunt Ellen about my dilemma with the Trazadone. She had worked at a psychiatric hospital in Huntington for 25 years. She hated the use of Trazadone for patients with depression. It's an old drug, and she was glad that I was off it and also told me that she was impressed I eventually recognized that it was hurting me. I worked like a banshee in the yard on Saturday, weeding two mulch beds that had grown out of control.

All of a sudden, I felt this calm and coolness, like an ocean breeze, envelop my body. I no longer had this gnawing sensation in the pit of my stomach. I felt like I had turned the corner. Ellen had told me it would take a few days for the Trazadone to clear my system, and that in her opinion 75 milligrams was way too much. I should have only been given 25 milligrams to get me to sleep. In her opinion, it was as though they were treating me for depression, not insomnia.

I had an unfortunate incident with Samantha during which I may have overreacted, but maybe I didn't. In retrospect, it's hard to say whether I was right or wrong. We had been out to dinner, and I was driving Will and Sam home. Will had some stomach cramps and he needed "Home Field Advantage" as quickly as I could get him home.

As we drove, Samantha said, "I call the first floor bathroom when we get home, and I don't care if you need it right away." I went berserk on Samantha and yelled at her that, of all the things I had to deal with, she had the gall to add the use of a bathroom to my list of issues.

When I got home, I sat her down and I explained to her that she had no idea of what it was like to be me and to have my responsibilities. She was being selfish and self-centered, just creating problems over something as silly as a bathroom.

"This is crazy!" I shouted. "We have five bathrooms in this house. Will was having a personal emergency, and you decided to make a big deal out of it."

I told her it was her job to "Help the dad, help the mom!"

That was the new saying I invented on the fly to try to get her to make my life easier. I knew the effects of the Trazadone were still lingering in my system, but she really sent me over the edge.

I went on to explain to Samantha that I loved her very much, but I had one singular mandate and that was to do everything I could to help save her mother's life.

I told her, "Samantha, I do love you, but you've got to understand that I have a mission, and if somebody gets in the way, and I don't love them or care about their feelings, I will run them over like a trucker runs over a frozen deer in his headlights. But in this case, you're someone I love, so if you're in my way I will set you to the side and come back to fix it later. This is all about the mom, so don't put it past me if you continue to be selfish and make things more difficult I will send you back to Ohio just like before, even though it's something I really don't want to do."

I had made my point. It was about the third time in a week Samantha had gone out of her way to make things more difficult, so I felt like I had to fix it, even though I really hated having to say the words that had just come out of my mouth. For the rest of the time, I had nothing but cooperation and helpfulness from Samantha.

My tirade worked, and she took over as the little lady of the house.

CHAPTER 33

University Place

On Saturday, Karen made a remarkable request. She asked that her father spend Father's Day evening with her in her room overnight. I found this to be a very poignant request, and my mind immediately envisioned myself never having to do the same with my own little Samantha. Karen's request was helpful to me personally because I had been burning the candle at both ends. I was spent. Tom didn't actually spend the entire night in the big blue lounge chair. He had a room at University Place and he slept there for a few hours. Periodically, he would come over to check on his "Little Kare." Tom was honored and grateful for the opportunity to spend the evening with his daughter. The thought of two cancer survivors—Tom, who spent the last year dealing with prostate cancer, with his daughter, Karen—spending Father's Day evening together, well, the irony of this scenario brought a lump to my throat.

After I got home I wrote the following entry:

Sunday, June 20, 2004 10:04 PM

Thanks to Tommy, Karen now has a laptop with dial-up capability to the Internet in her room so she can see updates to the guestbook as you update this website. She does take frequent naps, but she's psyched to see more words of encouragement. Previously, we would print off the most recent entries and read them to her due to the trouble she was having with her vision, which is now vastly improved.

She definitely has her rally cap on! I finally saw that the fire, grit and determination have returned in those beautiful Irish eyes. Seeing her children in person has her really pumped up and she knows it's just a matter of time until she comes home.

Please send a donation to caringbridge.org

They're trying to raise $75,000. With the number of hits I've seen on Karen's web page alone, I'd say we could raise that amount by Tuesday.

Our donation goes out Monday. This website has been truly inspirational and is a convenient vehicle allowing us to keep people, literally all around the world, posted on Karen's continued progress.

Will threw out his first runner attempting to steal second base and no, it wasn't some big, fat, slow, chubby kid either! He threw it on a line, on one hop, right on the bag just like Johnny Bench.

I'll never forget Father's Day 2004.

We had a very important meeting on Tuesday morning with Dr. Cripe. We were all fearful that he had decided to switch Karen from the arsenic trioxide to the same corrosive forms of chemotherapy used two years ago because her white count was continuing to climb. Dr. Cripe had been hinting that the big switch might be made. This made me very uneasy because, up to this point, we had been hearing that the colleagues he had been corresponding with, including Dr. Tallman, whom he had mentioned several times, had advised against switching the protocol.

This bothered both of us, and this possibility kept me tossing and turning at night. Dr. Cripe and Katie walked in and much to my dismay; my seven carefully prepared questions, assuming he was going to make the switch, were rendered moot. Here's why:

Tuesday, June 22, 2004 12:50 AM

This morning we had a long conversation with Dr. Cripe regarding Karen's prognosis. In all honestly, given the high white blood count we were prepared to consider the possibility that Dr. Cripe had decided to change Karen's protocol. We were concerned that a switch to the more invasive idarubicin was inevitable to bring down the WBC, which is still in the low 200s, and all of us were mentally prepared for this reality. We had even formulated a series of questions for Dr. Cripe given this assumption.

This proved not to be the case!

Dr. Cripe stated that even though Karen's WBC is extraordinarily high (the highest ever recorded for a person with this subtype of AML), the arsenic trioxide is doing what it's supposed to. However, the process is just taking much longer than he expected. Then he stated this is not a concern, it's the Blast that really counts and at this point the Blast is at 25 based on a recent visual inspection of her blood smears. The Blast has varied over the course of the past few weeks: 86, then 97 for quite awhile, then zero, then 70 and now 25. What a roller coaster ride!

He went on to say with the all the appropriate caveats, meaning no need for ongoing medical support (i.e. no around the clock monitoring and continuous transfusions of platelets, kryo, whole blood units etc…), that on Friday of this week they will make the determination of whether Karen can COME HOME on Monday, June 28, 2004. At this point she will rest at home and continue to receive her arsenic trioxide treatments, blood analysis and periodic EKG's on an outpatient basis. Again, if she requires continual around the clock support of numerous transfusions and monitoring, then it will not make sense to continue treatment on an outpatient basis. The WBC will eventually come down, however this is a long process and will require at minimum another six to eight weeks of continued treatment until remission is achieved.

Once remission occurs, then we will consult in person, probably in early August, with Dr. Cripe's colleague and expert on this type of cancer. His name is Dr. Tallman and he conducts his research at Northwestern University in Chicago. The purpose of this consult will be to determine the optimal procedure for an eventual bone marrow transplant (BMT). The type of transplant performed depends on numerous factors that I don't fully understand at this point in time. But you all know, it's just a matter of time until I acquire at least a general understanding of this aspect of Karen's case. I thought I was done, or should I say helping, with homework once school let out.

Dr. Cripe sketched out a decision tree regarding the various paths that may be taken and it is not a foregone conclusion that Tommy's bone marrow will actually be used for the transplant. There's also the possibility that Karen's own bone marrow will be used depending on a "molecular assessment" of Karen's bone marrow.

She's still having some vision problems with some blurring in the right eye only. We believe this will clear up in due time. This condition may well be attributed to continue post-op swelling related to the brain surgery performed almost two weeks ago.

This news was a little hard for us to comprehend at first, but talk about heart. An hour later Karen walked the hall a few laps and ate a complete helping of Stouffer's macaroni and cheese. She realized it's time to work at getting her strength back, and she now understands this will be an ongoing battle. She's sitting in the lounge chair most of the time instead of lying in bed, and she wants me to bring sweatpants and sweatshirts—no more nighties. This is good—the woman has spunk!!

Her dad is on his way back to Ohio and a special thanks to Karen's cousin Alice for her time and input the past day and a half.

The bottom line is that there is a very good chance our girl will be returning to Garden Gate Way very soon.

Tie a Yellow Ribbon round the old oak tree, or in this case pear tree Miss Kimmie.

Time for another Hail Mary.

Karen's cousin, Robert Smith, from Huntington added this inspiring message on the website. I found this message to be very poignant and full of great insight.

Hey Karen,

It seems too easy and convenient to be able to wish you well and say hello over this print. I know that you are in a tough fight, and I wish that everyone in the family and I'm sure a few of your friends would be happy to share in the pain and uncertainty that you face on a constant plain of thought. And to a certain point, we do. But you are the one that is really in the battle. Endurance athletes are admired by their ability to suffer. You make that statement seem very inappropriate. I have used much of my life to see what kind of pain I can tolerate. But you have succeeded in making that aspiration seem very ridiculous. I realize that I do not wish for TRUE pain and suffering. That's just silly I guess. A man once wrote, "I do not climb Everest to die, I climb to live." I guess you have to go through this to live whether it's your choice or not. I have a hard time believing things happen for a reason but you have given everyone a reason to be inspired.

We all love you and talk about your recovery constantly. And mostly we believe in you.

Robert
- Wednesday, June 23, 2004 4:11 PM

I was elated. Karen might be coming home before the end of June.

Over the day on both Wednesday and Thursday, Karen continued to progress.

Thursday, June 24, 2004 9:53 AM

Since our last update Karen continues to make baby steps

towards remission. Her latest blood work as of 2:00 a.m. this morning shows the WBC down to 158,000, hemoglobin at 8.7 and platelets at 82. I do not have a Blast number and visual inspection is superior to any machine generated calculation. I'm sure Dr. Cripe will review the blood smears yet today.

She's still somewhat weak and had a restless evening because she needed to use the "powder room" often. This evening they will give her something to help her sleep on request. She had some fluids in the lungs and her post-ox is now above 90, so it appears that she won't need the oxygen anymore while in bed. She's spending more time in the lounge chair and ate a PB&J on an English muffin with some hot chocolate. So add that to the mac-n-cheese as the food groups required to kick cancer's......

Dr. Cripe's team of oncologists just left and three new residents joined the group. I got to eavesdrop on their conference in the hall prior to talking with Karen and myself. They received the readers digest version of Karen's month of June. Her vision is still slightly blurred and is improving. They are going to begin cutting back on her pain medication and steroids; the latter will help decrease the WBC in time.

The bottom line is we're still thinking in terms of a return to Garden Gate Way on Monday. Dr. Metha is developing a strategy for this next part of the journey.

Karen plans to walk the halls and will venture down the hall out of isolation wearing the infamous duckbill mask to get a real shower. QUACK, QUACK, QUACK…sorry we don't mean you, doctor. I'm getting punchy.

Will and I are hitting the links, our new Father's Tradition that we were unable to keep due to his tripleheader on Sunday.

John Bird got to see Will play in a 6-5 win last night. He played the whole game: four innings in left and three flawless innings behind the plate, where he knocked down a few would-be wild pitches, even using his legs like a hockey goalie one time to keep the ball out in front of him with runners on second and third. Plays like that don't make it into the scorebook, but they're often the difference between winning and that other word we refuse to say.

Godspeed!

P.S. Pat and Aunt Ellen are back in town.

CHAPTER 34

St. Elmo's Steakhouse

On Friday afternoon I made my only entry into the guestbook. After thinking about it for a long time, I decided it was time for me to take a stab at writing Karen a letter, even though I was never one to put mushy love notes down on paper. Here's what I wrote to my bride.

My Beautiful Bride,

There are literally over 400 pages of well wishes and words of encouragement on your website. I have never made an entry into your awesome guestbook until today. I have always had the distinct advantage of being able to talk to you directly and it's been nice having a "blank check" to do so, whenever I please.

But on today, exactly two months before your birthday, I have decided to tell you in writing what you have demonstrated to me, not only over the past two years, but throughout our entire sixteen years of marital bliss. By the way, if things fall into place with your medical treatment, we are going to throw you one hell of a birthday party on August 24th. It won't be a surprise party, so I am just giving you fair warning now!

Bruce Springsteen and the E Street Band do private parties; they're just very expensive. But I can dream, can't I?

Here's what I really want to say to you and you know I've never been really good at writing mushy love letters; besides, this is on the internet for all the world to see:

Karen, you have taught me the virtue of patience, which is a virtue not necessarily found in many people of Italian descent.

Karen, you have shown me how to be the best parent I can possibly be to our three gorgeous children and have reinforced in our own family those values and spiritual well-being, instilled in the two of us by our respective sets of parents. At the same time, our immediate relatives and close personal friends have stepped up to the plate and shown us the true meaning of "family" as well.

Karen, you have motivated me to realize my fullest potential in my career endeavors and anytime I have said we're moving, you started immediately packing, well, actually you used the opportunity to have a garage sale first, then you started packing.

You always said, "I'll follow you anywhere, even if it's Erie, Pennsylvania," and have carried our family on your back to new opportunities four times.

And more importantly, over the past two years, you have taught all of us participating in this amazing story, the essence of faith, hope, courage, perseverance and most of all love.

It's very clear to me now that God picked you and you alone for this ordeal; despite the physical and emotional suffering, please always remember, this is why He sent you here, in this time and in this place with all of these loving and supportive people.

This was His divine plan long before you were ever born and all culminates in my mind in one brief statement that summarizes everything I am trying to convey here in simple words.

"My love, by your shining example, you have taught us all the true meaning of life."

God loves you and so do I, my beautiful wife!

I Pledge My Enduring Love Forever,

Volpe

Mark J. Volpe
Carmel, Indiana, The Greatest Country on Earth
Friday, June 25, 2004 10:11 AM

Late in the day on Friday, and unknown to me, two of Karen's best friends from her high school days flew into Indianapolis: Dr. Brian Wynne ventured over from Philadelphia and Tom Lambright, an architect, took the long trip into Indianapolis from Seattle just to be with Karen over the weekend. Their timing couldn't have been better because there was much debate as to whether Karen would be able to head home on Monday. Even though Brian is a not an oncologist (he is a respected medical researcher), he shed some light on Karen's condition and gave me some comfort as to whether she would be better off at home or in the hospital. They both lifted Karen's spirits immensely, and there were tons of stories about the old days. This unexpected visit really picked up Karen. She had spent 22 days in the isolation unit, and that coupled with the brain surgery were starting to wear her down.

Earlier in the day on Friday afternoon, I posted the following to the website.

> Friday, June 25, 2004 2:30 PM
>
> Karen's big decision day is here! Does she get to go home on Monday or not???
>
> Her WBC count is down to 139,000 and Dr. Cripe made it very clear she could return home Monday subject to several caveats. At this point, she is still having minor vision problems, lacks stamina and her breathing is still slightly labored. So the decision has been tabled for the weekend and depending on how she progresses on these fronts over the weekend will dictate whether Monday is the day she heads home or not.
>
> Bottom Line: Not a yes at this point for Monday; it's still a maybe.
>
> We will reassess the situation bright and early on Monday morning. So, we have approximately 42 hours to crack the whip. Aunt Ellen is perfect for the job; her resume fits this challenge to a T.
>
> What do I think? It really doesn't matter, because Dr. Cripe is the head coach and I'm just the QB; I'll run whatever play he sends into the huddle.
>
> Based on my conversations with Pat and Ellen, he's perfectly correct based on what he sees at this point.

I'm on my way south to IUMC in an hour.

Until later!

MJV

Throughout Friday, I pushed Karen to take more laps up and down the hall in order to demonstrate to Dr. Cripe that she was ready to take the arsenic trioxide treatments on an outpatient basis. I told her that it was like a job interview, and we needed to do whatever it took to get her back to the friendly confines of Carmel, after what was rapidly approaching a solid month's stay in the isolation unit. She was very down. At one point, I decided to pull out all the stops and try to deal with her psyche through song. I sat in bed with her and sang all the verses to James Taylor's ballad "The Secret of Life" from his old classic album entitled *JT*.

> *Any fool can do it, there ain't nothing to it*
> *Nobody knows how we got to the top of the hill*
> *Since we're only here for a while, might as well enjoy the ride...*

I was desperate to help her understand that this was a long process, a long fight, and there was no end in sight. Getting her back home would be a significant milestone while we inched slowly down the path back to remission. If we could get her mind focused on making it back north to Carmel, her body would eventually follow. After I got home on Friday night, I noticed there were fewer entries in the guestbook than usual. Kim Santucci told me that nobody wanted to dive back in and write after my entry. So I sat down Saturday morning at the computer and tried to motivate the people out there who loved Karen so much to resume making entries in the guestbook.

MARK J. VOLPE

Saturday, June 26, 2004 7:38 AM

So what's going on out there? Cat got your tongue? Is everybody lost for words?

Feeling a little intimidated by one little letter written by a guy who deals with a commodity that nobody can see and certainly wouldn't want to touch. Please don't be scared off by a man who's a part-time chauffeur, former computer programmer, baseball coach, a boring accountant/MBA type, who tries to play psychologist, and occasionally hits a golf ball outta sight, that once aspired to be a jazz saxophonist, or actor who also throws a mean Frisbee, enjoys drinking beer at the beach, would love to be a ski bum or travel all over the globe with his wife, of course, and even back in his teens was a rocket scientist.

Lately, I have been thinking about going to medical school at night school to earn some extra cash for the college funds. I have become interested in studying to become an oncologist, neurologist, ophthalmologist, or hematologist. I should already have a few credits for time served. I have already received several hours of on the job experience as a resident in the OB/GYN field having just stood there and watched while my wife pushed three beautiful children into this world, only to exit the maternity ward a few hours later to buy cases of Michelob and a few fine cigars.

Hey, come on out there, don't be shy. I want to hear some chatter! It's the weekend—don't tell me you don't have time, although I know most of you peek at this website when you're supposed to be working! You're all fired!

O.K. I'll shut my mouth now and tell you what you want to know.

Karen had a very restful night and is building up her strength. Dr. Metha told me she's doing fine and the main purpose of the weekend, besides Karen building back some strength, is to transition from the IVs to receiving her meds orally. He thinks she'll still be home on Monday.

I know what they're doing: Dr. Cripe is playing "bad cop" and Dr. Metha has the role of the "good cop." They're so sneaky! They think we're stupid just because we're not doctors, huh?

Actually, we still won't be certain until Monday morning's conference.

Mitchell and I visited for about three hours, and Karen's pace up and down the hall is getting much more rapid. She looked great, and I started bringing home items she doesn't need there anymore.

Karen, how was your stay?

It was too long; I'd just like to pay my bill and leave.

Leave it on my MasterCard.

Here's the room key!

Have a nice day.

I'm out of here!

Bye.

Mid-afternoon on Saturday I asked Tom and Brian if they wanted to dine at St. Elmo's Steakhouse, Indianapolis' most famous steakhouse, which has been around since 1902. St. Elmo's has the best steaks in town and their shrimp cocktail with the freshly ground horseradish makes your sinuses burn and your head hurt. We had a wonderful meal. I spent most of the evening trying to pick Dr. Wynne's brain regarding whether it was safe for Karen to head home. He said that based on what he saw there was no medical reason for her to remain hospitalized. Before my day began on Sunday morning, I sat down at the PC in our study and pumped out another journal update, complete with the tale of how my dad wrestled with a young opossum. It was one of the funniest things I had seen in all long time and I laughed and laughed.

For the prior two years, I did most of my crying in private, either in the shower or as I lay in bed in the middle of the night where my kids couldn't see my tears.

Sunday, June 27, 2004 6:50 AM

Glad to see more entries in the guestbook. I knew y'all could do it!

Pat, John and Ellen departed in the early afternoon for Akron and Huntington, W.VA respectively and our gratitude goes out to all three of them for being here at this important juncture in Karen's recovery. Pat's wounds are healing nicely; next time I'll have to push harder. Actually, I have a unique relationship with Pat. I seldom call her "Mom," because I've always felt this term should be reserved for the woman who actually carried me and brought me into this world.

By the way, my parents have been here since Thursday. The cuisine has been fantastic: Italian wedding soup, lasagna and my kids are very excited because I think tonight a roast chicken and the delicious angel hair pasta with white sauce is planned. I'm planning my day to not even be a second late. Anyhow, I digress, bottom line is Pat has always treated me like a son, and I know deep down in her heart, that I'm her favorite outlaw. I know Anne, Roger, Colleen and Diana will take no offense; this is just a fact. This is supposed to be a joke, O.K., so relax.

Here's the real news and sorry I couldn't get this update in earlier; I was outside in the yard most of the afternoon, and when I came in to update the site, I discovered a need to run Norton anti-virus, because some website Samantha hit sent our PC into a tizzy.

Karen has no Blasts and the WBC is down to, are you ready for this, 99,900. This was as of the wee morning hours on Saturday. I had forgotten Nora told me last week that two of Karen's good friends from way back Tom Lambright '78 (Another fine Walsh Jesuit alum) and Dr. Brian Wynne flew in from Seattle and Philadelphia, respectively. Their visit sure lifted Karen's spirits, and Brian's candid insight reassured my KareBear and myself that we are headed in the right direction. Her hemoglobin was a little low, hanging at 7.9 so she was given a unit of whole blood. This figure had been in the high 8s and low 9s as of late. This should help boost her stamina.

Dr. Metha met with Karen late Friday, and there are two other news bytes we wanted to pass along. The bone marrow transplant is likely to be performed in September, hopefully not on Sunday at 1:00 p.m. EDT (For those of you that know me even a little this is another funny little ha ha!) and Perfect Tommy's marrow will be used—"allogeneic" for those of you in the know on the BMT protocol.

Brian, Tom and I headed over to St. Elmo's Steakhouse, an Indy mainstay for over a century, for some red meat. Hey, Karen got her beef delivered by yours truly from another establishment famous for their beef, Wendy's. She ate every bite and this should help get her legs back.

Other notes from the week are the following:

Will continues to have a solid season with the Carmel Hounds' 7th grade travel squad making several outstanding plays behind the plate, in the field, at the plate and he even scored a few runs as well. His low point of the day came when he was a little too eager at the plate, striking out twice in the same inning. Anyhow, the Hounds won both games of the double header and now have a three game winning streak. Watch out, Devil Rays! I was really glad my dad drove him to some pasture out in Greenfield and got to see him play so well. Will and I also had our round of golf. The kid has turned the corner at least, with his driver hitting several balls over 210 yards. My big moment of the day came on the 16th, a 541 yard, par 5 at Brookshire GC here in Carmel.

A front was coming through and we were hitting down wind. I nailed the drive with Bertha and got the ball very high up into the wind. I explained to Will that a couple of weeks ago in a scramble that I only hit only one good 3 wood during the round, so I was really going to concentrate on the upcoming shot. I was all of 240 yards out and we were looking directly into the sun. I nailed it very high and straight, but we couldn't tell where the ball landed. I knew I was at least chipping from in front of the green for eagle. I told Will, given this was just a Father's Day round for fun, I was going to try my hardest to chip it in and make eagle. I had visions of my fourth career eagle running round my brain. The ball had made it all the way to the green on the fly and I was left with about 28 feet for eagle. I told him the old adage "100% of the putts that are short don't go in so I'm not going to leave this short." What happened???

As I hit the ball, I did scuff the green ever so slightly so I didn't think it had a chance, but it was rolling right on line, seemed to have enough speed and ended up just three rolls short.

Will said, "I thought you weren't going to leave it short, dad!"

The funniest, most comical scene occurred at dusk Friday night. When I walked in from the hospital, my mom said, "There's a critter problem outside, go help Dad!" There was a little opossum trapped in the large well leading to the egress window in the lower level of the house. My dad was trying to "fish" the scared little guy out with a fishing net. The varmint went down the drainage pipe in the well at one point, but eventually figured out it led nowhere and came back out. I picked up the large concrete down spout drain that runs the water away from the house. I then dropped it from about eight feet up right next to the drain thinking this will prevent the critter from escaping. My dad nudged me and said, "Nice shot except if you had broken the window, the thing would be in your house."

Melinda Bruggemann and her little girl Elana were watching the fiasco, as was Mitchell and I think Madison Jackson. Finally, dad had the varmint in the net, and as he pulled himself out of the well, the little guy started just scrambling and doing everything he could do to climb out of the net. By now the two of them were up on the grass, as Dad almost rolled over the long tailed animal and everyone was yelling, and it ran into the woods. It escaped, and we eventually ran him down again and got him into the net. Dad scrambled to the woods and threw the net into the edge of the tree preserve across the street. Smart animal, eventually he chewed its way out.

Then Miss Kimmie Wetzel from across the street came running over out with a big book. I said, "Never mind, Kimmie, we found something to cover the drain."

Kimmie said, "I know, I just had to go get out one of my old cookbooks to look up a recipe!"

Yummmy!!!!

Is KareBear coming home tomorrow?? Stay tuned. If I had to bet, I'd bet YES. I'm betting on Karen because she always comes through in the clutch and she's really sick of the place.

P.S. to Tom Thieme: Thanks for the mulch job, I'm sure the Jacksons appreciate it too.

On Monday nothing remarkable happened except that Dr. Cripe was taking a very conservative stance regarding whether she could come home. He had hinted that it might be better to keep her one more day, so Tuesday instead of Monday may be the day. This turn of events frustrated Karen, so I had to try and keep her calm. In the wee hours of the night, I updated everyone on Karen's condition and the prospects for her discharge.

Monday, June 28, 2004 1:25 AM

Karen's stamina remains as the next hurdle. From my standpoint and her friend Dr. Wynne MD, whose opinion obviously has relevance due to his background and having spent a good part of the weekend here, she is in good enough condition to continue this battle from home. I don't think there are any other medical matters, peripheral to the leukemia that would keep her in the hospital well into next week.

As she begins to get more aggressive in her walks, the overall pain, mostly to her head due to constricted arteries and blood vessels that are now being forced to expand, is the next hurdle. She had to take some oxycodone to subdue the pain.

Again, this is only my view, but I think she can take up this part of the recovery on the home front. A precautionary CAT scan shows the shunt to be intact and no residual bleeding can be seen. The ophthalmologists will see her tomorrow. Karen is having problems with her vision, but Dr. Cripe is treating this in parallel to the cancer, a two for one deal.

The numbers are pretty good except for the platelets. Still no Blast and her WBC is down to 58,900. Hemoglobin is good at 9.9 thanks to yesterday's transfusion. Platelets are at 39 and Dr. Metha said we must be at 50 for her to go home. These were the numbers as of early Sunday morning and more platelets were administered during the day, so I think this level will be fine come Monday morning.

If she is discharged tomorrow, I don't think it will be until the dinner hour as Dr. Cripe spends all day Monday in clinic, and it's his call. Besides, this gives us all day Monday to get her into tip-top shape.

Brian Wynne headed back to Philly and Tom Lambright took his little rental car over to Cincinnati to visit his sister. He's likely to stop back to see Karen on Tuesday in her beautiful home—God willing.

Have a great workweek, and if all goes well, I'll be back at the Midwest ISO solving problems and dealing with energy market issues on Tuesday.

I'd love to hit the alarm early Tuesday, take a shower and head off to work, only after I give my wife a quick kiss on the lips.

Those surgical masks really get in the way when it comes to kissing!

Before I close, I want to make an offer to any of our friends and family who are monitoring this website. A few months ago, I booked a week's stay at the El Quijote Inn in Mazatlan, Mexico, for Karen, Nora and Margaret Evans to spend some time together basking in the sun and taking in the numerous water sports. I saw this as a great chance for Karen to get some emotional and physical therapy with her close friends that backpacked Europe together back in the summer of 1982. The three ladies are obviously unable to use the accommodations, which are booked from July 3 through 10th and sleep four (1BR and a sleeper sofa for the kids if you have just a few). Margaret is headed to Indy and Nora said, "I'm not going without Karen."

I would cancel, however, the room is available as the result of a banked week Karen and I were unable to use for a timeshare we own in Vegas from when she got sick two years ago. This certificate is due to expire soon, so this is a use it or lose it proposition. The ladies had decided to spend the 4th of July celebrating the fourth with their families and then heading south on the 5th, so I even have a seat reserved in Karen's name leaving Indy on July 5 and returning on the 10th for $480 that I would need reimbursed for, and a name change can be made for, I think $75, for someone who might want to go from Indy. Someone out there may also have some frequent flyer miles to use that would make this getaway happen at a very low cost. Anyone interested drop me a line and we'll work out the details. If it's a close friend or family, the accommodations are on us, just take Karen and I out to dinner at someplace cheap to say thanks. I know this is short notice, but it doesn't hurt to try.

"Oh, Mexico, sounds so sweet with the sun sinking low, the moon so hot I forgot to go home, Oh Mexico." A little JT to light up the night.

Nighty night!

I got to the hospital at 2:00 p.m. and was pleased to find out that Karen would be released by dinner. We had spent the entire day getting the house ready for Karen's return. My mom worked very hard to have everything perfect. During this entire ordeal, my mom was pretty low-key, very prayerful and she tended to be more comfortable dealing with her grandchildren and handling the household chores. Karen's courage, hope and inner strength had changed her as well. She said her relationship with God was now very different because of Karen. Mom even told Karen she'd happily trade places with her, saying to her at one point, "I've already lived my life."

Our home was in great shape. The sheets had been changed, bathrooms cleaned, everything was dusted, the lawn was mowed and Samantha had adorned our house, trees, the flagpole, pillars on the front porch and most of the mailboxes up and down Garden Gate Way with yellow ribbons to welcome Karen home. Once we were headed up Meridian, Karen started wondering whether we had left the hospital too early. She did not want any fanfare when she returned to the neighborhood after her month-long ordeal.

The journal entry below describes the scene upon her return.

Monday, June 28, 2004 9:05 PM

Karen arrived home at 6:30 p.m. to a yellow ribbon-clad Garden Gate Way. A small crowd of well-wishers, many wearing LIVESTRONG yellow, quietly hung out at a respectable distance in the Bruggemann driveway while sipping wine and beer. Mitchell ran immediately to the car and opened the door for his mom. Amy Jackson and Kimmie Wetzel lifted their glasses and gently let out, "Welcome Home Karen. We Love You!" Her children then gave Karen a bouquet of yellow roses and a dozen Kit-Kat bars. Karen rested awhile and then dined on roast chicken, white angel hair pasta (my Mom's signature dish) and a little cranberry sauce. She made it all the way upstairs in short order, rested and then took a warm bath to thaw out in her Jacuzzi tub. Her room, #5827 at IUMC, was like an igloo all 27 days, even causing me the chills at times, even though I'm part polar bear after four years out on the prairie in Ada.

And that's the way it was!

There's No Place Like Home,

MV

P.S. A special salute to Mr. Scott Zigmond for taking the time today to call and check on me earlier in the day and most of all for motivating me to be a part of CRHP Team #16 two years ago.

After dinner, she wanted a bath. Karen was still cold from having spent a month in her freezing cold room, so I went upstairs and drew her a lukewarm bath in the Jacuzzi tub. The month of June in the hospital had taken a toll on her beautiful body, and she cried a little as I struggled to get her withered body into the tub. Her legs had atrophied severely, and even when healthy there is no easy way to get into the tub. I actually had to stand in the tub and help her get in one leg at a time.

She did warm up and got into her own fresh bed, relieved to finally be where she belongs, at home in her own bed with her three beautiful children at her side.

CHAPTER 35

Blessings

Karen's second encounter with cancer now moved on to the next step in what we knew would be a long process. For the rest of July and August, she was escorted daily to IUMC for her infusions of arsenic trioxide and any other whole blood or platelets she might require. Kim Santucci's children were away at camp the week of June 28th, so Kim volunteered to handle the driving back and forth for the rest of the week.

This allowed me to return to work for the bulk of the day, and for three days of the week Samantha would attend cheerleading camp sponsored by the new Blessed Theodore Guerin Catholic High School. The camp was from 9:00 to 11:00 a.m. Tuesday through Thursday at Our Lady of Mount Carmel grade school, not far from my office. I dropped Sam off, went straight to the office and got back into my routine. I picked her up and drove her home. Before returning to work, I quickly added the following update to the Caringbridge website.

Tuesday, June 29, 2004 11:20 AM

I never dished out Karen's stats as of her departure yesterday as we enter the next phase required to kick cancer's…..

6/28

W: 39.9
H: 9.7
P: 57

I am sure everyone has figured this out by now and I'll use this convention from now on as Karen gets her daily CBC. Karen is at the outpatient transfusion center and has yet to even get into the room to start her arsenic trioxide (ATO from now on) treatment even though she was down there at nine. Kim Santucci is doing the driving all this week and staying with KareBear.

I've noticed that a few very astute people have suggested that I write a book. Well, about ten months ago, I started on a rough draft while vacationing at Virginia Beach, having made the decision to write the story just about two years ago today when Karen and I were both experiencing varying forms of confinement.

I thought only God could write this script. I'm about a hundred pages in, and it begins with me going on a ski trip as my longtime friend Ed's roomie along with members of the Andrew Haas family and Nora Haas's best friend Karen Coyne.

It's January of 1987, and John Elway has just broken my heart with, "The Drive." At this point in the draft, I'm up to 2000 where I'm trying to assemble a Christmas present for Karen, Kathy and Pat that would take the three of them to the Windy City to see Oprah. I work on it in my spare time and back in May had decided that the last chapter would be entitled "Vail" with Karen still in remission skiing the Rockies with her husband and kids, and they live happily ever after. The name of the book is tentatively entitled "How Karen Conquered Cancer," but recently I thought a better title might be "The Months of June" or "Two Months Called June." I'd like some feedback on the title.

Q: Why are some of these entries so long and detailed?

A: Because they're all going in the book!

Also, note some select additions to the guestbook will also be included and kissing up won't help get you selected. For example, Julia Mattei's entry from last week talking about our Mitchell is in!! Don't worry, Aunt Ellen, we will put in the best of your best.

It's so nice for me to not have to be down at the hospital. Some get their strength from prayer, others poetry, others the Bible. For me, it's the lyrics written by the Boss. It's nice to not have to "make it through another Lonesome Day because It's Alright, It's Alright, It's Alright, ya, It's Alright, It's Alright." I hummed that one way too much, Bruce was speaking to me.

Today it's Glory Days.
MV

On Thursday afternoon, we reported out to everyone the latest white blood count numbers.

Thursday, July 1, 2004 4:12 PM

Karen is doing very well with the outpatient program to receive the ATO.

Her numbers continue to decline nicely with the WBC being as follows the past 4 days:

6/28 25.2 (at discharge)
6/29 11.2
6/30 11.1
7/1 7.9

Hemoglobin has been solid and platelets were recently administered when her count dropped below 30. She was at 21 a day ago. She's always tired after the ATO, but is doing very well.

Thanks to Kim Santucci and Pam Marske for doing the driving the last three days.

When I saw him on the cover of *SI* last week I knew it was time to also note that the Lance Armstrong Foundation and Nike have joined forces to collect $5 million for further cancer research. The program is named after Lance's mantra LIVESTRONG. Nike has pledged $1 million. Many of us here in Indiana and Ohio have joined on the campaign each paying $1 towards the goal and are wearing the yellow wristbands inscribed with LIVESTRONG. Jump on the bandwagon so someday a cure can be found for all forms of the disease. These are our rally caps!

Karen wears one, and so should you.

MV

On Friday, Victoria Hunt advised us not to come in on Monday, July 5th. I was skeptical. Regardless of the holiday,

Karen still needed to stick to the schedule and come in for the ATO transfusion.

"I want to see Katie or Dr. Cripe," I said. Not five minutes later Larry walked up and said to Karen, "Why don't you want any platelets? You're right on the border and going into the weekend. You need the platelets before you leave." We agreed, saying we wanted to come in despite what one of the nurses had said.

Karen was getting to the point where she wanted to make the journal updates, when she was up to it. I made this one on the holiday weekend:

Saturday, July 3, 2004 11:25 PM

Karen is resting comfortably and enjoying her two days off of the ATO. She has come to grips with having relapsed and is ready to get on to the bone marrow transplant phase. We will resume Monday. Her stamina and vision are improving, and she even saw some of the neighborhood's annual 3rd of July bicycle parade as the parade route went right by our house. Kevin and Tommy just arrived and will be spending the 4th here in Indy.

Thanks to Kathy for everything the past five days; it's nice having a sister again. You've also done a great job stepping in as Mitchell's godmother. This is what the true meaning of family is really all about.

The kids are wondering about our annual journey to Virginia Beach; I told them we'll all go, as in all five Volpes, only once Karen is able; they realize that it's not just about them and that the Mom is priority #1. Maybe we'll go to Orlando or some other beach in Florida.

Margaret will be here Monday, taking the long trip from Portland here to Indy.

Happy 4th of July to everyone!

Remember we're the only people on the plant celebrating Independence Day.

Stay safe if you just happen to be shooting off some fireworks.

God Bless America!

On the 4th of July, Kevin and Tommy were here tending to Karen and cooking on the grill. This allowed the kids and me to spend the day down at Mayor Bill's house for the neighborhood party. Mayor Bill did it up right. He had four sets of cornhole platforms set up, and there was a tournament. The sound system was cranking, and there were several coolers full of beer. The cornhole tournament was conducted in conjunction with the onset of the neighborhood's addiction to the latest fad in beer drinking fun. I was just happy I didn't embarrass myself, because my technique was not as refined as most of the guys in the hood who had perfected their soft loft shot, arching the bean bag onto the inclined platform. Everyone had his or her special team colors and logo on the cornhole set. There was LSU, IU, Purdue, Missouri, and OSU, to name a few. I have mine designed in my head, and one day, I'll get around to putting a set together. My design is pretty simple: all orange with a white racing stripe down the middle outlined in brown.

Margaret Evans arrived early the week of the 4th and spent some significant time with us. She always brings the best presents, and I have to credit Margot (Margaret goes by Peggy or Margot too) as being the person who got us all to jump on Lance Armstrong's LIVESTRONG bandwagon. The original plan was for Karen, Nora and Margot to rendezvous down in Mazatlan, Mexico, using one of our banked vacation weeks from our Vegas condo. Karen needed a little pampering that only a resort and spa type of facility could provide, celebrating meeting the two-year milestone in remission with the same two great friends she had traveled with throughout Europe 20 years earlier. But unfortunately, due to her relapse, we had to cancel the trip to Mazatlan, so Margaret came to Carmel, Indiana, instead.

Later on in the week, Karen resumed making entries in the journal:

Thursday, July 8, 2004 8:36 PM

Well………..

It's me!!!!!

Hard to believe, hard to believe a lot of things actually. I wanted to write to give my unending gratitude for all of the prayers and good wishes. This is such a humbling experience, and I am so thankful. I would have to say that it is just this week that I am starting to feel a little better and stronger. My mom always says, "If you're a little bit better each day, we'll get there".

The process is so long. I get so frustrated. They just keep telling me that they are not sure how long because this time, unlike last time, I have reacted very slowly to the drugs.

God is good, and he continues to carry me on my bad days. Being home makes the bad days fewer, however. These children and Mark are the light of my life. Leukemia the second time around is not for the weak of spirit. I know too much and the unknown is now more frightening.

We are taking it day by day here. We are so thankful for friends and family. We couldn't make it without you. God's blessings to the Starks…. You are in my daily thoughts!

Much love…Looking forward to health again!!

Karen

Karen continued her weekday routine of heading down to IUMC for her daily dose of arsenic trioxide and to have her blood work checked. July was going much better than June. She sat down late one July evening and wrote the following note to everyone.

Wednesday, July 14, 2004 12:39 AM

Hi to all! All is well here. At this point I am at the hospital right now getting my ATO. Kim Santucci is playing Florence Nightingale. I am so thankful for all those so willing to help us out! Dinners, driving, prayers, and your love and support. We count ourselves so blessed

My mom, friend Margaret, and sister-in-law Anne have just left. They cooked, cleaned, and made me laugh. It was great.

Thanks also to Pam and Grace for their limousine services!

Also, I want to let you know that the kids are OK. Those of you that have taken time to have them over, talk to them, show an interest or given them a hug, Thank You! They are my reason for fighting. Mark is officially back at work and that is a blessing.

My counts are good today and that is what we need as I continue to take the ATO for a couple of weeks. But now my body needs to start making platelets and blood on its own.

God has given me several good days lately. On Sunday, the family went to Spider Man. I wrapped myself in a blanket, wore gloves, and a mask. I looked like one of Spider Man's enemies. Great movie by the way. Love to you all!

Now we pray for counts to rise. 1, 2, 3, pray!

Don't forget about me!
Karen

Over the next few days, the saga continued. Karen "stayed the course," as George Bush, would say, taking her arsenic trioxide treatments on an outpatient basis. Karen also had a project she had worked on intermittently prior to her relapse and now she was able to get back to finishing this project she had been working on at SLDM with her friend, Pam Marske. Together they were opening a little gift shop called "Blessings" in Craig Willy Hall on the SLDM campus.

The shop would include Catholic-oriented items such as statues, crosses, Bibles, wall hangings, rosaries, cards and assorted books. They found the display shelving at a local business that was closing, and Karen spent a lot of time managing the inventory and cost of goods records, which she loaded on an old laptop. Just before the first day of school, "Blessings" opened.

While she was working on the gift shop that week, Karen took me aside and said, "I don't want you to immediately say no to what I'm about to say, but I want you to think seriously about taking the kids to the beach without me."

Karen knew how much it meant to the children to make their annual journey to the Virginia shore, and she wanted to make sure missing out didn't happen for the second time in three years. I had been saying, rather adamantly, that we would only go to Virginia or somewhere else warm only when all five of us could go. Will's baseball season only gave us a small window of opportunity before school started, and we also had to figure out a way to coordinate our trip with the annual family reunion the first weekend in August. After thinking about it for about five minutes, I agreed with Karen. When the kids were told they were going to Grandma and Grandpa's beach house after all, there was much joy in Hoosierville. Karen always thought of the children first.

Her next entry in the journal illustrates her frustration with the process and the toll it was taking on her family. For weeks, her white blood count had soared, and over time, the arsenic trioxide kicked in with her counts then plummeting. Now we were trying to coerce her bone marrow into producing healthy white blood cells and moving her counts back up into a normal range.

Sunday, July 18, 2004 11:49 AM

Sure hope that you are having a nice weekend. I kinda just slept all day yesterday. I find that I need the day to catch up after a week at the hospital. 5 weeks ago my white blood count actually hit 214,000. Dr. Cripe said that he needs to write a paper about it. Seems it was the highest documented ever. Wow, aren't I proud. As of Friday, my white blood count was .5. Now I seem to have gone in the extreme other direction, and they are anxiously awaiting my counts to climb. We want to get them somewhere in the "normal" range and then they will test to see if I am in remission. This is the path we are hoping to follow. No guarantees, ya know.

My dad will be coming to town this week, and my crazy and wonderful neighbors Amy and Kimmie will be driving me back and forth to IU Med Center. I'll keep you posted. It just takes sooooo long. Every step is so slow in coming. The summer has come and gone, and I'm not close to half way through this nightmare.

The following week we have worked out a plan so that Mark can take the kids to the beach. His parents have a place at Virginia Beach and the kids just love it. I have my babysitters lined up, but I will sure miss them.

The following is from my husband…..see ya next time…

I've been at back at work for a week, and I want to thank everyone at the Midwest ISO for their concern and support, but in particular Jim Torgerson, Steve Kozey, Ron McNamara, Jim Holsclaw, Lori Spence, Donna Dare, Michelle VanGordon, Heather Cain, Dorothy Shute, and Mary Lynn Webster. Also special thanks to Sally Clore and Jeff Sprague for holding down the fort while I was gone.

MV

A few days later, Karen's counts were still pretty low, but we proceeded with the plan to head off to Virginia Beach. I had to be at the FERC in Washington D.C. because an order from the Commission on our Energy Markets Tariff was due to be issued on July 28th, so I made a reservation at the J.W. Marriott on Pennsylvania Avenue just a stone's throw from the White House, figuring we could stop by and see "W" if his schedule allowed. Will's baseball team's season finally ended, with the Hounds going 18 wins and 24 losses on the season. Will had a very good season playing solid ball all summer. His catching was pretty good; the longer throw down to second was the big thing we knew he had to work on, but all in all, he hit good pitching pretty well, and defensively he was outstanding as he made all the plays all season, except one in left field where he tripped a little just as the ball hit his glove, causing him to pull a "Charlie Brown."

While we planned our trip, I made my own monumental decision. I decided it was time to replace the wedding ring that had been stolen during our move from Mason to Carmel. I found a great deal on a platinum ring that had a large solitaire in the middle, with a smaller diamond on each side that closely resembled the engagement ring and the diamond wrap wedding band that had disappeared from my dresser while our belongings were in storage. I started to plot how I'd give her the new hardware.

In late July, our good friend, Grace Hineman, was at swim team practice with her two kids. Dr. Cripe's children are on the same team. The good doctor's wife overheard Grace talking about Karen and she recognized the name, so she came over and introduced herself and asked Grace whether she was talking about one of her husband's patients that she had heard about.

They chatted and before they left, Grace added, "We pray for your husband, too, Mrs. Cripe, not just Karen."

"We have so much faith in your husband. We know he'll be able to save our friend," said Grace.

Mrs. Cripe walked away quickly, crying a little. This man everyone prayed so hard for is a wonderful doctor who concluded each visit with one word, "Godspeed."

At this time, I had also informed Karen that our medical insurance would only pay for one bone marrow transplant. She appreciated the information and thanked me for giving her all the facts regarding our medical coverage.

The following journal entry reveals Karen's inner thoughts, her strength and her misgivings about using her own bone marrow for a transplant.

Thursday, July 22, 2004 10:52 PM

I spend each day at the Hospital. 6 hours round trip is a quick day. I am on day 42 of the arsenic treatments, and I figure that I have at least have two more weeks. This was a good week, however, because we have signs that my bone marrow is "revving up." The platelets and red blood cells are holding their own right now with no need for transfusions. My whites are still dormant at .4. Germs are my enemy.

My dad has been in town and a great help. He took Sam and me today to the uniform store to make sure that Sam and Mitch have what they need for the new school year. Kelly Sventekis was our personal shopper, thank God!! Mark and the kids leave Tuesday for the beach. I have my babysitters lined up. God forbid I have a moment alone. Just kidding, I'm thrilled for the support.

I am now able to walk around my block. Soon I'll try for

two laps. This past Tuesday I got to pop into my CRHP group and say the rosary with them. It was difficult, but wonderful. They have been such a great source of prayer and support, and I am thankful for every one of them.

Don't really know what my future holds, but none of us do, right, Father Dave? I know that at some point, when my white count recovers, they will test me for remission. If I am able to obtain remission, discussion will begin regarding my bone marrow transplant. That will be scheduled in the fall somewhere I guess. My wonderful brother Tommy would be the obvious donor as he and I meet on 6 out of 6 requirements. However, there is serious discussion that they may extract my own marrow, wash it, and reinject it………Personally, I want nothing to do with my own marrow, if you know what I mean.

School will be here before you know it. The kids go back on August 18th. Sam can't wait, and the boys dread the thought. Typical. I am trying to be a parent. It is challenging when you are weak, tired and sick to your stomach. My mind is always wandering off somewhere. I hate that I have made this part of their childhood. Will came bursting into my room Sunday evening wide eyed and scared. "What Will?" I said," What happened?" He said "Mom, what if something happens to Dr. Cripe!" What will we do?" God Bless him. Still don't know the future but on this day, at this moment. The Volpe's are fine. One day at a time, right, Py?

Thanks for your unending prayers. I meet SO MANY sick people each day. I certainly am in good company, unfortunately. My love to you all.

God Bless,

Karen

The children and I got up on Tuesday morning, the 27th of July, and drove east to our nation's capital. We had some technical problems in the minivan with the Gameboy hooked up to the portable television. We couldn't get the AC adapters to work and one of the devices burned up on the way, so we stopped at a Best Buy in Columbus, Ohio, and tried to fix the problem. As it turned out, nothing worked, and we were stuck with just plain old movies for the road trip east.

Late in the afternoon, we finally made it to Pennsylvania Avenue and checked in at the hotel. Samantha was impressed with the magnificent chandeliers. We ate at the hotel and after dinner, we walked in a slight rain through the maze of security to look at the fountain in front of the White House. Will strained to take a picture with our digital camera that actually came out pretty nice, considering the lack of light. The next morning we all ate breakfast, and met up with my friend Anna McKenna, who had graciously agreed to supervise my children while I was at the FERC meeting.

Anna had just given birth to her second child and was on maternity leave after working diligently on the Midwest ISO's Energy Market Tariff filing. Anna is an amazing woman. She persevered on the tariff while dealing with her second pregnancy, she had a broken finger requiring surgery that had to be delayed because she was expecting. She also helped me, but I'd like to think we helped each other—she was also dealing with the emotional turmoil of her father's battle with cancer. He eventually passed away, having battled courageously for a long time. Anna traveled back and forth from Washington D.C. to Montreal several times until her pregnancy precluded her from travel.

She cruised in a little late, new baby in tow. I headed over to

FERC, because the tariff was scheduled as the first item up for discussion. But, when we arrived FERC announced there would be a delay, and the Energy Markets Tariff would not be on the agenda until later in the day. Five hours later the Commission pulled the tariff from the agenda. I called Anna to tell her that the tariff had been struck from the agenda. She had dragged those kids all over town while I waited with great anticipation for nothing. When we met back at the hotel, I finally had the pleasure of meeting young John Justin McKenna. The little guy had had a pretty rough day and was a little upset when Anna came in with my three monkeys and the stroller.

"What great kids," she said. And I said, "You have so much to look forward to as they grow up." The FERC's solid order approving our energy market was issued a few days later.

Then we hit the highway south before rush hour traffic and managed to get to the beach in three hours. We were just in time for an early evening swim in the Atlantic. Karen did not have the stamina to make the long drive over in the minivan and she also had to be downtown at IUMC for her routine blood work. There was a tentative plan for her to fly over for the weekend landing in nearby Norfolk, Virginia. She was scheduled to arrive late Friday night. This was a last minute decision. Just before she left, she made the following entry.

Thursday, July 29, 2004 9:46 PM

Hi all,

I met with Dr. Cripe today. My platelets and red blood are doing well but my white blood count is taking its "good" old time to recover. Dr. Cripe said that I am probably 10 to 14 days away from having another bone marrow biopsy. The results of this biopsy will pretty much decide for us the direction that we will take with the bone marrow transplant. We have options, all of them, a little scary. Still taking the arsenic on a daily basis at the hospital. I tolerate it pretty well. I am at 49 treatments to date.

Mark and the kids are at the beach. They are having a ball. I will leave tomorrow and meet them for the weekend.

Not knowing at the time what God had in store for me. Sam and I had started a little project that I was hoping you could help with. We have made trips downtown, and we have been surveying people on a topic that is important to us. I'll ask you all the same question, if you would please think about it for a minute and then answer the question, it would be greatly appreciated. We are hoping to put together a collection and raise money for cancer research. Here you go. WHAT IS THE BEST ADVICE YOUR MOTHER, GRANDMOTHER EVER GAVE YOU? The advice can pertain to marriage, cooking, raising kids, life…. My favorite so far is….

Wipe from front to back. (Sorry Aunt Patty and Alice)

Please help out. We would love to get some responses! Much love to all!!!!!
Our God is an awesome God………Right Lisa Roach?

Karen

The children had a great time back at the beach, and I was grateful that Karen had overruled me. One evening I took my daughter out on a date. We went to a local diner in called the Purple Cow and then we went to the mall to shop for CDs and clothes. Samantha was about to turn 12 and on the verge of entering womanhood.

At one point during the evening she turned to me and said, "Hey, dad, you know how you're always reminding me that I'm not allowed to marry a jerk? Well, who decides if he's a jerk or not? Is it me or you?"

I smiled at her and said, "I do."

She just shrugged and said, "Figures!"

The diamond ring I had bought for Karen had arrived, and while we were at the beach, I pondered how I'd present the ring to her. The obvious opportunity was at the family reunion, but how? I had sung "Thunder Road" to Kathy when she married Roger, and Anne when she married Kenny, and at the request of Karen's cousin, Katie, just a few months earlier at her wedding reception. I had never sung the great song to my own wife, so I decided I would give it to her after a rousing rendition of "Thunder Road". I knew all the words, but I decided to make some slight changes. I'd buy her three dozen roses, and I considered amending our wedding vows, instead of "in sickness and in health," I'd change the deal to read, just "in health," and leave it at that, because she had already had more than her share of sickness.

Karen arrived at the airport in Norfolk late Friday evening, totally exhausted after a long layover in Charlotte. I began to wonder if we had made the right decision—I wanted us to all be together, but not if it took Karen back a step. On Saturday, she made it down to the shore for a bit, and then we went to Rockafeller's for dinner after Mass. The boys polished off a couple pounds of crab legs at our nice private table on the porch overlooking the inlet. On Sunday, it was a little rainy, so we went to the mall to see a movie and then drove our mom back to the airport so she could return to Indiana and her chemo treatments on Monday.

A few days later she was scheduled to fly to Cleveland, so she could meet up with the four of us at the family reunion in Kent. She was not in a very cheery mood, and my plan to give her the ring turned out to be a total flop as I made a complete fool of myself in front of her entire family. I babbled on way too long about seeing Bruce Springsteen open the first concert that I had ever seen with "Thunder Road," and it went downhill from there. Karen just sat there with this look on her face that I cannot even describe. I felt totally rejected, but she did like the ring.

Later she said to me, "I know you love me very much, but it's as though you did this so you could cross another must-do item off your to-do list."

Our collective focus turned to the most important problem, the prospect for a successful bone marrow transplant. There were two options: either use Tommy's bone marrow and take our chances with rejection and graft-versus-host disease, which could result in death because the donor cells can actually attack the internal organs of the recipient, or use Karen's stem cells for transplant, assuming she had attained molecular remission. Under the latter scenario, the possibility of rejection was off the table, seemingly increasing the odds of a cure. Karen, however, was not enamored with the idea of using her own marrow, despite the odds.

"My bone marrow sucks! I'd rather have Tommy's," she said.

We were at a decisional crossroad.

I was in a funk and a little down, so I bought a car. On a whim, I purchased a beautiful blue 1997 Jaguar XK8 from a used-car lot. I saw it, I liked it, and two hours later it was in my driveway, with Karen's blessing, of course. I had been talking about getting a new car for a year, and finally I saw this slick blue convertible with a camel leather interior at a price I could afford. The six-CD carousel was immediately loaded with nothing but Bruce. Never could I have imagined what joy a material object might bring me. This car is awesome—it was made for me.

The purchase of the Jaguar was a minor distraction; our main focus remained on Karen. The arsenic trioxide treatments continued until she received her 60th bag.

A week before her bone marrow biopsy, she laid out the pros and cons of using her stem cells versus Tommy's bone marrow in the following two journal entries:

Tuesday, August 10, 2004 8:54 PM

Hi all,

Doing pretty well. My blood counts are starting to behave. My white count is sluggish, but we pray it will soon kick in. I am tired all the time, but I am not letting that stop me too much.

On Monday, I have a bone marrow biopsy scheduled for 10:45 a.m. That's where they drill a hole into my hip bone marrow to take a sample. Within 24-48 hours, we should know if I am in remission. From there, we will have decisions to make regarding my bone marrow transplant.

There are two ways we can go. Both have heavy pros and cons. One way would be to use my brother Tommy as a donor. We match on 6 out of 6 points. There is a high probability of rejection all the same. But, if I don't reject, I could be cured. The second way and the one that the Dr. is hoping for is that I use my own marrow for the transplant after they extract and clean it. Rejection isn't a problem here but getting Leukemia again is an obvious risk and one that absolutely sickens me.

Please pray that we make a good decision. Love to all.

K

Thursday, August 12, 2004 1:23 PM

CORRECTION....CORRECTION

Here is an update because dates and times have changed.

On Tuesday, Aug 17th, I have my last round of Arsenic, #60. At that time, they will also pull my jugular tubes.

On Thursday, August 19th, at 10:45, I will have my bone marrow biopsy in Dr. Cripe's office. By Friday, we should know if I am in remission. I could seriously use your prayers. We are getting down to the scary decision making part.........I pray that the answers come to me!

Much Love and thanks,

Karen

August 19th was Samantha's 12th birthday, but our focus was on Karen's long-awaited bone marrow biopsy. Dr. Cripe performed the procedure with which Karen had become all too familiar. He had told us that Karen's best odds were with achieving molecular remission, thus allowing use of her own bone marrow for the transplant. Dr. Cripe had also told us that after the results of the bone marrow biopsy were known that Tommy, Karen and I would consult in person with Dr. Martin Tallman in Chicago at Northwestern Memorial Hospital. Dr. Cripe had been consulting with Dr. Tallman throughout Karen's case, but this was the first time we realized he was just three hours up the road in the fabulous Windy City.

When Dr. Cripe performed the bone marrow biopsy, I saw the way the marrow immediately appeared in the syringe as he pulled back and knew that Karen was in remission. The first test, called a "FISH test," was performed in Indianapolis. The results were ready the next day. Based on Dr. Cripe's, and especially Katie Hincher's body language, I could tell they were pleased with what they saw, and there was a very good chance Karen was in full molecular remission.

Of course, we had to await the lab analysis and visual inspection of the blood smears for the official results, which could take as long as a week.

The next day, Karen called to tell me that Katie Hincher had confirmed what we had suspected. "You were right, it's just like you said yesterday. I'm in remission."

Karen ran to the PC and typed away.

Friday, August 20, 2004 11:56 AM

I want to share my GOOD news right away!!

My oncology nurse, Katie, called at 10:30 this morning to tell me that I am in remission!!! That means that right this minute, there is no evidence of cancer!!!! I feel great and am thrilled.

The next step will be on Tuesday when we will receive

an additional report from my bone marrow biopsy that I had yesterday. This report will tell us if I am in "molecular remission." We are hoping that I am because that will open up my decision making process for my bone marrow transplant.

I will then have two options for the transplant both of which have their positives and NEGATIVES. We will meet with Dr. Tallman at Northwestern on August 31 at 10:00 a.m. Then, we will make our decision. Please keep us in your prayers. As Dr. Cripe said yesterday, "I wouldn't want to be in your position to make this decision." I pray the answers will come to us.

The way I see it, we are at the half way mark. The transplant will require a month in the hospital. We still have a lot to learn about it.

God Bless,

Karen and Mark

Karen celebrated her 44th birthday on August 24th. We were confident she would celebrate at least another 44. I picked up a fountain for the back patio for Karen's birthday present—no wrapping required.

How did Karen celebrate? She sent flowers to the ultrasound technician who had told us the truth about the condition of the yet-to-be-born Mitchell back in 1994. This was classic Karen.

The next day Karen updated the website.

MARK J. VOLPE

Wednesday, August 25, 2004 4:31 PM

Thank you for your birthday wishes. Your thoughts and prayers mean so much.

No news from the molecular remission test yet! I guess no news is good news, right? I should say that I am losing my mind but quite frankly that is old news. I wish I knew the future so I could make decisions about today. I hear it doesn't work that way though…..

I'll send news as soon as I get it!! Keep the faith!!!!

Karen

CHAPTER 36

Northwestern

Right before we left for Chicago, Karen received a brief phone message from Victoria Hunt, "You're in total remission."

On Monday night, August 30th, Tommy, Karen and I sat outside at McCormick & Schmidt's Steakhouse overlooking the Chicago River. Karen could hardly get to sleep. She had so much running around her sweet little brain.

I leaned over to her and said, "There's going to be bumps in the road, and there's going to be good days and bad days. No matter what, you've got to remember you are going to live. I know you are going to outlive me. That's just the way it is and I'm not going to die anytime soon."

I couldn't imagine what it was like to live with what my wife had to deal with on a daily basis. She's simply amazing.

The night before our meeting with Dr. Tallman, we jointly penned a quick update on a tiny laptop at the Apple Computer store on Michigan Avenue.

Monday, August 30, 2004 6:24 PM

This is Karen and Mark live from downtown Chicago. Tomorrow we meet with Dr. Tallman and from there we'll learn enough to figure out the next step in this long and crazy journey. We are confident everything will go well and the next time we're here it will be to see Navy Pier, the Aquarium, Sears Tower and Wrigley Field with our children.

Love to all,
Karen and Mark

When we entered the bright little room overlooking Navy Pier with a fabulous view of Lake Michigan, we immediately took a liking to the surroundings. How could you not? The hospital was very state-of-the art and very well organized, a total first-class operation. Dr. Tallman was not intimately familiar with Karen's case, so we gave him the entire history in bullet-point form. At one point, Dr. Tallman asked what Karen's platelet level and white blood count were at the onset of the disease and Karen said, "I don't remember, I was so out of it when I was admitted."

Finally, I had a chance to add something to the conversation.

"Back in June 2002, when the disease originally set in, she had a white blood count that immediately escalated to 77,000 with a Blast of 97, and her platelets were low, ranging day-to-day from in the teens to 45, as I recall."

With this Dr. Tallman looked up at us and said, "These two parameters would be indicative of what we would refer to as a high risk of recurrence."

At that, his pager went off and he looked at it and said, "I hope you don't mind, but I just took my oldest to Princeton this weekend. My first daughter is off to college, and if she calls, I'd like to take her call if that's okay."

Of course we found this to be a laudable attribute.

Later Karen would say, "That was just so cute. How could you not love that man? He's so genuine!" After just a few minutes, I could tell this was no ordinary doctor. He was brilliant.

Then I asked Dr. Tallman the following question, "If there was a high probability of relapse with a high-risk case like Karen's, then why don't we perform bone marrow transplants upon achievement of the first remission?"

Dr. Tallman peered at me over the top of his glasses and said, "You just hit on the subject of my next paper. I need to get with Dr. Cripe and get more details on your bone marrow biopsy results. I'm especially interested in the results of a PCR test which takes some time, but if you are indeed in molecular remission, my preliminary advice would be that you have an autologous stem cell transplant where we would use your own stem cells, based on the premise that you are in molecular remission. I believe the probability for success is much higher, because if I do a bone marrow transplant using your brother as the donor, there is a 15 to 25 percent possibility that you would reject his bone marrow, and at that point, there would be nothing else we could do; you would die, and we can't go back and use your stem cells at that point."

Then he added, "Do you have the results from the PCR test related to your bone marrow biopsy that would prove conclusively if you are in a complete molecular remission?"

"I don't know," Karen replied. "All I know is I got a call from Victoria, Dr. Cripe's assistant in the clinic, saying you are in molecular remission. And the only test I know about for sure is the FISH test."

"I'll talk with Larry and find out about the PCR test. I'm sure they did one," Dr. Tallman replied.

Then he added, "You mentioned that your insurance company will pay for the procedure to be done here at Northwestern. If that is the case, I would be happy to take full charge of your case should you decide to come up to Chicago, and I will also be happy to coordinate your transplant from here if you go with IU, although I'm not familiar with their doctors or their protocols, and that would make it harder."

As we walked to the elevator, Tommy who had been quiet throughout the conversation, said, "To me it's simple. You have it done here with this doctor, he's unbelievable, and if your insurance will pay for it here, then you just have to do it."

I almost hugged Tommy on the spot because he said out loud exactly what I was thinking.

Karen said, "Fine, but we have our consult with Dr. Schwartz at IUMC tomorrow, and I want to hear what they have to say. I have the fullest confidence in IUMC, even though it won't be Dr. Cripe in charge of my case."

The next day we met with Dr. Jennifer Schwartz, the bone marrow transplant specialist at IUMC. The process was different at IUMC than at Northwestern. At the Indiana University Hospital, once a patient was in position for the transplant, the patient was transferred to the Bone Marrow Transplant Unit, and in our case, Dr. Schwartz. At Northwestern, the patient had the same oncologist from start to finish. Dr. Schwartz was lovely and very knowledgeable. She said many of the same things Dr. Tallman had said the previous day, also recommending the autologous stem cell transplant using Karen's own bone marrow.

Karen really liked her and said, "We have a tough decision to make. I like her too, and I have full confidence in her. Besides, I don't want to inconvenience the family any further with the expense and distance involved in getting back and forth from Chicago."

Convenience was not a factor in my mind. The deciding factor came from Dr. Schwartz herself when she said during our consult, "And if you should decide to go with one of the world's foremost experts up at Northwestern in Dr. Tallman, we will not be insulted. We will do whatever we can to support you after you return if you decide to go to Chicago."

On Friday, Karen called Dr. Tallman and told him we were coming up to Chicago for the autologous stem cell transplant consistent with the plan he had outlined.

The next day Karen relayed the details of our consult with the very impressive Dr. Martin Tallman.

Thursday, September 2, 2004 10:50 AM

We met with Dr. Tallman at Northwestern. The hospital is right downtown, just a block off of Michigan Ave. He is a wonderful man and said that he intends to cure me. Gotta love that. We have YET ANOTHER test result that we are waiting for. Then the decision. We are pretty sure at this point that it will be an auto transplant, where I use my own marrow; this of course, depending on the test result.

I will be in Chicago for 2 to 3 weeks, then a prisoner in my home for a few months. Juggling life and sickness is getting old. We really just want this behind us. The old saying of "The joy is in the journey" was not talking about Leukemia, clearly.

The first step will be to harvest my stem cells and then they will start chemo. This will be the strongest chemo yet because now they will not have to worry about too much destroying my marrow. Now they don't care because they will have the harvested stem cells to inject back. I'll be bald again but that is the least of my worries. Sorry that I am rambling. Once we have dates, I'll let you know. It will be soon......

ALL my love and appreciation,

Karen

We went up to Cedar Point for our annual Labor Day weekend date with all of the roller coasters, sponsored by Karen's dad. This year Mitchell was the grandchild who decided which color T-shirt we would all wear in order to easily spot members of the Coyne entourage. My Mitchell did me proud as he picked his dad's favorite color, orange. A few weeks earlier on a visit to see Karen at IUMC, I decided Mitchell was old enough to be told about his mother's courageous efforts back when she was pregnant with him almost 10 years earlier. Mitchell certainly understood, and I don't think he'll ever forget it. He knows he is a very special child because of his mom's heroics.

Early the next week, we found out we had a problem. Apparently there were no test results available for the PCR test that Dr. Tallman absolutely needed to see before being able to proceed with Karen's treatment protocol. The laboratory in California did not perform a PCR test, and they needed a fresh bone marrow specimen in order to perform the test. This meant Dr. Cripe would have to drill into my wife's rump again to get another sample of her bone marrow. Karen was not very happy and Katie Hincher was immediately in contact with the lab out west to make sure the specimen was rushed through the process, and that we received the results as quickly as possible. We were sure Dr. Cripe had filled out the paperwork properly and that the lab that had dropped the ball. In any event, this was another timing setback, and while Karen was in remission she wanted to move as quickly as possible toward the stem cell transplant. And now there was another bump in the road.

She didn't really care about placing any blame. "Let's just do it and get it over," she said.

Thursday, September 9, 2004 9:39 AM

It appears that I am in a "hurry up and wait" mode at this time…..

Dr. Cripe called yesterday morning. The bone marrow biopsy that was done two weeks ago was not completely processed. What that means to me is that to determine whether or not I am truly in molecular remission, the test has to be done from my bone marrow. Not from a blood sample. So, I need to go back in for another biopsy, ouch.

Additionally, there has been an ongoing concern that due to my brain surgery and headaches early on, I need to rule out that my central nervous system is clear from cancer. To do this, I will require a spinal tap. Both of these tests need to be done before I can proceed with any kind of transplant.

I am so anxious to just get on with IT and get IT over. That is not meant to be. After the tests I will have to wait again. In time, baby steps….

I am feeling OK. Our family took their annual pilgrimage to Cedar Point last weekend. My dad plans it yearly and treats us all to a very special day. There were 27 of us and the kids, and Mark, the biggest kid, had a ball. I did too! I did need to sleep for the following three days to make up for all the walking. I went on a merry go round and I had to do the Blue Streak with my sister. We do it as the last ride every year. What memories!

The kids are great. Will is trying football for the first time. He's quarterbacking for our CYO team. He is also playing fall baseball. Sam is busy with her gymnastics. 18 hours in the gym each week. She loves it; I hate her being gone so much. 2 days ago she was at the top of the climbing rope and lost her grip and slid all the way down. Rope burns you can't believe. Mitch is awesome. Cute as the devil. School is easy for him so he is getting into the socializing more than he should, if you know what I mean. Girls have noticed him in a major way, good Lord.

Mark and I had a dinner party here last night for Mark's office for 40 or so. The big project that will keep his market going has been recognized and accepted by FERC. It looks like we will be here awhile. A time for celebration. He works with such amazing people.

I am planning on getting these tests out of the way yet this week. Gotta keep this train-a-movin'.

My love to you all and my constant appreciation for your prayers.

Karen

On Friday, September 10th, we were back at IUMC for another bone marrow biopsy, and Dr. Cripe seemed very bummed out about the situation, but Karen's attitude was let's just move on.

Dr. Tallman had asked IUMC to perform a precautionary spinal tap to make sure there was no infiltration of the any leukemic cells into the spinal fluid given the manner in which the leukemia had manifested itself in June. On September 14th we were back downtown again for a spinal tap. Dr. Cripe performed the procedure without a hitch and with great dexterity. The diameter of the instruments used for the spinal tap was about an eighth in size compared to the tools used for the bone marrow biopsy, so for Karen this procedure was a piece of cake compared to the pain of a bone marrow biopsy. The small test tubes were then set aside for further analysis.

Karen described her first spinal tap below. You can feel her anxiety.

Thursday, September 16, 2004 5:40 PM

My spinal tap on Tuesday was a lot of fun. Then I had to lie there and not move my head for 5 hours. It was worth it though. The call came today that all is clear and I don't have cancer in my central nervous system. Like I need that like I need ANOTHER hole in the head.

NO NEWS yet on my PCR test. Yes, I am losing my mind. I am anxious to start planning for the transplant before I lose remission. I promise to send out word as soon as I know. I was told that tomorrow would be the earliest that I could expect a result. Please keep us all in your prayers.

Yikes............

Karen

We finally received word from Katie Hincher regarding the test results of the PCR test. This test was negative, too.
Good news travels fast on the net!

Friday, September 17, 2004 10:46 AM

THANK YOU DEAR GOD

I got a call from Katie Hincher an hour ago. My PCR is negative. I am definitely in molecular remission. I will be doing an auto transplant, a transplant without a donor. It will be a three-month process now instead of a year long, process. I won't be as sick for as long. A blessing at this point I can tell you. I will be doing the transplant in Chicago at Northwestern.

I am busy with details now…appointments, insurance, planning. Busy for me is WAY better than waiting! When I was SO sick back in June, Dr. Cripe drew a diagram of all the possibilities that my case could bring. His chart included everything from cure to death. He drew a little dotted line and said that it would be difficult, but that we needed to stay on the dotted line he had drawn as my way out of the maze. So far, I'm still on the line. We are no longer discussing mortality. Our concern at this point will be that the auto transplant doesn't cure me for some reason and that the Leukemia could come back.

For the transplant, they will remove some of my bone marrow. Then I will get 10 days of intense chemo, very intense, designed to kill EVERYTHING. Then they will reinject my own bone marrow back into me without the fear of rejection. This PCR test result that I just got today makes us feel confident that the sample they remove to reinject back into me will be cancer free.

Praise God…………..I still have a lot ahead of me…. but I feel like I am ready for the task. This is the first time since I have been sick that I'll actually get to pack for the hospital!! I am going in feeling good instead of full of cancer. Please keep me in your prayers. I can see the end of the tunnel, but no light just yet.

Love,

The Volpes

We visited with Dr. Tallman again at Northwestern to drill down into the details of the stem cell transplant process. She would be hospitalized for five days, receiving eight rounds of high dose Ara-C over four days. This form of chemo would serve three primary purposes. First, it would consolidate her remission. Second, it would cross over to the central nervous system and attack any leukemic cells present in the brain fluid, and third, and most importantly, the Ara-C would drag down her bone marrow to the point where Neupogen would be administered eventually resulting in a mobilization of her stem cells to the point where they spill out of the bone marrow and into the peripheral blood. Then the stem cells would be able to be harvested on an outpatient basis over the course of several days. She would come home and rest a few days before going back to get two forms of chemotherapy, probably busulfan and cytoxan, over the course of several days before transfusing the harvested stem cells back intravenously.

After explaining the process, Dr. Tallman looked at us and asked, "Did Larry inject any methotrexate when he did your spinal tap?"

"I don't think so," Karen said.

I concurred, adding, "I watched the entire procedure and nothing was injected."

Then Dr. Tallman called Dr. Cripe. All we could hear was

Dr. Tallman asking questions. "He should have injected methotrexate," Dr. Tallman said.

It was déjà vu all over again. She had to have a second spinal tap to add methotrexate as a precautionary measure. This second spinal tap was on the heels of a second bone marrow biopsy. Then there was another bad turn of events.

"I'd admit you today and start the Ara-C, but I don't have insurance approval yet, so I can't admit you," Dr. Tallman said.

Karen cried. There was so much red tape and balls were being dropped all over the place. Nothing seemed to be coming together.

At the end of the meeting Dr. Tallman stated with confidence, "This procedure will result in a cure. In fact, I'm 99 percent sure you will be cured once we have successfully harvested and transfused your stem cells. There is very little risk. This will work."

We were still on the ideal path Dr. Cripe had charted for us in June.

The next hurdle was an unbelievable go-around with the insurance company. They required us to provide documentation that Karen needed the stem cell transplant. This was the same insurance company that had paid hundreds of thousands of dollars in claims related to Karen's case while she was under Dr. Cripe's care at IUMC, but now she had to prove that the same Karen Volpe, with the same case of leukemia, had elected to have this phase of her treatment done at Northwestern Memorial Hospital in Chicago. All of this was required in order to get the preadmission approval through the unbelievable bureaucratic insurance process.

After we got home from Chicago, an obviously frustrated Karen spoke to her fans again.

HOW KAREN CONQUERED CANCER

Wednesday, September 22, 2004 8:47 PM

What a frustrating experience we have had today. Mark and I have been to Chicago and back. It wasn't very productive. We got there only to find out that the insurance forms are not in place. I am approved for IU, but not for Northwestern? There have been plenty of screw-ups with our trying to transfer now. I am hoping that we are doing the right thing.

Of highest priority is to get the insurance thing fixed. Then they will admit me immediately, probably Friday or Monday. Then I will be in for 4 days of chemo. I will then come home for 10 days and then go back for the harvesting and the transplant. That should take 2 1/2 weeks. The first week will be chemo and the remainder will be trying to get my marrow to grow back again. It can't happen soon enough for me. Patients with my APL tend to relapse in the central nervous system so they will be hitting me with chemo for that too as soon as I am admitted.

I will be in downtown Chicago, 1 block off of Michigan Ave on St. Clair. Shopping, anyone? They have discounted rooms available for family so that will help.

Thank you for caring enough to check in on the web site to keep up with the continuing saga of "Karen has cancer." So sorry that it couldn't be more interesting.

I appreciate you. God Bless…God Bless…

Karen

On September 27th, Karen spent the day at IUMC doing all sorts of tests to document her case and the need for the stem cell transplant. She had to get a Letter of Necessity, Current H&P, A Protocol Description from Dr. Tallman, a MUGA, PFT's, radiology results, bone marrow biopsy results, labs including viral titers and a test for hepatitis, CBC, chemical profiles, liver function, phosphatse, renal status to include BUN and creatinine, and a psychosocial profile that Dr. Theobald provided on very short notice. Finally, everything was in place, and Karen received word in writing from the insurance company that they would pay for the stem cell transplant at Northwestern.

I threw a quick news flash out on Caringbridge.

Sunday, September 26, 2004 11:55 PM

Karen will begin her consolidation chemotherapy Monday, October 4th, at Northwestern University Hospital in downtown Chicago and not tomorrow as originally planned. She still has a handful of tests and procedures that will be done here at IU yet this week prior to heading north. The basic plan outlined in the last journal entry remains the same.

Have a great week!

The Volpe Family

Finally, a second spinal tap to inject methotrexate was scheduled, but this one didn't go as smoothly as the first. Dr. Cripe accidentally hit the spinal column causing Karen to uncoil and with major discomfort. He did manage to inject the chemo agent and Karen lay still on her back for a couple of hours. Grace Hineman came down to visit and brought us some food. She was wonderful and stayed with Karen until she was ready to go home, allowing me to return to work.

After dinner, Karen left a very upbeat update out on the website.

Tuesday, September 28, 2004 6:50 PM

God, I have really enjoyed hearing from everyone. I've let this mess get me down but your words of encouragement are awesome. All is well. My head is in a good place (I sound like I'm in the 60's). I just keep telling myself that I am NOT sick. I am IN REMISSION. I have been feeling good. Not napping all day, but playing all day. It's been great. I was only off of chemo for three weeks when I relapsed in June. But I didn't feel good. I have been drug free for a month now and I have found energy that I had forgotten about. I'm officially back on the drugs as of today. Dr. Cripe did a spinal tap and injected Methotrexate. They have a concern that I will relapse in the central nervous system. The old feelings came back quickly. Dull headache, burning eyes, tired…

I AM NOT SICK. Repeat 3 times as needed. Just want this to be over. I can't get to Northwestern soon enough. Love your love. Love your prayers. Looking forward to a successful CONCLUSION to all this DRAMA. I am so not a drama queen and this has all been way too much. Please pray for all the sick and suffering. There are so many in need right now……

Looks like Monday is a go. I'm gonna miss gymnastics meets, football games, soccer games, birthdays (Will). You know how I hate that…..Thank you for your calls and cards (Jackie Mewborn) and prayers. It will take me the rest off my days to pass on my *"Pay It Forward."*

My Love,
Karen

On October 4th Karen was finally admitted to begin the stem cell transplant process. This would prove to be a logistical challenge for me as I was heading over to Cleveland for a Browns versus Redskins match-up with Chris Miller, a good guy from FERC, who was on a two-year assignment at the Midwest ISO. This was planned for months and it was the only time I'd see the orange helmets in person this season. We headed over to Cleveland on Saturday night, and my parents were coming over to Carmel to hold down the fort while I was in Chicago with Karen, so we stayed at their empty condo. On Saturday night, Ohio State was playing at Northwestern and the Wildcats upset the Buckeyes in overtime. I saw this as a sign: Northwestern Memorial Hospital beats Buckeye Girl's Cancer Over Time.

Chris was as much a Redskins fan as I was a Browns fan. His grandfather worked at Gate A when he was a kid, and he'd be at the gate on game days. He saw Sonny Jurgensen, Billy Kilmer, Joe Namath and Presidents Nixon and Kennedy come through Gate A over the years. His family still held 16 season tickets for the Redskins. D.J. and Paula met us to party before the game. They threw a wonderful tailgate party featuring filet mignon and a wide selection of beers from the Great Lakes Brewery. The Browns won, and at halftime, the Buckeye marching band on their way home from the prior night's loss to Northwestern did the famous "Script Ohio" and I went crazy. They were playing it for my Buckeye Girl.

Chris agreed to allow me to sleep in the back of the Bonneville during the five-hour ride because once we were back in Carmel, I'd grab my pre-packed luggage and head north with Karen to the small apartment building called the Worchester House that Northwestern made available to patients for a nominal fee. Karen's father, Tom, would arrive on Monday.

We left at about 9:30, thinking we would arrive just after midnight. Things were going very well. The show was finally on the road and then I had to bring the minivan to a grinding halt. We didn't move for 20 minutes, and then we got word from the truckers who radioed each other on their CBs that the contents of a truck about a mile and half ahead were on fire. An hour later fire trucks finally made their way past us and a few other emergency vehicles passed by on the shoulder. Then the teenage girls in the car behind us tapped on the window as I tried to rest my sore eyes. Their car's battery was dead, and they were looking for a jump. Karen told them we had battery cables, so we did a five-point turn and spun the Montana 180 degrees pointing straight south in the northbound lane. We quickly got the little compact car started, and I disconnected the jumper cables.

Then I noticed the car I had just jumped had a very quiet engine. I went to the window and said to the young lady, "What happened?"

She said, "I turned it off."

I said, "What did you do that for, you need to leave the engine on to charge the alternator?"

She said, "I'm sorry, I'm new at this."

So I reconnected the cables and jumped the car again. I was concerned that they didn't have enough gas. Finally, after two hours the cars ahead of us slowly began to move.

We finally checked into the simple little apartment, after parking in a garage a couple of blocks away. I set the alarm for 6:30 a.m. because we needed to check in at admitting at 7:00.

Our heads finally hit the pillow at 3:30 a.m. It was a long day, and we had little sleep, but it didn't matter. We were finally on our way toward a cure.

Once we settled into Karen's room the next morning, I used the trusty laptop to dial up the Internet and add the following journal entry.

Monday, October 4, 2004 11:07 AM

We have finally been admitted to Northwestern University Memorial Hospital in downtown Chicago. Karen's room overlooks Lake Michigan and Navy Pier. This is a wonderful state-of-the-art facility. For the next four days, Karen will undergo consolidation chemo using a drug called high dose Ara-C. She will then return to Carmel for ten days while her stem cells are mobilized. Then she'll come back for the actual harvesting of her own bone marrow which will be followed by several rounds of chemo prior to the actual transplant which we understand will be done intravenously. We just met briefly with Dr. Aurora, the bone marrow transplant fellow who works with Dr. Tallman—everything's a go at this point. This is an amazing facility. We're very fortunate to be here.

It took us five hours to get here last evening because a tractor-trailer just a mile and half in front of us caught on fire. We had to jump start some poor teenager's car whose battery needed a jolt. Our heads didn't hit the pillow until 3:30 a.m.

Tom is on his way and brother Kevin is flying in tomorrow.

Have a great week; we're starting into the homestretch and thanks for the thoughts and prayers.

Mark and Karen

The next day Karen took a stab at updating the website.

Tuesday, October 5, 2004 10:25 PM

Chicago is my kind of town.

Sure would like to see more of it though. Great room, staff, food and surroundings. The chemo is pouring in. The countdown is on. This time I am not sick and I am not post-surgical. Sure makes it easier.

If anyone has seen my children and can write with an update, I sure would love to hear it. I miss my kids...

Any Vegas stories you would like to share? Our neighborhood went to Vegas for the weekend and I have not yet been briefed?

Looking forward to the upcoming CRHP weekend. Hope I can make it cause I want to be there to support you all. Having a group of strangers coming together for a common purpose is hard and you have done it and I am thrilled.

They have enough drugs running into me right now to knock out a horse. It is finally getting to me.

Good night, Will, Sam and Mitch. Mommy loves you....

The four days of administering the high dose Ara-C went smoothly. Tom made it over on Monday and he found a great parking spot right out in front of the apartment. He also brought his bike, allowing him to have a wonderful time peddling around Lake Shore Drive, downtown and out to Navy Pier.

One day he came in after a ride and said, "Sinatra was right; this is my kind of town."

I spent the majority of time with Karen and had time one day to jog around the running track between the hospital and the apartment while returning work-related phone calls. I also talked at length with Kim Santucci.

Dr. Tallman was wonderful and he stopped in to see Karen early every morning.

He was very confident and always reassuring and at one point remarked, "We love patients like you that are on auto pilot."

His resolve never changed and he soundly reiterated on more than one occasion that Karen would be cured.

On Thursday afternoon, we visited the Rube Walker Blood Center where the stem cells would be harvested using a process called apheresis and then fought our way south through traffic and made it back to Carmel, When Karen left the center, she was not very happy.

"It's very small and very crowded. Besides the machine they will hook me up to, in order to spin off my stem cells, reminds me of some sort of diabolical form of dialysis. It's so gross," she said

My parents drove over from Ohio to deal with our kids, playing taxi service for all of their activities and taking them out to eat while we were up at Northwestern. Karen was home for about 10 days and then she went to IUMC just about every day to have her blood checked. Her white count was still very low despite the numerous shots of Neupogen she was taking in order to mobilize the over production of stem cells pushing them out into the peripheral blood. As of Saturday morning, her counts were still in the low hundreds for her white blood cells, which indicated to me that she had not experienced the explosion of white blood cell production necessary to saturate her peripheral blood sufficiently for stem cell harvesting. Dr. Tallman had said that ideally we wanted to harvest five to ten million stem cells and then they would be frozen before the transplant.

On our 16th anniversary, I updated the website after we returned from celebrating at Dodd's Steakhouse.

> Friday, October 15, 2004 8:58 PM
>
> A week ago today, Karen left the hospital in downtown Chicago and walked the four blocks to the car. Over the course of the week, the eight rounds of high dose chemotherapy (Ara-C) started to take hold and slowly dragged her down.
>
> She's been to IU three days this week for blood work and today she had to take on some platelets as her numbers have dipped as designed, her WBC is down to 200. She has been taking shots of Neupogen to help spur the production of new stem cells. Bright and early on Monday morning she'll be back in Chicago, on an outpatient basis to have a port installed into her jugular vein and then the process of harvesting over 5 million stem cells, that have hopefully been mobilized sufficiently to be pushed out into her peripheral blood, will begin. Her wonderful mom will be there to guide her along the way.
>
> Today's our 16th wedding anniversary. I'm a lucky man!
>
> LIVESTRONG!
>
> The Volpe Family

On Sunday, October 17th, Will was playing in his last CYO football game of the season. He would miss the last game because his friend, Corey Erickson, and his family had invited Will to tag along with them over fall break on a six-day jaunt down to Atlantis in the Bahamas. We had received Will's passport a few weeks earlier and he was excited about heading out. We gave Will a cell phone as an early birthday present. Let's face it, the 14-year-old leads a very charmed life. In August, he spent almost two weeks at Virginia Beach, then the Bahamas, and we had also planned on all five of us vacationing down at the Marriott Grande Vista Resort in Orlando as soon as the cancer was behind us. I was looking at trying to find a deal on airfare for Karen. I figured she would be feeling up to a big family celebration over Thanksgiving week after being done with the stem cell transplant. In order to save some cash, I thought Karen and maybe one of the kids would fly, and the others would drive down to Orlando and meet up. We invited Kathy and her family to join us, but they couldn't make it so we were planning on going solo.

This trip would end up being postponed until April 2005.

Pat had driven out to Carmel and was helping Karen get to her appointments at IU. The plan was for her them to catch Will's game and then take off for Northwestern for the harvesting process.

Will's team, the SLDM Cardinals, had suffered through a very long season. Will had played most of the season at quarterback. He also played linebacker and did the long snapping for punts. He knew the game well and played great considering his size. When I asked him how he knew the game so well, he said, "You've been making me watch 12 quarters of football every Sunday since I was born." I was the special teams coordinator for the inaugural addition of the Cardinals. These 14 young men were pioneers; they were the first 7th and 8th grade team ever at SLDM. We had never won a game or even scored in our first five games.

Karen went straight to IUMC after church on Sunday before the game, figuring she could easily make it to see Will play. The weekend crew was very slow, and it took them over 4 hours to do the blood work and transfuse one unit of platelets. The previous day it had only taken an hour to do the same set of procedures. She called and was lost because I had given her such lousy directions. I felt awful. My wife had been through so much. I had my misgivings about her prospects of actually being able to harvest stem cells on Monday because her numbers remained so low.

When she arrived at the game, Will was limping and the Cards were getting whooped again, 34-0.

I yelled over to Eric, the offensive coordinator, "Hey, Will's mom is here! Can you call a pass play?"

Eric said, "I'm way ahead of you."

Will dropped back and completed a short pass out in the flat for a nice gain. The clock was down to five minutes, so Eric continued to send in pass plays with Will scrambling for a nice 12-yard gain. SLDM actually had a nice drive going. He then completed a deep out pattern for about a 25-yard gain, and then he hit the tight end for a gain of eight. Will's buddy, Chris Presley, a distant relation to Elvis, from the Volunteer State, made the catch. Then Will hooked up with Chris Brown for a nice gain inside the 10. They ran the ball to the four and took a timeout with four seconds left.

Eric called for a sweep and I said, "It's only second down. Tell Will to throw a quick pass, and if it's incomplete, we'll still have time for one more play."

Will threw an interception to end the game and the season.

He had thrown for 80 or 90 yards in less than one quarter of a CYO game. It was amazing! Our fans were going nuts. We almost scored and we had actually made some first downs. For me it was a very emotional moment. I was very proud of Will and his teammates. Someone had to start the SLDM football tradition.

All of the Volpes and "MaMaw," as the kids fondly refer to Pat, made our way to the minivan. It was time to go our separate ways. I was glad I was wearing my sunglasses because I was losing it. We held hands and said an Our Father, as a family, standing in a circle. Every one of us hugged and kissed Karen, and then she was off to Chicago with her mom to harvest some baby stem cells. I went home and watched my Browns kick the crap out of the Bengals, even though they turned the ball over four times in the first half. You've got to love TiVo.

Karen and Pat had a frustrating few days in Chicago, although they did manage to find a few good sales on Michigan Avenue's Magnificent Mile, especially at Anne Taylor. They also found a wonderful Italian restaurant called Joey Buona's very close to the hospital. The hostess's name was Fawn and after they were there the third time or so, Fawn came over and told Karen they could tell she was going through a very difficult time, and they were all praying for her. Karen explained she was there to harvest her stem cells for an eventual transplant. Fawn gave Karen a big hug and a VIP card good for 25 percent off each visit. Joey Buona's would become a major refuge for our family members over the next six weeks.

I made the following entry on the website based on a phone conversation I had with Karen.

HOW KAREN CONQUERED CANCER

Tuesday, October 19, 2004 6:39 AM

Karen's new port, which is required for the harvesting process, was put in yesterday morning. Her numbers remain very low, only 500 white blood cells, hemoglobin is in the 8's and her platelets are still low. The bottom line is that this set of factors indicates it's unlikely that a sufficient level of stem cells are present in the peripheral blood, so today there will be more blood work to see if her bone marrow is starting to produce on its own. The harvesting will not begin until tomorrow. Some people just take longer after the high dose Ara-C to turn the corner in producing the stem cells. The Neupogen shots, designed to spur the production of all of these blood products, just haven't kicked in enough to get her marrow moving in the right direction.

I'm sure Pat and Karen will find something to do out on Michigan Avenue's Magnificent Mile.

The kids are good, although Mitchell stayed home with a low-grade fever yesterday, so he did the Ferris Bueller deal. Will made the travel baseball squad and he threw for a hundred yards in his final CYO game. He heads down to the Bahamas tomorrow for some R&R. Samantha has a minor foot injury that has kept her off the basketball court and away from her gymnastics, but we think she'll be able to get back to sports soon.

We'll move forward, all in good time. Now it's time to get the kids off to school.

MJV

In the meantime, Karen's white count remained very low, creeping up slowly from 400 to 800 and then 1,500. Marina, the lady in charge of coordinating the stem cell harvesting, sent Karen back home to Indiana. The Neupogen shots hadn't sufficiently kicked in, and her marrow was moving along rather sluggishly.

The lack of progress was conveyed out on the website in a quick report.

Thursday, October 21, 2004 10:50 AM

Karen's WBC has increased to 1,200, but at this point in time her bone marrow has not produced a sufficient level of stem cells for harvesting. She's on her way back to Carmel and will return to Chicago on Monday contingent on blood work results from Saturday at IUMC. She's very upbeat and looking forward to coming home.

Keep The Faith!

Karen didn't do anything on Friday. She didn't even go down to IUMC for her customary blood work. She was bummed out and frustrated that the process had bogged down, resulting in another delay. Only this time, it was her body that wasn't cooperating. On Friday night, Melinda Bruggemann came over and gave Karen another shot of Neupogen because Kathy and I were both miserable failures at administering the shot without causing Karen significant pain.

On Saturday morning, Karen and Kathy headed downtown to IUMC. Melinda must have had the velvet touch because Karen's white count had exploded to 12,000.

The results were faxed to Chicago. Northwestern did not perform outpatient services on the weekend, but Miranda called and told her, "Get up here quickly tomorrow, and we'll slip you in to do the harvesting and then handle all the paperwork on Monday." Karen's explosion and the opportunity to harvest the stem cells that had been mobilized in sufficient volume to push out into her peripheral blood had happened on a weekend.

The news flash read as follows:

Saturday, October 23, 2004 6:38 PM

Karen's white blood cell count jumped from 1,500 to 12,000 indicating her stem cells are finally ready for harvesting. Her sister Kathy will drive her to Northwestern University Hospital early tomorrow morning and the process will begin mid-afternoon. Hopefully, Karen will be ready to come home Tuesday. Then Karen will go back to Chicago and begin her FINAL round of chemo treatments on November 1st, prior to receiving her stem cell transplant.

Another step forward towards a cure!

The Volpe Family

Kathy and Karen cruised up to Northwestern. They were done harvesting on Tuesday, October 26th, having harvested and frozen approximately 6.4 million stem cells which were split into two batches, documented, tagged, frozen and guarded closely by the transplant team. Another significant milestone had been reached. I drove up to Chicago and picked up Karen, so Kathy could make the long drive along the Indiana and Ohio Turnpike back home to Stow. Will arrived home from his fun in the sun the same night. He had a great time, and Corey's father did well at the poker table, so everyone came away happy.

Karen let everyone know how she was feeling in her next update.

Wednesday, October 27, 2004 9:48 PM

This girl is overwhelmed. I am loving your support and hating being sick. I am thankful for my family and angry that I have to leave them. I have wonderful doctors and nurses and I never want to see them again.

When they went to remove my central line I panicked and started questioning them. Are you SURE that you have all the cells that you need? Will you please check to make sure that they have been stored correctly? How can I be sure that you have not harvested leukemic cells too? I have grown rather paranoid and protective out of necessity. Also, I am a pain in the ___.

Can't wait to take move on to the next step and I am scared to death to take it.

The kids are OK. This has been hard for them, but they are truly amazing. St. Louis de Montfort Catholic School and Church is my personal gift from God himself. Fr. Dave and Fr. Tim are amazing and they are 150% when it matters most. Because of germs I have stayed away. I will look to the day that I can come back and enjoy Mass.

I leave on Sunday night and I will be gone for about 3 weeks. It all has to do with how quickly I respond. I hate that I am away when our friend Tom Stark needs us. I will be in good hands and I know that Tom will be too!!

Much love and thanks,

Mark—The Adventure Continues....

Karen

CHAPTER 37

We Are Marshall

Karen's wonderful Aunt Ellen was lined up to take Karen up to Northwestern for the stem cell transplant. Marina had set up Halloween as the admit date for Karen to begin the final chemo treatments prior to the transfusion of her stem cells. Karen was delighted that the process was finally moving forward; she had been overly patient, and the transplant was finally on the radar screen. She had mixed emotions because she would miss the big neighborhood party prior to Trick or Treat. The Thieme family was hosting the early evening events this year. The kids all dressed up in their costumes and all the neighbors would be gathering to drink Coors Lights, eat hot dogs, slurp some chili and then head out into the night. Some of the houses on Garden Gate Way, especially Miss Kimmie's home across the street, were well decorated for the occasion. In order to hit the party and also be home to celebrate Will's 14th birthday, Karen and Ellen were going to head up to the Windy City at 8:00 in the evening. In any event, she ended up having a very good time on Halloween and she continued to bide her time, wondering if she was ever going to make it to transplant.

Before heading to the office, I updated her website:

Monday, November 1, 2004 8:06 AM

Karen was supposed to head up to Chicago today to begin her final round of chemo today, but due to some confusion regarding a spinal tap that was performed a month ago she will not be admitted until Wednesday. Aunt Ellen will be escorting Karen up to the Windy City. Karen's a little frustrated, but she was able to celebrate Will's 14th birthday with the entire neighborhood on Halloween.

Next Monday she will receive a transfusion of her stem cells!

Vote for "W"—The President

The Volpe Family

Then Karen called me the next day from Chicago with more news. This time she was really, really pissed to the point of tears. Apparently, the final spinal tap performed by Dr. Cripe when he injected methotrexate directly into Karen's spinal column indicated some abnormality that nobody noticed until mid-day on Friday, the 29th. Dr. Tallman tried desperately to contact Dr. Cripe by phone, but Dr. Cripe was unreachable because he was out of town with his family enjoying fall break. I had done the same, taking Samantha and Mitchell up to South Bend to climb the sand dunes at Indiana Dunes State Park and to visit Notre Dame. The night before visiting the campus, the cursed Boston Red Sox won the World Series.

Hell had frozen over and pigs could fly!

Karen worked all day Friday to try and find out what the story was, and at the end of the day, Marina did the conservative thing and rebooked everything for Karen clear out to Wednesday, November 3rd, the day following the Presidential Election. Dr. Cripe finally talked to Dr. Tallman and everything seemed fine. Dr. Tallman insisted that another spinal tap be performed in Chicago as a precautionary measure. Karen agreed to undergo the procedure. She was concerned the delays would result in her losing her remission, although Dr. Tallman did not share this same concern. He did understand that Karen wanted to move on with her life. Before they left for Chicago, Karen repeated to me the same message she had been telling our children.

"I can't lose! If the transplant works, and we have every reason to believe it will, I get to be here with you, and if it doesn't I go home to heaven to be with Jesus."

On Election Day, Karen and Aunt Ellen drove up to Chicago to make sure no dead people, especially if they were registered Democrats, voted for our least favorite flaming liberal John Kerry. There was so much at stake, and we were concerned the vote in Ohio or Florida might swing Democratic and give the presidency to the anti-life, poor excuse for a Catholic, Senator John Kerry. I had booked a very nice room at the Courtyard Marriott, and naturally Ellen and Karen managed to make it to a few stores and over to Joey Buona's for dinner. We were all delighted to find out early Wednesday morning both Ohio and Florida remained as Bush states, and "W" would remain in office for four more years. All of those people voting for Kerry must have been confused. They must have thought they were getting Springsteen as their President.

Early Wednesday morning after several delays, Karen was finally admitted and Aunt Ellen was there every step of the way. The two main procedures that were performed were the addition of another Hickman line into her jugular dedicated to the chemotherapy she would receive later and the precautionary spinal tap.

I was upset when Karen told me about the new heavy-duty Hickman line when she stated, "The line I have now will melt if they use it for my chemo."

My mind immediately shot back to when she was scalded in 2002 with the duanorubicin literally burning her from the inside out. My heart sank as I could only picture more unbearable suffering for my beautiful bride who had already been through so much trauma.

Karen was also upset when she found out that they had changed her treatment protocol. Initially she was told she would be given 16 rounds of the oral chemo agent called busulfan; concurrently with the intravenous chemotherapy that Dr. Tallman had told us would be cytoxan. Instead of these substances being administered concurrently, they were administering the busulfan over four days followed by three days off before giving her one round of a powerful form of chemo called VP-16. The chemotherapy would be followed by the transfusion of her stem cells soon thereafter, depending on her counts. She was mad as hell about another delay. Karen then told me the trip we had planned for Orlando was very unlikely. After a couple of days, I called and cancelled.

I put the following update out on the website.

Thursday, November 4, 2004 9:55 PM

Karen was admitted early yesterday morning and soon after her arrival she found out her two chemo treatments would not be given concurrently. Instead, she will do the entire set of oral medications first, and then wait 72 hours before doing the intravenous chemo. I believe the new oral meds she has started is busulphan (I'm sure I spelled this wrong), but I'll follow up with her on this. Our phone conversations have been pretty brief; she's getting tons of attention. She said, "Volpe, they beat me up pretty good today."

Today was a long day for her. In addition to the chemo, she had some tests done to make sure her respiratory system is able to deal with the chemo and everything with her breathing is fine. She had a second line put in. This line will be dedicated to the IV chemo treatment once this part of the process begins early next week. She also had her third spinal tap in order inject more methotrexate into her spinal fluid. Dr. Cripe did the same thing over a month ago. This is being done purely as a precautionary measure, just to make sure. There is no evidence of any leukemic cells anywhere. Karen remains in remission and nothing has occurred to suggest otherwise. There was never any infiltration of the central nervous system with the leukemia dating clear back to June. This was done purely out of an abundance of caution.

Karen is pleased with Dr. Tallman. He knows what he's doing and even though it will take more time before she receives her stem cells, which is now scheduled for Wednesday of next week, she's now moving full steam ahead.

Her address for cards only is as follows; remember, no flowers, please.

Karen Volpe
c/o Northwestern University Hospital
251 E. Huron St.
Chicago, IL 60611

Also add Room #1523 in the lower right hand corner.

Aunt Ellen will remain with Karen into the weekend and then her mom will be there. I'm flying in from Washington D.C. on Monday and will be there a day or two.

Keep the prayers rolling; she's doing fine even though today was pretty tough.

MV

The entry I made on November 4th contained one significant error. Aunt Ellen called me the next day saying was a problem. She was not alarmed, and more importantly Dr. Tallman was not discouraged, just surprised. The precautionary spinal tap did reveal a very small number of leukemic cells in the spinal column, so Dr. Tallman had to inject methotrexate into Karen's spinal column. This was the second round of methotrexate administered to her central nervous system. My first reaction was to jump in the Jag and head straight north, but Aunt Ellen and Karen both felt this was unnecessary. Dr. Tallman was working on a plan to address the situation. He saw this as only a "bump in the road" and more importantly, this turn of events did not change the plan to infuse her stem cells the following Thursday or Friday.

Karen and I decided not alarm the children with this latest setback. It was the first time in this almost two-and-a-half-year ordeal that we had decided not to be totally honest with Will, Samantha and Mitchell. We agreed that one day we would tell them, but only after there was closure. Karen was devastated!

All of a sudden cancer was back on the table.

The plan was for Pat to fly over on Saturday to relieve Aunt Ellen who was grabbing a flight back to Huntington, West Virginia, the home of the Thundering Herd from Marshall University. Marshall's entire football team was lost in a horrific plane crash back in 1970. The football program returned the following season, led by the student body's inspirational battle cry—"We Are Marshall."

I held steady with my plans and went to Washington D.C. for a quick meeting with FERC. Then I flew directly to O'Hare, where I jumped the train to "The Loop." At this point I was attempting to do a delicate balancing act: Karen, our children and my career. This wasn't always easy: Karen had great support in Chicago. Family and neighbors helped with the children, so I tried to be as productive as possible at work.

Karen was in major pain. She was severely nauseated from the 16 rounds of oral chemo that had just been completed. Plus, she had a severe headache. She could barely get her head off the pillow and moving the eight feet to the bathroom took all the strength she could muster. Early on Monday morning, Dr. Tallman stated the headache was not from the chemo and was more than likely caused by a continued seepage of spinal fluid. This was a classic spinal headache, and there was a relatively simple procedure called a blood patch that Dr. Tallman felt should be performed to alleviate the headache. By the time I maneuvered my way to her room, she was off to interventional radiology for the blood patch.

Earlier in the day, Karen had received the final intravenous chemotherapy treatment. It was not cytoxan as we had originally been told. Instead VP-16 was given as Karen's last blast prior to the stem cell infusion. This was without a doubt the nastiest chemo Karen was administered. It leveled her and it would take a long time for her body to recover. We both realized this was a necessary evil prior to the stem cell transplant.

When Karen returned, Pat was delighted to see the almost instantaneous positive results of the blood patch. As they wheeled Karen back, I turned and washed my hands as they unloaded her from the transport gurney. When I turned around, I surprised her, and she exclaimed, "Monster," one of her pet names for me. She was able to move, and her color looked good.

Pat had prepared me for a much worse-looking Karen, but she was already rallying.

Over the next couple of days, prior to the stem cell transplant, our focus was on figuring out a way to give Karen the chemo treatments for central nervous system in the least invasive manner as possible. We did not want to do a spinal tap every time to inject the chemo if at all possible, so we searched for an alternative. Dr. Altman worked closely with a doctor from neurology named Dr. Addleman. Our attention centered on exploring use of the existing shunt Dr. Witt had installed months earlier in Indianapolis, and he was consulted to find the exact specifications of the shunt. Dr. Addleman theorized the shunt may be used instead of having to inject through the spinal column. I was lobbying for this option because I wanted to avoid numerous spinal taps and the associated headaches. Dr. Tallman had decided to alternate between injecting two chemo drugs, methotrexate and Ara-C, to address the handful of leukemic cells in Karen's spinal column.

On Tuesday morning, I updated Caringbridge on my laptop from Karen's room.

Tuesday, November 9, 2004 8:47 AM

Karen spent the better part of the weekend and well into Monday battling a nick that allowed spinal fluid to continue to leak after the spinal tap performed on Thursday of last week. Finally, late in the day yesterday, Pat got Karen some resolution as interventional radiology performed a simple procedure called a "blood patch" that quickly sealed the leakage and provided Karen instant relief from the constant headaches that had been making Karen very drawn, listless, nauseated and unable to even make it out of bed. Dr. Tallman had said very early in the day this procedure would fix the problem; the issue was getting the people in anesthesia to respond. Special thanks to Dr. Jessica Altman for getting the procedure done around quitting time.

Today, she walked down with me to the second floor to the cafeteria for breakfast. She ate very well and managed to make it all the way back up to the 15th floor, taking only one little break.

We're still on course to transfuse the stem cells on Thursday as Karen received the final dose of chemo, VP-16, which was administered intravenously yesterday. So she has a couple of days to rest, but she has big plans to traverse the halls a few times each day.

Today, she'll be able to read the guestbook entries on the website.

She's simply amazing!

On Wednesday, the team of doctors studying Karen's predicament with the cancerous cells decided they would take a chance on wasting a round of Ara-C and Dr. Altman injected the liquid into Karen's shunt in her brain while Dr. Addleman held the valve closed by pushing on the instrument that had been surgically inserted just under her skin.

The next morning at 7:30 a.m., Karen went to Nuclear Medicine to run a test that would prove whether the shunt would work for our purposes. Dr. Altman explained that the chemo had a half life of four to six hours, and if the valve on the shunt was opened, then the chemo would just go right down to her stomach instead of simmering in the spinal column as desired. For the test, they would inject radioactive beads into the shunt and then they would take what appeared to be time-lapse photos of Karen starting at her head and traversing downward toward her torso.

The people in Nuclear Medicine had very little bedside manner. They never told Karen when she could move from lying flat on her back in the freezing room. They refused to tell her how long the test would take, and Karen had to beg for a bathroom break. With all the liquids constantly being injected, her bladder was full all the time. After an hour or so, they called me in to calm her down. It was the first negative experience we had at Northwestern, besides Pat's frustration with getting the blood patch procedure performed.

A little while later the same day, the moment we had all waited and worked so hard for finally became reality.

Thursday, November 11, 2004 2:10 PM

Karen received her long awaited stem cells at 2:10 p.m. central time.

The cells had to be thawed out first and were given intravenously.

Karen had us take a picture of herself, the whole crew of hospital staff, Pat and Mark to commemorate the big event.

Prayers Do Get Answered!

It only took 20 minutes for the transfusion. We called a number of family members to let them know Karen's baby stem cells were on their way back to her bone marrow. They used a preservative with the stem cells that smelled like a can of corn. The aroma lingered for several days.

Karen coasted for the next few days, but then the side effects from the chemo started to set in. She had to deal with diarrhea and vomiting, as well as numerous mouth sores. Tommy surprised her on Saturday morning walking right up to her in the cafeteria. It was a very happy moment for Karen. Her mom had been there for the long haul, and now "Perfect Tommy" who always makes Karen laugh, was there, too. Tommy's daughter Riley and wife, Diana, were with him. Karen's father had arrived on Friday, and then on Saturday, he headed to Carmel to deal with Samantha and Mitchell.

Pat had been at Northwestern for 17 consecutive days, literally sequestered in the hospital with her daughter for over two long weeks. A mother's love for her child is amazing. I had seen Karen do whatever it took for her unborn Mitchell years earlier. Now Karen's mom did the same, doing everything humanly possible to give her daughter a chance for life.

On Monday morning, Dr. Tallman came in, and it appeared to him that everything was going as expected. The devastating side effects were all part of the process as the chemo was expected to continue to work inside Karen's system and eventually level her bone marrow.

"You have to go through 10 more days of this agony for 50 more years of life," he told her.

These types of bold statements were exactly what we needed to hear. Her counts had gradually descended from Day Zero, which was the prior Thursday when she received her stem cell infusion at which time her white blood count was 3,200. On Friday, her count was up to 5,400. On Saturday the 13th of November, her white blood count declined to 2,700. And by Tuesday her numbers had plummeted to 800 and then as of Wednesday half again to 400.

Karen made the following lengthy update on the PC located right outside the cafeteria at Northwestern.

Saturday, November 13, 2004 8:53 PM

I JUST found out that I have computer access!!! I am so excited. Soon I may not be well enough to check my site, but for right now, I am thrilled. So far, all is well. My counts are dropping like a rock. Gloves and mask will go on tomorrow for a week or longer. Trying to stay healthy. Tired all the time. My family and friends are amazing. I am sitting here now with my brother Tommy. He and his wife and daughter came into town to visit. Mom is still with me. Thank God. World's best Mom and nurse. Except for Aunt Ellen, she, my friends, is quite a nurse too and hysterical to boot. Dad just left here today to take care of the Volpe critters in Carmel. Mark's mom and dad just left Carmel today. They have been on Carmel duty all week and the kids are all so happy. We are going to make it through this. I can feel it. Just some more time.

Kathy comes next week, also Kevin and Colleen and I are expecting my friends from St. Louis de Montfort as well.... I BETTER start feeling good. It is hard being away from the kids. Mark is going to try to get them here somehow too.... We'll see, just taking it day by day.

They just found leukemic cells in my brain stem 2 days ago. Not sure exactly how we are going to handle that yet. It seems that I am registered case #31 to have my leukemia cross out of my bone marrow. Oh Lucky me. They tell me not to worry and that they are on top of things...

My love and prayers go out to my father's family, the Coyne Family. Last evening our Aunt Elaine died after a lengthy battle with ALS. Ricky, Mike and Marty, you are all in my prayers. I said a rosary for Aunt Elaine last night. Uncle Don will be so glad to have her back.

My love to all. So glad I have been able to get to your messages!!!

Karen

The next day, she made another update. I left this one exactly as she typed it while wearing her awkward latex gloves. Usually I'd go through and edit the entry before adding it to the book, but this one was so cute, I had to just leave it alone.

Sunday, November 14, 2004 9:21 PM

I am down off of the caffeteria in my PJ's with my n=mask and gloves. Just wanted to check for messages. Have been feeling very ICK today. My white count is at 1.7 and will continue to drop over the next 3 dys. Fun Fun.

I have been checking in at home and all is well. Thanks to each and evertone of you that is there with a smile, hug, ride, dinner.......

Mark went to the Browns game today. Steelers won..... Story of our married life!!!! He took Will ans a friend anf they had a ball.

Time passes slowly here. Real slowly. Not looking good for being home for Thanksgiving right now. My Dr. said that maybe by the weekend.. We'll see.

Feelin so like crap that I asked my visitirs not to visit, yet. How's that for be antisocial. Need to just take this time a lay like a pancake till my energy comes back.

Love you tons,
God Bless,
Karen

Her platelets had dropped from 115,000 to 11,000 as of Wednesday the 17th. She called me on Monday and said she really missed me. I was concerned about getting the children up to see her and planned to take them out of school to see her on Wednesday, but Karen said she didn't want her kids to see her this way, saying, "I've already scarred for life them enough. I don't want to do them any more harm."

So I headed up to Chicago on Tuesday, as she requested. She was pretty good on Tuesday and things seemed to have calmed down, but on Wednesday the nausea broke loose. As Karen attempted to eat, we found that even yogurt didn't stay down. Her weight loss was a minor concern, and she received antibiotics to counteract her compromised immune system. Mouth sores and irritation down her esophagus set in and the woman could hardly talk or swallow. For the remainder of the week, Karen remained at rock bottom. She could hardly lift her head off the pillow. Finding the words to describe the total annihilation of her body as a prelude to the stem cell transplant is difficult, but she took it on and hung tough despite her agony. The white count had hit the low of 100 on Thursday, followed by 300 on Friday and then 200 on Saturday.

I let everyone know how Karen was doing on the anniversary of an unforgettable day in U.S. history.

HOW KAREN CONQUERED CANCER

Monday, November 22, 2004 9:23 AM

Karen is beginning to feel better, but her throat is still very irritated. She is resting and has made laps around the 15th floor. Her white blood count had been very low as expected, but as of this morning it's up to 500. We have been told that she can come home when her count gets up to 2,000.

There is a possibility she may be released at the end of the week, as early as Friday or as late as Sunday. She will still be neutropenic at that point, and we will need to take all necessary precautions upon her return.

Pat returns to Ohio today. I can't say enough about her extraordinary love and the special care she has given her daughter over the past two and half weeks. She has literally lived in the hospital with Karen this entire time.

Light at the end of the tunnel?

Stay tuned.

Kenny was in town Wednesday night. He took Pat and me to Shaw's Crab House for dinner. John Bird cruised over on Friday, and on Saturday, Karen's sister arrived. I was still wondering what to do for Thanksgiving. There was a remote possibility Karen could come home over the Thanksgiving weekend, but at the same time I didn't know whether she'd be feeling up to having her kids up for a visit. I hoped that her body would turn the corner and she would at least be able to see her kids over Thanksgiving. The doctors explained we would eventually see her bounce back once her stem cells had successfully graft to her bone marrow. At that point, her stem cells would start to produce white blood cells, red blood cells and platelets on their own. In the meantime, Karen had to live with total discomfort and wait. She received a transfusion of platelets and whole blood. They did their best to boost her immune system with antibiotics, and she continued to get medications such as Ativan and Dilaudid to help with the pain. For the continued bouts of nausea, she received Compazine.

Unfortunately, she also had to deal with the affects of being weaned off morphine, which included some mild hallucinations.

CHAPTER 38

The Holy Land

Pat went back to Akron with Kathy's husband, Roger, on Monday, and Kathy remained at Northwestern. I had given Karen zero odds of being home on Thanksgiving Day. Even Dr. Tallman felt she'd be going home after the holiday. I pegged Friday or Saturday as the more likely day.

On Wednesday, Karen called. "They're releasing me tomorrow!"

I was shocked, but I shouldn't have been surprised. The woman had always beaten the odds, so why should this situation have been any different?

Kathy took a flight back to Cleveland on Thanksgiving morning, and I got up very early to drive up to Chicago. An ice storm had hit northern Indiana, and I was determined to make it up without a problem. Karen was anxious to get home. When I arrived, she was still on an IV of potassium, which took an hour and a half to finish. By 11:00 a.m., we were heading home. It was a challenging ride home; Karen was still seeing things that weren't there, but she did recognize a McDonald's sign and said, "I want some fries!"

Karen was lucky to be released. She had hardly slept, primarily because infection in her esophagus was causing mucositis, a miserable condition that caused her to constantly spit up a thick, sea foam-like substance, making sleep nearly impossible. But, her white blood count had surged to 1,500 and then 1,900 on Tuesday and Wednesday, and Dr. Tallman had said she could leave once the count reached 2,000. The rest of her medical care could be carried out in Indianapolis.

We were just happy she was coming home and I made the following update to the website upon Karen's arrival back home.

> Friday, November 26, 2004 9:11 AM
>
> Karen returned home on Thanksgiving Day after a successful stem cell transplant procedure at Northwestern Memorial Hospital in Chicago. She went to her Aunt Patty and Uncle Bob's for a brief visit early in the evening. Her spirits are good and she still needs to recover from an overall lack of sleep due to the constant side effects related to the chemo and transplant.
>
> The Kevin Coyne family is on its way, and we will celebrate the most memorable of Thanksgivings over the weekend. I just got back from Kroger's and I think I have everything we need.
>
> The children are elated to have their Mom back home where she belongs.
>
> There's No Place Like Home!

For the next several days over the Thanksgiving weekend, we celebrated the fact our mom was home from a successful stem cell transplant. It was a quiet celebration, but the children were elated their mother was finally home after being in the hospital for more than three weeks. Kevin and his family came over on Friday, and on Saturday we celebrated Thanksgiving at our home in magnificent style. Colleen cooked, cleaned and did all laundry. I can't say enough about all that Colleen did throughout this challenging time. She was in Carmel multiple times and she always took great care of the kids and she also spent many challenging days and nights with Karen at IUMC.

We had put up the Christmas tree and the front of our house was adorned with lights. As we were putting the ornaments on the tree, I came across a little angel holding a banner that read "Karen's Guardian Angel." The ornament had a magnet on the back, so I put it on the front of the fridge where it would remain long after the decorations were taken down. For me it felt more like Christmas than Thanksgiving.

A home nursing service visited every other day and monitored Karen's progress. The nurse's name was Jean, and she was absolutely wonderful. She was always on time, and she was very good at her trade. We could tell she enjoyed her work. It was also nice to have her come by to draw Karen's blood, and in a matter of hours, we had the results. The blood work confirmed that the stem cells had taken hold and were producing. The mucositis had cleared up; she was able to eat, and more importantly, sleep. Over the course of two days, there was a noticeable difference in her energy level and in her eyes. On Tuesday, November 30th, we reported on Karen's progress and thanked several people who had helped us make it through November.

As I hit send, I hoped and prayed this would be my last entry on Karen's website. It was only fitting that she would have the last word.

Tuesday, November 30, 2004 4:24 PM

Karen continues to make progress as her CBC numbers indicate her stem cells have definitely taken hold and are producing new platelets, white blood cells and red blood cells. Her platelets have increased from 17,000 on Thanksgiving Day to 116,000, while her white count has increased from 2,100 to 3,500 over the same time period. Her hemoglobin has increased from 8.2 to 10.6. Late yesterday and into today, she was somewhat dehydrated and she took on some fluids which immediately helped. We have a great home nurse named Jean who has been very diligent and helpful. Tomorrow, Karen has a checkup in Chicago with Dr. Metha. We understand Drs. Tallman and Cripe are at conference, and they will be discussing Karen's case in person. At some point soon, Dr. Cripe will take full charge of Karen's case.

Pat and I want to express our gratitude to everyone who traveled to Chicago to help with Karen's stem cell transplant, so I hope I don't miss anyone. Aunt Ellen started everything clear back on Election Day, then her dad, Tom, visited before cruising down to Carmel to help with his grandchildren. Tommy, Diana, Riley and John Bird all drove over for a long weekend. Kenny stopped in for a few days and Kathy put the icing on the cake leaving the big city just before I arrived to pick Karen up on Thanksgiving Day. Again, I want to personally thank Pat for being there for over almost three weeks. Karen is so blessed to have so many heroes, and we know the neighbors on Garden Gate Way and all our friends from SLDM are waiting in the wings.

We all want to thank everyone who helped with Will, Sam and Mitch in Carmel as well. Aunt Ellen was over for the weekend prior to heading north, sometime back around Halloween. My parents, Marilyn and John returned for another round of fun. Tom was in for almost a week. Colleen, the awesome Mom, was here for the better part of a week; then she returned again the day after Thanksgiving with her husband Kevin and their kids: Sean, Katie and Timmy. We all celebrated a very special Thanksgiving on Saturday, and Karen's very good friend Nora Wilson is here in Carmel now, and Pat will be back in Indiana next week.

I hear there's a job opening in Cleveland.

Karen continued to coast; her white count had picked up to over 4,000 and her platelets were above the 90,000 level. She was still having trouble eating, nothing tasted good, she was always cold, and her skin had been trashed by the last round of chemo. One of the more bizarre things that happened during that time occurred when Karen received a Christmas present in the mail from her Aunt Elaine who had just passed away after suffering a long time with Lou Gehrig's disease or ALS. It was so hard to imagine that in her last days she had thought of Karen and sent a very thoughtful present. Imagine receiving a Christmas present from someone who had just passed on.

On Pearl Harbor Day, I went out to her website while I was at work, and I saw the update Karen had made the previous day.

I had to shut the door to my office. I didn't want anyone to see me cry.

Monday, December 6, 2004 3:20 PM

Well, I've been to hell……. Don't plan on going back.

Thank you for all of your prayers and good wishes. I don't know what we would do without you. I was too sick to pray. I never thought that would happen, but it was so comforting knowing that other people were praying for me when I could not. That is a true friend.

I am starting to feel human again. That is a huge statement. Last Wednesday at my doctor's appointment in Chicago, my Doctor said that it was a science to give me enough chemo to kill the leukemia, but just short of killing me. The side effects are disgusting. My body is still covered in chemical burns and the taste buds have been burned out of my mouth. Bald, pale and very tired. God must not be done with me yet because here I sit.

Mark and the kids are doing fine. I am trying to get out a little; I need a reason to go on. Lying in bed isn't doing it for me. I want my life back……. It is definitely going to take some time. Standing wears me out.

Prayer is a powerful tool; it's why I am still here. Thank you one and all.

Karen

For the next week or two, I prepared for an arbitration case that was taking place in Chicago, of all places, from December 13th through the 15th. The plan was that I'd get done in time to be with Karen at her last appointment with Dr. Tallman. Karen's dad was superb. He arrived on Sunday just after I had left to drive up north. On Wednesday, he drove his daughter to her appointment with Dr. Tallman. Karen's numbers were great. Her white count was up to 5,700, but we were concerned about her platelets, which had hit 119,000, but then dropped to 59,000. Dr. Tallman was not perturbed by the drop in her platelet level, and offered no viable explanation. He was heading off to the

Holy Land for the holiday season, and we were anxious to get a plan in place to address the troublesome handful of leukemic cells found in her spinal fluid at Northwestern.

A few days later, I penned the following e-mail to Dr. Tallman in the hopes of spurring a dialogue between Northwestern and Indiana University Medical Center regarding the issue of the leukemic cells infiltrating the central nervous system. We had never closed the loop on this pertinent matter.

> Dr. Tallman,
>
> I am writing this on behalf of my wife Karen Volpe who has been a stem cell transplant patient of yours the past several months. We are concerned regarding follow up and defining a course of action with regard to the leukemic cells in Karen's spinal fluid. The specific purpose of this correspondence is to get all relevant parties involved and coordinated as to how we should proceed.
>
> Here's what Karen and I understand. On November 10th, 2004, at Northwestern Memorial, Dr. Jessica Altman and a Dr. Addleman from neurology injected methotrexate into the shunt that had been installed by Dr. Thomas Witt at IU in June of this year. The next day Karen had a series of tests done in nuclear medicine at Northwestern using radioactive beads to determine whether the shunt could be used for the purpose of treating the leukemic cells in the spinal fluid. It is our understanding the reviews on whether this methodology was correct are mixed. At one point we heard the shunt could be used for this purpose, and more recently, we were told the shunt would not work. In any event, we understand a spinal tap procedure could also be used to inject the necessary agents.

Dr. Tallman, please take whatever action is necessary to develop and coordinate a plan with your counterparts at IUMC, especially Dr. Cripe, as to how we are going to proceed. Drs. Altman and Addleman can be consulted as to exactly what they did on November 10th. Dr. Raizer and Dr. Witt need to be included as well before an overall game plan can be communicated to Dr. Cripe and Katie Hincher at IUMC.

Thank you for your assistance in coordinating this course of action.

Karen & Mark Volpe

After our journey to Chicago, Karen made the following entry on the website. With just 10 days of holiday shopping left, Karen really wanted to take the entire family back to Chicago to enjoy the big city lights. In her website update, I thought it was really cool how she put the word "FAMILY" in all caps at the end of her entry. Karen has always been all about family, and it shows as she writes about our friends the Starks.

Wednesday, December 15, 2004 9:12 PM

Christmas is almost here!!

I am feeling a "little bit" better every day. I guess that is progress!!

I was in Chicago again today. We are trying to plan the next steps. Looks like my treatment at this point will be continued at Indiana University. My blood counts are fluctuating wildly and have given me a little cause for concern.

I will go to IU on Monday, and hopefully the counts will have adjusted, otherwise….a bunch of tests…AArgh.

Mark and the kids are doing great. Everyone needs a break from their daily grind.

Please keep our friend Tom Stark in your prayers. He is a wonderful man and needs our strength right now. He has another surgery scheduled…

Thank you for your love and support. Sometimes I feel like I am just watching my life instead of living it. This entire mess just doesn't seem real.

Thank you dear God for the gift of your son.
Merry Christmas,

The Volpe FAMILY

On Monday, December 21st, we met with Dr. Cripe and Katie Hincher. It was so wonderful to be back closer to home. They did the customary blood work, and Karen's white count had gone up a little more to 6,100. We were pleased with this trend, but still concerned with the low platelet level, which remained at 64,000. Dr. Cripe explained why the platelet count was so low.

Clinical data had revealed that many autologous stem cell transplant patients would never have total recovery of their platelet counts. Many of these patients had platelet counts in a range between 50,000 and 70,000 because the vast majority of the transplanted stem cells were devoted to the production of white blood cells, the major goal given this subtype of acute myelogenous leukemia. Finally, we had an explanation for the low platelet count and Dr. Tallman's non-reaction to this number. This left the little villains in her spinal column as the last issue, besides getting her back to her playing weight.

Dr. Cripe went over the plan for dealing with the leukemic cells in her spinal column, and he drew another decision tree. This one was pretty simple:

If there was no further evidence of any leukemic cells, we would do six monthly injections as a preventative measure, alternating between methotrexate and Ara-C. We would also alternate between use of a traditional spinal tap and the shunt or; if there were leukemic cells, we would do a similar set of injections, twice a week over a much more aggressive six-week timeframe.

We went to lunch and then reported to the hospital for the spinal tap. A small amount of fluid was drawn, sent off to the lab, and methotrexate was also injected. Everything with the spinal tap went well, and then we went out with the neighbors to celebrate Christmas. Karen's appetite was definitely picking up. She ate plenty of pizza at Bucca de Bepa. Katie Hincher promised to call as soon as she received word on the analysis of the spinal fluid. On Wednesday, Karen received a call from Victoria Hunt, of all people. It would be the last time we heard from Nurse Hunt.

"There are no leukemic cells in your spinal fluid," she said, like a robot. Then she hung up.

Later that evening, Karen made the following announcement on the website.

Wednesday, December 22, 2004 11:41 PM

MERRY CHRISTMAS TO ME!!!!!!!!

God is good.......Your prayers are powerful......

I got a call today that "the results from your spinal tap show no evidence of leukemic cells in your central nervous system." How's that for a gift? The likelihood of this happening was so small that I dared not even hope! I felt like opening my window and screaming!

The relief is overwhelming. The plan is that I will have a spinal tap each month for the next 6 months. They will test the fluid each time and inject chemo each time just as a precaution. At this moment in time…it appears…I am without cancer. Thank you, dear God. My kids have been so celebratory, wound up and giddy. The pressure is off them too. Such adult worries for these little ones.

Santa will be here before you know it. Our Christmas was today.

Thank you for your love and prayers. God listens. I am humbled.

Merry Christmas,
Love,
Mark, Karen, Will, Sam and Mitch

At Mass on Christmas Eve, the Starks were already in the pew when we arrived. Karen led her family in and took her place next to Tom. He was also amazing and during the times when he was in pain, while battling with his cancer, he prayed that God would transfer Karen's pain and the suffering his young nephew, who was also dealing with leukemia, over to him. They chatted briefly as the choir sang the traditional carols before the Mass began. The opening song was "O Come, O Come Emmanuel," and as Father Dave made his way up the aisle to the altar, I looked over at Karen. She was wearing her red Adidas baseball cap and the black mink fur coat I had given her the previous Christmas. A winter storm had hit the Midwest. It was very, very cold, and Karen was still having trouble staying warm. She was slightly pale, had no body fat and very little hair. Her skin was still very dry and arid. A few tears streamed down her face as the entire congregation loudly sang the final verse of the traditional song. I then looked up at the statue of Jesus Christ nailed to the cross and fought hard to choke back my own tears. It was the night of nights; we were celebrating the birth of Christ, sent to us in a most humble manner, born in a manger. I knew in my heart our long and tumultuous ordeal was finally over.

As promised, Karen would have the last word on her website.

Tuesday, January 4, 2005 10:58 PM

Some day, I hope that this will all make sense to me. For the time being, we are great. The transplant went well. Now I need to regain my strength, and I continue to do so daily. I look like a plucked, skinny chicken, wouldn't feed a family of four. No hair growth yet. I am waiting patiently...

We had a wonderful Christmas. We spent considerable time with the Volpes and the Coynes, and I slept a lot. The kids ran crazy with cousins and enjoyed all the snow in Cleveland!

Dear, dear friends and family, you have worn holes in your jeans praying for us. We needed each prayer. This has been a very trying time. Thank you. It is our sincere hope, that we "live" our appreciation. Daily.

I can say, however, loudly and clearly, that I am the luckiest woman that ever lived. I have no regrets. It is my sincere hope that God is done testing us for a while. I need a break…I knew and continue to know that I have an amazing husband and that my children are exceptional. This experience has only proven me correct. I love being right!!!!

Dear God-
Please help each of us learn to value our health. To appreciate the passing of time, and to have confidence that we are where we are supposed to be at this very moment.

I was telling my mom how thankful I was that it was me that was ill and not one of my children. I told her that I could not have handled that. Mom waited a minute and then said, "Now you know how I feel."

This will hopefully be my last entry. I will hopefully never be sick like this again. I will hopefully get to hug my grandchildren. I will hopefully always remember how your prayers got our family through this cancer nightmare. I will hopefully be there for you when you need me.

I love you,
Karen

CHAPTER 39

The Tunnel of Love

We have finally been able to move on, but there will always be the constant reminders and remnants of what we have been through. Mismatched pieces of miscellaneous Tupperware from the numerous meals friends and family brought in can be found in the lazy Susan in the Volpe kitchen. I'd bet Karen's Aunt Patty and her daughters, Alice and Sarah, brought in more than 20 meals, so most of the Tupperware probably belongs to them. Pat had told us that Aunt Patty and Uncle Bob were originally asked to be Karen's godparents when she was baptized, but weather precluded them from traveling that weekend back in 1960. I will always think of Aunt Patty and Uncle Bob as Karen's godparents; the role they played in supporting us throughout this ordeal was extraordinary.

There are literally pounds of medical insurance-related paperwork stuffed in desk drawers. It's hard to thank everyone who did so much. Our good friends Kim Santucci, Amy Jackson, Kimmie Wetzel, Grace Hineman, Shelly Thieme, Pam Marske, Julie Thompson, Julia Mattei, Pat Rocap, Linda McLaughlin and Melinda Bruggemann brought in numerous meals as well. One of our SLDM friends, Jackie Mewborn, continued to send Karen some very funny and uplifting cards well into 2005. There were days when as many as eight cards from Jackie would arrive in our mailbox. Jackie often couldn't decide which card to buy, so she bought them all.

Karen was asked by Kim Santucci, who was one of the co-chairs for the 2005 Mardi de Montfort, to be the master of ceremonies for the big event in February. As Karen made her way to the podium to introduce the assorted dignitaries, I was very proud of her. I had been worried about what she would say when she got up to the microphone, where one can feel seemingly alone on an island with those long pregnant pauses.

In reality, my fears were not well-founded. She was surrounded by members of her family, numerous friends and neighbors who had been there with her for the past few years to witness and support our entire family throughout this remarkable journey. During the evening she was very funny, totally natural, and very much at ease, even though she was totally bald under the silk scarf she had glued to her head. Not many women head out for an elegant evening with lipstick and a glue stick in their little black purse. It's hard to fathom the hours of prayers and number of rosaries said on Karen's behalf just by the people in the beautifully decorated and hardly recognizable school gymnasium.

One of the high notes of the auction was when the yellow Labrador puppy we had donated was put up as the last oral auction item. One of my CRHP brothers, Dave Ritter, took the adorable little guy home to his family for a mere $2,000 tax deduction. I had brought home a female from the same litter a week earlier with the intention of donating her to the big event, but Samantha immediately named her "Peanut," and she was ours. She reminded us of our old dog Calgary, so I went back to the breeder, bought the brother and placed him for adoption at the auction.

Some history is good history that needs to be repeated.

Karen had a few more spinal taps early in 2005, all of which proved negative, although, during one tap in February her spinal fluid dripped way too long, causing Karen to have a classic spinal headache for the rest of the week.

On a Saturday night a week or so before St. Patrick's Day, we were with a group of our neighbors at the Claddagh Irish Pub. The local distributor for Guinness was sponsoring a St. Patty's Day Guinness Toast Contest. Karen's impromptu toast won the local toast off, so the following week we went downtown for the finals. Karen finished second to a fat chap from Ireland who sang this long traditional chant for his toast. He didn't even say "Guinness" in his toast as required by the rules. As we left the bar, Karen ran into a group of guys who said they couldn't hear Karen's toast, so she recited it again.

> *Here's to our country, the U.S. of A.*
> *Here's to the friends, we drink with today*
> *Here's to Guinness, dark and strong*
> *For today to the Irish, we all belong*

They said they couldn't understand why Karen hadn't won.

"I just couldn't get the male vote because they all thought I was a lesbian because my hair is so short. But actually I've been fighting leukemia for well over two years," said Karen.

Then the conversation stopped.

"My little brother just died from leukemia two weeks ago," said one of the guys at the table.

Karen welled up with tears and left the bar very upset.

One of the things that bothered her most about her illness was that she knew of only one other patient with leukemia who had survived. We had become aware of many other people, especially children, who also struggled with the disease. None of their stories had a happy ending except for Karen and Sally Neff, a survivor she had met through Team-In-Training, the Leukemia Foundation's mini-marathon group. Sally gave Karen hope.

For the 2005 Mini-Marathon, Karen was bound and determined to make it all 13 miles again. She wrote the following letter, which helped her raise more than $5,000 for the Leukemia and Lymphoma Society.

Dear Friends,

This is a difficult letter for me to write. We have been through so much as a family these past years since my diagnosis with Leukemia. Soon, it will be three years that we have been battling, fists up, game face on. I lost my remission this past June. The fight was on again. It decided to come back in my brain this time. Surgery was required to stop my brain from swelling so that I could regain my vision. Yes, it has been hard. But the payoff is extreme. Getting to spend the days with my family is all that I can ask.

Last year was my first year to do the mini for Team-In-Training. Hindsight being 20/20, my husband and I realize that the blinding headache I had while completing in the mini last year was to soon prove to be the reappearance of my Leukemia. Last year I was honored at the spaghetti dinner as an award winner for the "Celebrating Life Award." Do I celebrate life? Absolutely!

I received a bone marrow transplant in November. I spent the month in the hospital and began my recovery in December. It is a very long road to recovery. The transplant was THE most difficult part of the process for me physically. But how blessed I was and how thankful to all those that have come before me, that have raised money for cancer research. Those that have TESTED the drugs that I could take with confidence that saved my life. Research and prayer are our only options. Blood cancers can't be radiated or surgically removed. There is no time to waste. We need to find out how to save these precious lives. At times, I can feel so guilty for being among the living when so many worthy souls around me have lost their fight.

My children and my husband and I hope that we can look toward the future. I want to go to weddings and hold grandchildren. I want to travel and laugh and spend time with family and friends. I don't know what my future holds, and neither do you. We need to take it upon ourselves to make a difference. Funds raised through Team-In-Training will go to research as well as supporting patients and their families. Thank God the help is available. I hope that you never need it.

I am asking you to contribute toward my personal goal of $5,000. This is your opportunity to change the future of the next patient diagnosed with Blood Born Cancer. Please donate whatever amounts that you are able, $10, $50, $100 are just suggested amounts. Any gift will be smiled on and greatly appreciated. Your contribution is also tax deductible. Checks should be made payable to The Leukemia and Lymphoma Society and mailed to my address below by March 17, 2005.

Thank you so much, and may God watch over you.

Karen Volpe

Karen walked the 2005 race with her dad and Samantha. She had an iron-on transfer on the back of her purple Team-In-Training jersey. Karen had one message for the entire world to see on the back of her shirt.

SURVIVOR

Janet Dorger, a friend of Karen's from SLDM, also ran with Team-In-Training, with the following message on the back of her jersey:

<u>Volpe Victory</u>
Karen 2 Leukemia 0—
Karen, You Are My Hero!

The next day was Mother's Day, and while we were driving home from taking Karen out to dinner on Sunday, the day after the race, Mitchell pulled the card he made at school out of his book bag. "Sorry, I forgot to give this to you earlier," he said.

He had drawn a picture of his mom, with hair of course, wearing a green Nike shirt. On the right he wrote in cursive:

May 8, 2005

Happy Mother's Day!

Mom when I think of you, I think of…

Diet Coke…Oprah…kicking a soccer ball…ER…sewing…socializing…the phone…E-mail…caring…nice…TV…joyful…Mini-Marathon…Virginia beach…skiing…walking the dog…roses…errands…driving a lot…helpful…loving…grilled cheese…colorful…good personality…homework…smiles…fun to be around…hyper…funny…Survivor.

Love ya,

Love,

Mitch

As I looked back over what I have documented, I felt like this extraordinary odyssey needed closure. After the Christmas holiday in 2004, we all became acutely aware of the devastation the tsunami caused. The pictures defy description with more than 220,000 lives lost in just moments. All of us were right in the middle of the joyous Christmas season when we were forced again to understand and be reminded again how fragile life really is.

Dealing with cancer had become part of our daily life for more than three years. With the tsunami, thousands of lives were swept away quickly. Due to the outbreak of disease and lack of a clean water supply, many more were likely to perish. Some of the things happening in our lifetimes are simply beyond comprehension. We were given the luxury of time and were able to realize the benefits of all the years of tireless cancer research and the care from the world's most dedicated doctors and nurses all focused on helping us conquer Karen's leukemia.

The Caringbridge website for Karen had more than 45,000 hits. A wealth of love and concern was heaped upon Karen from friends, family, sports celebrities and even strangers from all corners of the world.

It's time to end this remarkable story.

Back in April 2004, Karen and I had a date, and we went to

see Mel Gibson's documentary, *The Passion of the Christ*. I say "documentary" and not "movie" for a reason. *Spiderman II* is a movie; Gibson's controversial work that he funded on his own, in my opinion, is a realistic and accurate depiction of Jesus Christ's last hours on Earth. We saw *The Passion* right before Karen's loss of remission in June.

I remember the scene when Jesus falls the second time, and he turns to his Mother Mary and says, "See, it is happening as it is written, I make all things new." I clenched Karen's hand very tightly. Keep in mind that at this point in time, Karen was very near the end of her two-year maintenance program. She was still in remission, but I still had lingering doubts that it was really over. The odds were not on our side, and we both wanted time to hurry up and get us through the two years. As I looked up at the screen it dawned on me. If she had died, she would have been granted the promise of the power and glory of the Resurrection; she would be born anew in her new life with Christ. This would occur because she believed. Faith gives us hope.

She had always told her children, "I can't lose, I either live here with you, or I live with God; I can't lose."

Karen was sent here to this place, in this time, with these people, to deal with this disease with courage, faith, hope and love. She battled with the leukemia not to die, but to live and go on with the rest of her life as a survivor.

She taught, and continues to teach us all, the real meaning of life!

I knew I married a very special person, but I had no idea I was picking a partner for life who would become the most amazing person I would ever meet in this lifetime. Now, it is finally over, and I have no more lingering doubts.

The stem cell transplant was a success!

There are no more mutant leukemic cells hanging out in her spinal column. Her hair is slowly coming back and her internal organs are intact, despite the fact that she received 10 different types of chemotherapy throughout this saga.

"Why didn't I get the simple leukemia?" Karen wondered once.

She had the leukemia that also included multiple surgeries: the extraction of her female organs, the insertion of a permanent shunt into her brain and finally the infiltration of leukemic cells into her central nervous system. Karen endured in spite of all of these hurdles.

This is part of the great mystery we call life.

How do you know in your heart when the woman you love and the mother of your children has beaten cancer?

This moment occurs the minute you stop doubting God, stop doubting His Will and questioning the plan He has in store for each of us. He alone wrote this script long before we were born.

When I sit alone and meditate, I often remember and take time to ponder the last lines of my favorite artist's single "Brilliant Disguise" from *The Tunnel of Love*. Bruce wrote these lyrics when he was going through his own personal anguish of being married to one woman while in love with another.

Karen even commented long before she got sick that these words at the end of this song are "About as heavy as it gets."

These are the words that are a constant reminder not to doubt and to keep the faith.

My mind failed me early on during this ordeal, but now it is over and I'm a better man, stronger and still a full believer in my faith.

I know it's not good grammar to end this fabulous story with a preposition, but of all the words he has ever put to music, these are the most awesome and thought-provoking lines he ever wrote. This long chapter of our collective lives is now over. I'm sure, and have absolutely no doubt, Karen will have a long and happy life as a cancer survivor, but the essence of Bruce's words will never leave me.

Tonight our bed is cold

I'm lost in the darkness of our love

God have mercy on the man,

Who doubts what he's sure of.

CHAPTER 40

Bone Marrow Transplant Unit

Early June 2005—I had just sent my book to the self-publishing company for editing. I liked the fact that I had decided to end my story with a spiritual quote from Bruce, but in the end it would be even more fitting that Dr. Cripe have the last word.

Dr. Larry Cripe is a spectacular man and a brilliant doctor. He saved my wife's life and he will always be very special to us.

On one of those few warm summer nights when Will didn't have a game, it was after dinner and I was surfing the satellite looking for something to watch on the tube. As I scrolled through the channels, I just froze when I saw *Pay It Forward* was just starting on WTBS in Atlanta. I shrugged it off and remembered that it was a good movie, but for a moment in time, I flashed back to June three years prior.

Karen recently had a minor scare. She was coming back from a weekend trip in Ohio, and her mom was with her. Karen just didn't feel right, slight nausea and aching a little, so she went straight to IUMC and had her blood tested as a precautionary measure.

When her counts came back normal, with no Blasts, Katie Hincher said, "See, everything is fine, there's no reason to worry."

There was a reason to be a little nervous. It was June again, and historically, this had been a bad month for Karen. Leukemia had reared its ugly head in the early days of June in both

2002 and 2004. In 2005, everything was going fine and we were counting the days until the month was over. Her numbers as of her June 6th visit were right where we expected them to be and consistent with the prior five months. The platelets had always been low; however Dr. Cripe had explained the research data showed this had been the case with several autologous stem cell transplant patients. The platelets never quite fully recovered.

The kids and Karen gave me a really cool black mountain bike for Father's Day.

We went to Chicago to see Dr. Tallman for a follow-up visit complete with the customary blood work a few days later.

All of her key numbers had suddenly dropped.

Her white count had gone from 6,400 thousand to 3,900 and the platelets had fallen from 158,000 to 108,000.

"I'm not alarmed, but I want you to get it checked again next week," Dr. Tallman said, at least twice.

Because there were no Blasts, we took this to mean her bone marrow was just not putting out the same amount of blood products as were normally required.

Samantha and Mitchell took in Navy Pier. We cruised the Magnificent Mile before hitting Joey Buona's for dinner. Then we drove back home down I-65. Will caught both ends of a double header that evening, so he couldn't join in on the very fun one-day trip.

Later, I scrolled around the Internet and learned that the symptoms of low platelets and low white blood cell counts were a condition called neutropenia. This situation could easily be remedied with medication. We weren't worried—there were no little pests we had come to know as Blast cells. Everything was fine and she felt great.

On July 12th, she went back down to the Cancer Pavilion to see Dr. Cripe. I fidgeted at my desk waiting for her to call with her numbers. Finally, I couldn't wait any longer, so I called her cell. The numbers had dipped even further, with her white count down to 1,600 and her platelets plummeting to only 8,000.

My heart sank. Something was very wrong.

Our former babysitter from Stow when the children were very young named Kristina, who had sent us green sweatshirts which read "PROPERTY OF TEAM VOLPE—LIVESTRONG" a year earlier, had come over for a visit. She accompanied Karen for her monthly check-up and then headed back to Cleveland. I did not want to go because I didn't want to appear panicked, but deep down inside I was a mess.

Dr. Cripe conferred with Dr. Tallman, and the next step was obvious. A bone marrow biopsy was needed the next day to determine exactly what was going on. I emailed the latest numbers to Dr. Tallman, and in his reply, he expressed some confusion over the counts, but he felt the biopsy would tell us everything we needed to know.

The next day was July 13, 2005. Karen and I made our way back to IUMC and Dr. Cripe performed the biopsy. Katie was there first, helping Karen get prepped for the procedure we had come to know all too well.

"What if it's back?" Karen asked.

Katie promptly replied, "More treatment!"

Dr. Cripe had to probe around to extract the marrow and Karen was in some pain, but it wasn't at all like her first biopsy when the marrow could hardly be found. At the same time, it wasn't like the biopsies when she was in remission either. Those times, the syringe immediately filled up. This time it was somewhere in between. The syringe filled slowly, and a piece of bone was extracted. Dr. Cripe told us it would take him about 90 minutes to review the smears under the microscope. At least we didn't have to wait overnight.

We went back to the outpatient clinic, across the hall from the Bone Marrow Transplant Unit, where Karen had received numerous rounds of chemo and transfusions. A young college student was getting treatment for graft-versus-host disease, and when he left, he stopped by because he had overheard us talking. He explained that he had received an allogeneic bone marrow transplant a few years earlier from an unrelated donor. Then one of the transplant nurses who knew Karen stopped by to talk, and we explained the situation.

When we told her there were no Blasts, she said, "That's encouraging unless they're still packed in the bone marrow."

This possibility had never occurred to us; we thought if there were Blasts, they'd have shown up in her peripheral blood by now. Ten minutes later, Dr. Cripe and Katie arrived, and we started to make our way to a small private room so we could talk.

"This means the news isn't good," Karen said.

"No," Katie replied. "This doesn't mean that it's necessarily bad news."

A minute later, Dr. Cripe closed the door and said, "The news isn't good. About 60 percent of the cells were leukemic cells, identical to the ones we saw back in 2002."

We sat there in shock!

"How long do I have?" Karen asked.

"If you do nothing, it will be only one or two months," Dr. Cripe replied.

"Eventually the platelet transfusions will not help and most patients die from either bleeding or infection," he explained.

Dr. Cripe went on to say that if she resumed treatment, she could have a reasonable quality of life for maybe nine months to a year.

"If you achieve some quality of a remission, then it's possible to consider a bone marrow transplant using Tommy's marrow," he said, "but this is a wholly separate track, a whole different set of decisions. The first thing we need to do is resume treatment with the arsenic trioxide and the ATRA on an outpatient basis for at least five weeks to start. My job is still to cure you and Dr. Tallman and I both see this as curable, but if the arsenic isn't working for you, and you're miserable, it will be your decision whether to continue on with the treatment or not."

I couldn't believe what I was hearing.

Dr. Tallman had told us that Karen would be cured after her autologous transplant. We knew nothing was for certain. It also occurred to me that Karen's type of leukemia, APL or M3, was chemo-resistant, meaning there was the possibility that the arsenic trioxide might not get her into a third remission. Karen learned about this possibility while reading *My Sister's Keeper* by Jodi Picoult earlier in the spring.

Karen looked over at me and said, "Honey, what do you think?"

I thought for a second and then replied, "You handled the arsenic last year very well! I think you need to do at least the five weeks of arsenic."

"I know you'll have a long line of people willing to bring you down here each day," Dr. Cripe said.

"Okay, then that's what we'll do," Karen said. "I'll continue to fight."

A number of things shot through my mind. We'd have to tell the kids a third time the cancer was back, only this time Karen would be able to tell them herself. None of the research I had done on the Internet to learn more about Karen's illness ever mentioned a third remission.

We decided to keep this turn of events private—just our close friends and family would be told the bad news. We would not use the Caringbridge website.

Eventually the word got out; and the phone was ringing off the wall, so Karen finally made a journal entry on the website which simply read:

Tuesday, August 9, 2005 10:26 PM

I guess I need to make this short and sweet.

Yes, the Leukemia is back…

Yes, we are in need of your prayers…

We are all fine; unfortunately, this has become a part of the fabric of our lives.

I'm back on chemo and more chemo. We are trying to buy all the time that God is willing to sell.

I have felt pretty good today. One day at a time….

All OUR love,
The Volpe Clan

Karen asked Dr. Cripe one last question on that fateful July 13th visit. I hoped and prayed that for just once, Dr. Cripe would be wrong.

It was right before we left.

There was a prolonged and anguished silence; Katie was visibly upset and everything was just starting to sink in. The stem cell transplant had only worked temporarily, for 5 measly months.

Karen looked over at Dr. Cripe.

"Dr. Cripe, will I be there to dance at my daughter's wedding?"

He paused for a moment, just looking down at the floor.

Dr. Cripe exhaled and then slowly looked up at Karen and said very quietly, "Probably not."

EPILOGUE

Karen resumed the arsenic trioxide and ATRA treatments immediately after a bone marrow biopsy confirmed that she had relapsed a second time. In September 2005, she contracted a staph infection, from the PICC line (peripherally inserted central catheter) in her left arm that kept her hospitalized for most of the month. Despite her compromised immune system, she was eventually able to beat the infection with a heavy barrage of antibiotics.

On Thanksgiving, after another bone marrow biopsy we received word that Karen had attained remission for a third time, after over 60 rounds of arsenic trioxide. Dr. Jennifer Schwartz informed us right before Christmas that the quality of the remission presented "a window of opportunity" where Karen could undergo an allogeneic stem cell transplant using Tommy's cells. Even though there was a low probability of success and the fact that the procedure was wrought with potential complications, Karen decided to do the transplant under Dr. Schwartz's direction.

In early January 2006, she was admitted to IUMC and underwent 11 rounds of total body irradiation and cytoxan as a conditioning regiment prior to receiving a transfusion of Tommy's freshly harvested stem cells at the end of the month.

On Valentine's Day, she was put on a ventilator for a week in order to battle RSV, a viral infection that more commonly infiltrates the lungs of newborn infants. Five days after she was taken off the ventilator, she returned home. In early April, she had to be readmitted because graft-versus-host disease (GVHD), where the donor marrow attacks the patient's body, became more pronounced. In its harshest form, a Grade 4 case of GVHD, all by itself, can be fatal. Karen had a Grade 4 case of GVHD of the skin, gut and liver. After a few weeks she returned home and continued to recuperate at home. An antibiotic called grancyclovir was used to successfully fend off GVHD of the gut.

She continues to battle GVHD, taking a large array of immune suppression drugs. The key drugs being administered are methylprednisone and cyclosporine to deal with the persistent GVHD of the gut. A bone marrow biopsy taken in May 2006 revealed that the DNA comprising Karen's bone marrow was 100 percent Tommy. As of January 2007, a follow-up bone marrow biopsy confirmed the DNA makeup remained 100 percent Tommy and there was no evidence of any translocation involving chromosome 15 and 17. The allogeneic stem cell transplant, despite its risks and potential complications, has been deemed a success, although none of the doctors are using the word "cured."

How did Karen conquer cancer? I believe the real reason Karen beat cancer is simple. The answer can be found on the front cover of this book. Modern medicine and her enduring spirit certainly helped, but Karen absolutely refused to leave her three children. The thought of not being there as they grew up and started families of their own was more than she could bear.

Karen visits the Bone Marrow Transplant Unit at IUMC regularly for assorted treatments to boost her new immune system and for the ongoing monitoring of her blood. She would rather not have to make the trips downtown, but she is slowly getting her life back. Karen recently decided that she had to make a choice: either fear or faith.

HOW KAREN CONQUERED CANCER

I don't think I have to tell you what she choice she made.

Made in the USA
Lexington, KY
21 September 2019